Advance praise for
Turtles All The Way Down:
Vaccine Science and Myth

"We have found the book to be well written, serious, scientific and
important... We sincerely recommend it as a scientific, medical, and
public 'must read'. This book should be central to a scientific, rational,
logical, skeptical, and critical discussion on routine vaccination... The
authors should be congratulated on their vast scientific in-depth
endeavor as well as on their courage to think outside the 'establishment box'."
—**Nati Ronel, Professor of Criminology, and Eti Elisha, Senior
Criminologist, in *Harefuah Medical Journal*, Sep. 2019**

"This is a wonderful book – indeed, a masterpiece – and one that
really needed to be written. Clearly written and very comprehensive,
it is an invaluable source of knowledge for all truly interested individuals, parents as well as physicians. The title may seem puzzling at
first, but once you read the book you'll realize it is a stroke of genius.
I congratulate the authors on a work extremely well done."
—**Russell L. Blaylock M.D., Neurosurgeon, Author of *The Liver
Cure***

"In the complexity of the modern world, where media manipulation is ubiquitous, it can be difficult to discern fact from fiction, truth from propaganda. To truly understand an issue, we can no longer just trust what we are told, we must first verify through our own research and exploration. This is your opportunity to research and explore a topic of enormous importance to society. There is powerful truth told in this book, rigorously researched, meticulously documented, and written with impeccable integrity. History will judge *Turtles All The Way Down: Vaccine Science and Myth* as an important anchor to truth at a time when so little of what we read and watch can be trusted."
—Beth Lambert, Author of *A Compromised Generation* and *Brain Under Attack*

"I strongly recommend that you read the most important book ever written about vaccines. The book presents hundreds of facts, backed by solid scientific references, which will leave you speechless. The authors present an unprecedented analysis of the world of vaccines. The book shatters myths that we grew up on, one by one. And it does so elegantly and logically. It reads almost like a fiction thriller – when I read it, I could not put it down. It presents everything the medical establishment knows and does not want you to know. An entire world is about to be revealed to you. It is no exaggeration to say that this book is about to start a revolution."
—Dr. Gil Yosef-Shachar M.D.

"*Turtles All the Way Down: Vaccine Science and Myth* is a well-documented and persuasive guidebook to vaccination. The book could be, and should be, a game changer. I congratulate the authors on a work well done!"
—Neil Z. Miller, Medical researcher, Author of *Miller's Review of Critical Vaccine Studies*

"This impeccably researched and documented book formulates a cohesive and clear view of the vaccine science that is scattered in numerous scientific papers and government documents. It is a real

eye-opener, guaranteed to change your thinking. You may find it hard to believe what you read, but with the documentation right there, in front of your eyes, the conclusions are inescapable."
—Patricia Lemer M.Ed., Licensed Professional Counselor, Author of *Outsmarting Autism: Build Healthy Foundations for Communication, Socialization, and Behavior at All Ages*, Chair Emeritus, Epidemic Answers

"Turtles All the Way Down: Vaccine Science and Myth is an extraordinary book, as its name implies. This is a must-read for anyone who wants an in-depth introduction to the subject of vaccines to make informed decisions for themselves and their family.
The authors deserve many compliments for their comprehensive and thorough work, based mainly on sources from the scientific literature and the websites of health authorities. The book presents its arguments in clear and easy-to-understand language so that a medical education is not required in order to read it and benefit from it. However, I also strongly suggest that medical professionals of all fields delve into it. Personally, I learned a lot from reading the book and I highly recommend it."
—Dr. Haim Rosenthal M.D.

"While the media is saturated with messaging that vaccines are 'safe and effective,' an increasing number of parents are growing skeptical of this narrative. This book is a comprehensive and exceptionally well documented look into the 'science' behind vaccine safety, exposing the fact that most of the supporting evidence is based on shoddy research biased by vested interests. This is arguably the most thorough and persuasive book on the market on this important topic."
—Stephanie Seneff Ph.D., Senior Research Scientist, MIT, Author of *Toxic Legacy*

"Turtles All The Way Down: Vaccine Science and Myth is an important book, because it fills a gap that has long begged to be filled. It explains the science behind vaccines, distilling down a huge amount of litera-

ture, making a solid understanding of the science accessible to any committed reader. Until now, books on vaccines were either too technical for the average reader, or too simplified, or were not up to date on the current issues facing the vaccine enterprise. Every parent should have this book in their library."
—**Meryl Nass M.D.**

"If you are in the habit of quoting CDC as an authority on vaccine safety and efficacy, this book will break you of that habit. Our society is engaged in an existential battle between those willing to acknowledge the evidence on vaccine safety and those who make claims based on falsified and fraudulent data. In just over 500 pages, the exquisitely referenced 'Turtles' presents reality-based fact after fact, demolishing false claim after false claim made by vaccine proponents until the truth becomes inescapable."
—**James Lyons Weiler Ph.D., IPAK-EDU.org**

"This book is a phenomenal resource for parents navigating the decision-making process about whether or not to vaccinate their children or for any truth-seeker daring to journey down the rabbit hole of vaccine science. Extraordinarily well written and organized, this book is the perfect primer to quickly empower the reader with a clear understanding of how the public has been bamboozled with the scientifically meaningless claim that all vaccines recommended by the CDC are 'safe and effective'. Anyone who reads this book will come away with a firm understanding of the gross inadequacies of vaccine studies and the institutionalized corruption that enables the so-called 'public health' establishment to sustain the illusion that public vaccine policy is evidence-based."
—**Jeremy R. Hammond, Independent Researcher, Journalist, Author of *The War on Informed Consent: The Persecution of Dr. Paul Thomas by the Oregon Medical Board***

"This is the book we've been waiting for."
—**Lisa Joyce Goes, The Thinking Moms' Revolution**

Turtles
All
The
Way
Down

Vaccine Science and Myth

Editors

Zoey O'Toole

Mary Holland

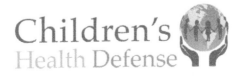

Download the References document for the book from: https://tinyurl.com/TurtlesBookEngRef

Or scan this QR code:

The book may be purchased in bulk.
Contact the publisher: **turtles.all.book@gmail.com**

ISBN: 978-965-598-104-9

To MS, GK, and HB

To Asura

CONTENTS

FOREWORD

By MARY HOLLAND, J.D.

In January of 2020, the world began hearing rumors that a deadly virus was wreaking havoc in Wuhan, China. Shortly thereafter the virus made its way around the globe, causing the most pernicious pandemic since the influenza pandemic of the early 20th century, over 100 years earlier.

Governments around the globe invested heavily in the development of vaccines they hoped would relegate the disease named COVID-19 to a historical footnote. The FDA fast-tracked these vaccines, skipping large segments of the usual testing process before authorizing several different brands for emergency use in early 2021. Some of the new products, including those sold by Pfizer and Moderna, used technology never before applied to vaccines: Messenger RNA (mRNA) temporarily hijacks cells in the recipient's body, forcing them to make the "spike" proteins that enable the SARS-CoV-2 virus to invade human cells. Why would vaccinologists want the body to make the most problematic protein of a noxious virus? The intent was to provoke production of antibodies that would selectively bind to the spike protein, neutralizing the virus whenever it was encountered and rendering it harmless to human cells.

Never has vaccine development been followed so intently by the general public as it has for COVID vaccines. Suddenly, people who had never exhibited any prior interest in vaccine science or technology began debating the relative merits of the novel mRNA technology over conventional live-virus vaccines and dissecting the formal stages of the vaccine approval process. Many, including some well-known vaccine proponents, expressed concern and skepticism about the safety and/or effectiveness of the rushed COVID vaccines.

Despite purportedly putting science in the driver's seat, governments and health authorities in the US and around the world enacted COVID policies that were, more often than not, anything but science-driven. This was especially true when it came to the vaccines.

Some of the most egregious actions health agencies and pharmaceutical companies collaborated on during the testing of COVID vaccines include

- Rushing to market vaccines that were insufficiently tested in clinical trials.

- Concealing and withholding crucial clinical trial data from the medical community and the public.

- Recommending vaccination of vulnerable subpopulations (pregnant women, children) although the vaccines were not adequately tested in these groups.

When it comes to monitoring the safety of COVID vaccines the same parties have been guilty of the following:

- Employing superficial and inadequate monitoring of post-marketing vaccine adverse events.

- Dismissing post-vaccination injuries out of hand as "unrelated to the vaccine".

- Providing no tools for medical personnel to identify, diagnose, or treat vaccine injury.

- Discouraging doctors from reporting vaccine injury.

- Sponsoring virtually no science seriously investigating reported vaccine injuries.

With respect to public discussion of COVID policies in general and vaccine policies in particular, these agencies and corporations colluded with mainstream media and social media moguls to

- De-legitimize criticism and open debate, labeling critique from senior scientists, doctors and the public as "misinformation" or "anti-science".

- Promote the false notion that COVID vaccines provide herd immunity in order to pressure the public into vaccinating "to protect others".

- Initiate, publish, and promote bad science to support the lucrative vaccine agenda.

- Artificially inflate the market for COVID vaccines by smearing and banning safe and effective, over-the-counter medications (such as ivermectin and hydroxychloroquine).

Seeing how ineffectively and dishonestly the COVID pandemic was handled (particularly in the US, which fared worse than any other country but Brazil), many people around the world grew disillusioned with their governments and health agencies. At this point, however, most of the disillusioned restrict their criticism to the mishandling of the COVID crisis, and relatively few extend their critical analysis to vaccines in general, or to the childhood vaccines. Perhaps the majority are unaware of the grim broader reality of vaccine science or they fear being labeled "anti-vaxxers" (which would be understandable, as that epithet is thrown at anyone who dares question any aspect of vaccine dogma). Even now, in 2022, after all that has transpired in the last two years, vaccines are still the "sacred cow" of medicine that should always be defended and never doubted.

But is such reserve justified? Was COVID just a one-off, with the all-encompassing folly we have witnessed born of the need to do something and to do it quickly? Or did governments and their health agencies simply take their modus operandi to extremes in order to exploit a worldwide health crisis to advance their agenda and benefit their collaborators?

In the wake of the COVID fiasco, it is time for a deeper look down the larger vaccine rabbit hole: Are childhood vaccines so different from COVID vaccines? Are they safer? Were they tested any better? Are their injuries better documented and investigated? Are medical professionals (or anyone else) allowed to question them any more than they were allowed to question COVID vaccines? And the most important question of all: Can we entrust our babies to vaccines produced, tested, and marketed by the same agencies and corporations, doctors and government officials, researchers and high-tech moguls that failed us so miserably over the last two years?

You are now holding the book that answers all those questions, and answers them definitively. This book dissects the CDC's recommended childhood schedule with respect to the issues I highlighted above: the clinical trials, adverse event reporting, recognizing and treating vaccine injuries, vaccination recommendations that are not supported by science, science censored and contorted to support the vaccine agenda, mainstream media vaccine propaganda, and more. Throw in a thorough rebuttal of three foundational vaccination myths, and there you have it – everything you ever needed to know about vaccines, but were afraid to ask.

Turtles All the Way Down: Vaccine Science and Myth was first published in Israel in early 2019. Later that year, it set a worldwide precedent for a vaccine-critical book when a mainstream medical journal published a positive review of it. The article in the September 2019 issue of *Harefuah* (*"Medicine"*), the leading medical journal in Israel, was authored by a pair of senior academic criminologists, Nati Ronel and Eti Elisha. To the dismay of the Israeli medical establishment, Ronel and Elisha "found the book to be well written, serious, scientific and important", offering "a comprehensive view of the issue." Though heavily criticized by some vaccine doctors as "only" criminologists who should stay in their lane, their appraisal of the book still stands today, unscathed: In the three years since its (Hebrew) publication, no medical or medical science professional has succeeded in refuting the book's claims. Unable to demonstrate that the book or its *Harefuah* review actually contained any errors, critics – doctors as well as lay people – chose instead to target the review's authors. The fierce personal attack on Ronel and Elisha for merely reviewing the book served to illustrate one of the major points in their article, that the science and medical establishment resorts to aggressive personal attacks to cover-up inconvenient truth: "It appears that science and medicine are becoming hostile to criticism in ways that are historically associated with the violence of fundamental religious orthodoxy or even inquisition committees similar to those of the Middle Ages. They are convinced they know the 'truth' and reject every attempt to question this 'truth' as heresy."

One academic, Daniel Mishori, Ph.D., a senior faculty member specializing in ethics and philosophy at the Department of Environmental Science at Tel Aviv University, was so disturbed by the lack of discussion of the book's arguments that he offered a cash prize ($4,000 donated to the hospital ward of choice) to anyone who could refute them. Since *Turtles* is over 500 pages and contains more than 1,200 references, Mishori declared he would settle for a proper rebuttal to the harsh conclusions drawn in the first chapter of the book. To this day no one has been able to meet his "Turtles challenge."

Clearly, the main reason no one has been able to refute the book's arguments thus far is that the authors made a very conscious effort to rely exclusively on publications available from "kosher" sources such as mainstream scientific journals and leading government agencies (CDC, FDA, WHO, etc.). The book contains virtually no references to studies, articles, or even quotes by anyone who has been painted as an "anti-vaxxer" by the media at any time, regardless of their quality or scientific validity. Thus, it has proved impossible, until now at least, for even the most venerated vaccine experts to refute conclusions that were based upon savvy and accurate analysis of scientifically sanctioned sources.

You may have noticed this book does not list an author. That is because the book's authors have chosen to remain anonymous, and they have some good reasons for doing so. If you're already familiar with the vaccine debate, you are probably aware that whenever someone questions any part of the official narrative surrounding vaccines, no matter how minor the point or reasonable the argument, that person is immediately attacked – to the point that well known, dedicated scientists in numerous countries have lost their careers for challenging vaccine dogma. The authors of *Turtles* are from Israel, a small country where, if someone were deemed enough of a threat to the powers that be, it would be quite simple to make their lives, as well as those of their family members, a living nightmare. This abysmal state of affairs was not lost on Ronel and Elisha, who found it disturbing that such a worthy scientific book had to be published anonymously, noting "The fact that the authors chose anonymity invokes criminological questions on the decision making processes by the medical establishment and on the issue of medical ethics surrounding the heated debate over vaccines."

Another good reason the authors chose anonymity, and perhaps the more important one from your perspective as a reader, is to "immunize" the book against ad hominem attacks, a favorite tactic employed by the pharmaceutical industry and the medical establishment. When they can't disprove an argument scientifically, vaccine loyalists typically resort to personal attacks against the people making it, following the notorious PR motto of "smear the authors – kill the book." However, this "shoot the messenger" tactic only works if there is someone to shoot. Thus, *Turtles*' authors artfully disarmed their antagonists, taking the smear campaign option off the table.

Personally, I sympathize with the authors and fully understand their motives. I have witnessed many smear campaigns targeting advocates of vaccine safety. One noteworthy example is my colleague Robert F. Kennedy, who was a well-known environmental lawyer, when he looked into the long-term negative effects of repeatedly injecting mercury into infants' bodies. Before he published *Thimerosal: Let the Science Speak*, about a mercury-based preservative that was present in many childhood vaccines until someone in the FDA actually added up how much mercury infants were receiving, his media connections made it easy to get on television to talk about whatever he wanted. He could present the dangers of environmental mercury in any other context and the media would cheer him on, but mention the word *vaccines* and suddenly no one in mainstream media wanted anything to do with him. Despite the fact that he made it clear he was steadfastly in favor of vaccines as long as they weren't laced with a neurotoxic metal, he was increasingly vilified in the media, called everything from "anti-vaxxer" to "crazy and dangerous." But if his arguments were simply "misinformation," as the media implies, why would they need a smear campaign? Wouldn't it be better from their point of view to invite him to a public debate where their hand-picked "experts" could crush him into a fine powder? When it comes to *Turtles*, a scholarly analysis with no author to attack, the so-called experts' only options are to debate the book's content or be silent.

While character assassination can be an effective public relations strategy, it has no place in the search for scientific truth. When it comes to science, it shouldn't matter who is making the argument. All that should matter is whether or not the argument is valid. In other words, good arguments should stand – or not – on their own merits, not on the credentials or popularity of the person making the argument. Albert Einstein was a patent clerk when he published the Theory of Relativity, but his dull job and lack of academic standing obviously didn't stop him from having brilliant insights in physics. If the more established scientists of his day were allowed to shout down his theory because its originator lacked credentials, science would have lost one of its brightest lights.

The information on vaccine science contained in this magnificent book is far too important to be allowed to be co-opted in this way. Our children's lives depend on getting this right. The authors of *Turtles* don't want you to take their word for anything. They want you to read the arguments in this book and verify the references and quotes they are based on (which the authors went out of their way to make accessible). And they want you to think about what you read – not about who wrote it. In this day and age, it seems that the only way to keep the focus on *what* is said in a vaccine-critical book, and not on *who* is saying it, is to say it anonymously.

So that is what they did.

With that, I challenge every physician and scientist to read *Turtles All the Way Down: Vaccine Science and Myth* and make your best effort to shoot holes in the arguments it makes. I suspect that for the vast majority it will be an eye-opening experience. If you choose not to take the challenge because you don't have the guts, then you have no place in the vaccine debate. In other words, speak now or forever hold your peace.

INTRODUCTION

"I can only show you the door. You're the one that has to walk through it."

Morpheus, The Matrix

If you are reading this introduction, we can safely assume that you are aware, at least to some extent, of the controversy surrounding vaccines. On one side of this prominent public debate stands the health establishment with its many representatives repeatedly assuring us that vaccines are safe and effective. Opposing them is a large and growing group of parents claiming that vaccines can, and do, cause severe side effects, and even their efficacy is exaggerated.

Due to the inherent complexity of its underlying subject, the vaccine debate challenges medical professionals and scientists alike – and, to an even greater extent, the average parent. In order to attain even a moderate level of expertise on this topic, one needs to have at least a basic understanding of numerous and varied medical and scientific disciplines, which are described and noted in parentheses below.

To begin with, one has to have a good grasp of vaccine-preventable diseases (expertise in *infectious diseases*). Some of these illnesses are specific to infants and children (expertise in *pediatrics*), while others are common to all age groups (*family medicine*). Next, one has to understand how vaccines for these diseases are developed (*vaccinology*): First, one must identify the causative agent (pathogen) – typically a bacterium (*bacteriology*) or a virus (*virology*) – and study its interaction with the body's immune system (*immunology*). Furthermore, researchers need to investigate the pattern of disease in various populations and how a vaccine may affect disease dissemination and severity (*epidemiology*).

Along with any potential health benefits, vaccines are also liable to have undesirable side effects. Vaccines are composed of a multitude of diverse biological and chemical compounds, some of which are considered toxic (*toxicology*). To diagnose adverse side effects, assess their severity, and find suitable treatments, one needs considerable knowledge of clinical medicine, with the specific fields depending on which organs are affected and the level of harm sustained (*neurology, gastroenterology, dermatology, allergology, rheumatology, autoimmune diseases*, etc.)

The above is by no means an exhaustive list. Vitally important aspects of the vaccine debate lie outside the domain of medical science, and one must also devote time to those as well in order to truly understand this complex issue. One must learn how vaccine research is conducted and vaccine policy is formed in the real world – where power, money, and politics shape the rules. Vaccines are manufactured by corporations intent on maximizing their profits. As is the case for every other business sector, vaccine company executives are first and foremost obligated to their shareholders, rather than to the health and well-being of the general public. Licensing, regulation, and marketing of vaccines are all carried out by governmental entities, which are influenced by political and financial considerations. Supposedly objective and impartial, scientific research dedicated to vaccines and vaccination practices is mostly funded by these same governmental entities and vaccine manufacturers whose considerations and interests may be at odds with the interests of the general public.

Vaccine research is published in scientific and medical journals which are, in every sense, also commercial enterprises endeavoring to maximize profits for their shareholders. Physicians and researchers working in the field of vaccines (or related areas) operate inside a confined system with strict rules, both formal and informal, that limit their freedom of investigation and expression. Media coverage of vaccines is also not immune to bias and conflicts of interest. Media outlets have financial relationships with some of the entities mentioned above, and these relationships shape their reporting on the subject of vaccination.

Legal and constitutional matters, especially with regard to severe vaccine side effects, occasionally crop up in courts across the globe. And ethical questions arise from legislative initiatives to compel immunization by law. Every one of these aspects (and this is still just a partial list) is an essential piece of the intricate tapestry that is the world of vaccines. It is impossible to grasp the whole picture without understanding how each of its diverse parts fits into it.

Thus, some knowledge in all the aforementioned academic and non-academic disciplines is required if one is to gain a comprehensive understanding of all the issues surrounding vaccines. Vaccination, then, has to be one of the most complex issues – if not *the* most complex – to be publicly debated over the last few decades. It's safe to assume there isn't a single person on Earth with expertise in all of these fields, even among those celebrated as "experts" on vaccination and those responsible for shaping vaccine policy. Despite the extreme complexity of this wide-ranging topic, at the end of the day it is you, the parents, who have to make vaccination decisions: Get vaccinated or not? Vaccinate your children or not? Vaccinate on schedule or space them out? Skip some of the shots or get them all?

Like everyone else nowadays, when you need information in order to make important decisions, you go to the Web, launch Google, and type in some relevant search terms, hoping the results will help you make an informed decision. But after surfing the Web in search of the answer to the to-vaccinate-or-not-to-vaccinate dilemma, you realize in short order that nailing this one will be anything but easy. A vaccine war is raging out there: Proponents and critics, parents and doctors, authorities and executives – all are stirring an enormous cauldron of... controversy soup. You'll find a dizzying variety of material – photographs, videos, testimony, articles, quotes, opinions, arguments, explanations, proofs, and rebuttals – an endless assortment of information, interpretations, and conflicting opinions being published 24/7. And, as you delve deeper, it just gets more and more confusing.

So, where do you start? How do you put all this chaos in some kind of order? How do you collate all the seemingly random pieces of information floating around the Web into a logical and coherent mental image? How do you reconcile the contradictions between the different positions? Do you really have to spend years diligently reading in WhatsApp or Facebook groups and carefully analyzing multitudes of scientific papers in order to make decisions about a procedure that, up until a few years ago, wasn't questioned by the vast majority of parents? Is it even possible to make informed decisions without proper medical training? And who should one believe – the parents who warn against the harms vaccinations inflicted upon their children or public health experts staunchly asserting that vaccines are proven safe and effective?

Who in heaven's name is right?! Come on, we have to make this @#$& decision!

Take a breath. You can relax. You have come to the right place.

After spending a few days reading this book, your question – Who is right? – will be answered. The answer to this question that troubles millions of parents around the world is out there, its pieces scattered across hundreds of cyberspace locations – visible to all, yet hidden in plain sight for the vast majority of the public.

The purpose of this book is to reveal that answer and shine a spotlight on it for everyone to see.

Who Is This Book For?

This book is intended, first and foremost, for parents, those who are taking their first steps into the confusing world of vaccines and those who want to deepen their understanding of the field. Please note: This book does not provide comprehensive information regarding vaccine-preventable diseases, nor does it directly discuss questions concerning vaccination, such as *Should I vaccinate? Which vaccines should I give?* and *When should I vaccinate?* Instead, the book focuses on decisively answering the all-important question at hand: Who is right in the vaccine debate – vaccine proponents or their opponents?

In addition to parents, the book is intended for medical professionals, as well as medical researchers, who are interested in approaching the hot topic of vaccines from an unconventional, non-dogmatic, perspective. (Pro tip: You might want to think twice before taking this book to the office.)

Finally, the book is also intended for all those professionals whose work sometimes touches on vaccine-related topics – reporters, politicians, government officials, lawyers, teachers, social workers, therapists – and anyone else who cares about the health of their country, most notably, its children.

How to Read This Book

The book is replete with citations and references backing up its claims. The referenced documents are drawn almost entirely from mainstream sources, with a handful of exceptions. These sources include medical journals, publications and websites of health authorities (such as the US Centers for Disease Control and Prevention and the World Health Organization), vaccine manufacturers' publications, news stories and articles from mainstream media, and history and science books.

References are marked in the body of the text by a superscript number (like so[1]). For each reference, the exact quote to which the text refers is provided (if possible or relevant), including the page number (if applicable), the document name, its main author, year of publication, and a link to the original text on the internet.[a] Since there are more than 1,200 references, in order to reduce costs and avoid unnecessary waste of resources, we chose not to include a "References" section in the printed version of the book. An electronic PDF document that includes all the references, arranged by chapter, can be downloaded for free from the internet (see the link and QR code on the book's back cover or first pages). For convenient access to the references while reading, we recommended that you read the book with your favorite screen display by your side and the reference document open to your current chapter.

Whether you are a medical professional, medical science researcher, or a parent who wants to make the best choices for your child's health, we urge you to spend some time browsing through the references, at least reading the specific quotes the text alludes to or cites. In addition, we encourage you to read as many of the original documents as you can. Since it is unlikely that you'll have enough spare time to fully explore all the book's references, we advise starting with those references that apply to any claims that seem particularly far-fetched to you. For each such reference, you might want to verify where it was published and who its authors are, making sure that the quotations used are accurate and that they faithfully represent the spirit of the original document (that is, are not taken out of context). Moreover, you are more than welcome to challenge your contacts in the medical profession – your family doctor, pediatrician, friends working in medical sciences, etc. – with the claims made in this book (making sure to attach the relevant references). Ask them to provide you with evidence that contradicts the book's assertions, but make sure they cite proper references from credible sources.

---

[a] Some of the papers in scientific journals are not accessible to the general public (access to the full text requires payment of a fee, which is usually quite high).

In addition to numbered references, the book also includes footnotes, denoted by superscripts of lower-case English letters ([a], [b], [c]...), that usually provide a little more detail. Unlike the references, you can find the footnotes at the bottom of the page where each appears.

And Finally: A Warning and a Recommendation

There are two possible answers to the central question in this book. If the answer is the one you'd expect, that vaccine authorities are right, you will just go on with your week somewhat better informed. If, on the other hand, the answer is that the parents are right, the earth beneath your feet may start to tremble.

Thus, you are now standing on the verge of an intellectual adventure that has the potential to violently rock your world. Once you pass through the gate, there will be no going back. You won't be able to "un-know" what you already know.

If you choose to continue reading, you will have to gather the courage required for a journey to the other side of reality, courage to face new facts and examine them objectively, courage to ask hard questions when you are expected to merely obey, and courage to stand your ground in the face of pressure from family, friends, doctors, government officials, and what will probably feel like everyone else.

If you aren't brave enough to get through this book, you might want to put it down, at least for now. Give it to someone else that you think is ready for the challenge. Come back to it in the future, when the time is right.

If, however, you choose to accompany us on this journey, you might want to make yourself a cup of coffee, get a smartphone or tablet and download the reference document so you have it next to you, and get comfy before we embark on our odyssey to the godforsaken corners of the vaccine version of Wonderland, where nothing is quite as it seems.

PART I

VACCINE SAFETY

Vaccine safety lies at the heart of the public debate on vaccines. Although prominent in many discussions, vaccine efficacy is only of secondary importance. The chief motivation driving vaccine-awareness advocates is the conviction that vaccination causes serious health harms in some recipients, and that this grim truth is largely concealed from the public. Had vaccines been perceived as completely safe, like health authorities claim, the animated public debate about them would never have gained traction. A vaccine with side effects that are mild and transient, that only causes serious or permanent damage extremely rarely (the proverbial "one in a million"), is unlikely to make any parent climb a virtual soapbox and preach to the cyber masses – even if its efficacy is less than ideal.

The public entities that promote vaccines – health authorities, physicians, researchers, medical societies and organizations – all echo a unified message: Vaccines have been tested more than any other medical intervention and are completely safe. This categorical claim, however, stands in stark contrast to the firsthand experience of thousands of parents who insist that their children suffered serious vaccine-related health harms. With the exception of a very small number of cases compensated by the government, the health establishment's response to parental claims of vaccine injury is utter dismissal and complete denial. Parents are told that they got it all wrong, that their child couldn't have been harmed by vaccination. Any temporal association between vaccine administration and subsequent deterioration in health is merely an unfortunate coincidence. The safety of each vaccine, they are told, was thoroughly vetted before it received marketing approval and is constantly monitored thereafter. Science has spoken – and science must prevail. Any negative impressions about vaccines are false and should be discarded; any misgivings should be put to rest. Vaccines are safe! Vaccines are effective!

The medical establishment's claim that [all] vaccines are

completely safe is based on activity in three distinct domains: a) clinical trials every new vaccine must undergo before it is approved for general use; b) computerized vaccine adverse event reporting systems that monitor post-marketing vaccine safety on an ongoing basis, and c) ad hoc epidemiological (population) studies that explore various aspects of vaccine safety. All of these will be scrutinized in the chapters that follow.

The first part of the book will thus explore the critical question of vaccine safety, examining in detail the institutional claims that vaccines are extremely safe and that their safety has been established by rock-solid science.

1

TURTLES ALL THE WAY DOWN: VACCINE CLINICAL TRIALS

According to a well-known story in the scientific community, an elderly woman approached a famous scientist shortly after he concluded his lecture on cosmology and the structure of the solar system:

> *"Your beautiful theory about the earth being round, and rotating around the sun, is very interesting, young man. Unfortunately, it is also very wrong. I have a better theory," the woman told him.*

> *"And what would that theory be, madam?" the scientist responded.*

> *"Well, what you call 'planet Earth' is not round at all. Actually, it is kind of a large, flat disk that rests on the shoulders of four giant elephants."*

> *"And what do these four elephants stand on?" the scientist inquired.*

> *"They stand on the back of a giant turtle," the elderly woman answered.*

> *"And what does that turtle stand on?" the scientist asked with an inquisitive grin.*

> *"On another, bigger, turtle."*

> *"And what does the second turtle stand on?"*

> *"Well, my dear man," said the elderly woman with a victorious smile, "it's turtles all the way down!"*

Even today, approximately 150 years after it first appeared, the story of the scientist, the elderly woman, and the turtles remains quite popular in scientific circles. Its appeal appears to be due not only to the paradoxical punchline, but also to the way it portrays the relationship between scientists and laypeople: On the one hand, the wise scientist, rational and calm, and on the other the simple-minded elderly woman confusing scientific knowledge and reality with myth. By emphasizing the wide intellectual chasm between expert and layperson, this amusing anecdote reinforces scientists' deep-seated expectation that science be unanimously recognized as the arbiter of objective Truth. Standing on their high pedestal, scientists, at least in their own eyes, are both worthy and capable of making final judgments on matters of public interest related to their expertise.

This paternalistic tendency is evident in long-standing attempts by scientific and medical entities to portray the public conversation on vaccines as a lopsided dispute. On one side of the debate, we are told, stand doctors and researchers who draw their moral authority from years of academic training and work experience and whose arguments are backed by solid scientific evidence and validated by the medical establishment worldwide. On the other side, they tell us, stand a multitude of parents and activists, who lack formal training, follow charlatans and quack doctors, and feed on fake news spread through social media.

Yet, as will become clear in the following pages, the surprising truth – which becomes self-evident when one devotes enough time and energy to researching vaccines – is that the roles are reversed: The elderly woman (the parents in this case) anchors her claims on bedrock science and displays a deep understanding of scientific methodology, while the medical establishment bases its position on… "turtles all the way down".

Vaccine safety lies at the heart of the long-lasting and intense clash between those that support universal vaccination and those that oppose it. Health authorities' argument that *Vaccines are safe!* is based, first and foremost, on the presumption that each new vaccine undergoes a meticulous process of testing and approval. This process includes a series of clinical trials, which purportedly utilize the most advanced scientific tools and techniques available and adhere to the highest safety standards. Once a new vaccine successfully passes these hurdles, it is considered safe by all relevant medical bodies.

This chapter, then, examines the methodology used for testing vaccines' safety as part of their pre-licensing approval process. Are new vaccines really rigorously scrutinized, as the public is routinely promised, in keeping with an uncompromising commitment to the highest possible safety standards?

Not only is the answer a flat "no", by the end of this chapter you will learn the inconceivable secret the medical establishment has concealed from the public eye for decades: **Clinical trials of vaccines are rigged to hide their true (and high) rate of side effects,** which means the medical establishment's longstanding claim that vaccines are safe has no scientific merit.

It sounds improbable, doesn't it? Impossible to believe!

By the time you finish reading this chapter you will know it's true.

Before we explore the methods employed by medical authorities to conceal vaccines' inadequate safety testing, we must familiarize ourselves with their pre-licensing approval process and its principal tool – the randomized controlled trial. Armed with this knowledge, we can then peel off, one by one, the protective layers that enfold the hidden, abhorrent, and nearly unbelievable truth.

The Vaccine Approval Process

Medical "biologics" (such as vaccines) undergo a lengthy and tedious approval process, replete with bureaucratic forms, documents, and reviews. The process is determined by the authorizing body – most commonly the US Food and Drug Administration (FDA) or the European Medicines Agency (EMA) – and includes, in addition to endless paperwork, a requirement to conduct a series of clinical trials[a] that demonstrate the effectiveness and safety of the product submitted for approval. This required series of clinical trials is divided into three *phases*, with each phase commencing only when and if the preceding phase has been successfully concluded. If the product does not prove safe or effective in any one of the phases, it will not win the coveted approval. Consequently, its development is likely to terminate, and the (usually considerable) funds invested in it will go down the drain.[1]

The first hurdle a new vaccine must leap is the "pre-clinical phase", in which the product goes through a multitude of laboratory[b] and animal experiments.

The next step in the series is a *Phase 1 Clinical Trial,* in which a small trial group (typically dozens of subjects) is given the new vaccine in order to determine how the human body responds to it. The underlying assumption is that, despite its success in animal experiments during the pre-clinical phase, the vaccine could still prove to be harmful to humans.[2] Therefore, in this stage, researchers attempt to identify particularly salient or severe side effects, such as severe allergic reactions, disability, early symptoms of a chronic problem, severe illness, or death. Due to the limited number of subjects, a Phase 1 trial cannot provide a complete picture of the extent and variety of side effects (adverse events) that could potentially be caused by the vaccine.

If the vaccine successfully passes Phase 1, the next experimental phase – the *Phase 2 Clinical Trial* – is performed on a larger group, typically several hundred people, and the vaccine's

---

[a] A clinical trial is a research study with human subjects (as opposed to animal studies). The word *trial* indicates artificial (deliberate) conditions specifically designed for the study's purpose (unlike studies that do not interfere with subjects' daily lives). The word *clinical* implies that the study involves some kind of intervention (for example, vaccination of subjects), as opposed to observational studies which only collect and analyze information. More on this topic in chapter 4.

[b] A laboratory experiment is an experiment made with specialized equipment outside the living organism (e.g. in a test tube or Petri dish). It is termed *in vitro*.

effectiveness is evaluated in its designated population (e.g., adults over 65 or diabetic patients under 18). This stage is also when the effects of varying the vaccine's dosage and delivery timing on efficacy and safety are examined. However, the absence of a control group (see the *Randomized Controlled Trial* section below) and the relatively small number of subjects in Phase 2 trials, preclude the attainment of definite or final answers regarding the vaccine's efficacy and safety. Those await the next testing phase.

Phase 3 Clinical Trials are conducted in several thousand subjects, sometimes even tens of thousands. These trials are designed to assess and validate the vaccine's effectiveness, to compare the new treatment with existing treatments (if any), and to collect information that will allow the vaccine to be used safely. This is the final experimental phase before the approval for commercial use, and it is of paramount importance in determining the efficacy and safety of the experimental vaccine. Phase 3 results will be published in the manufacturer's package insert and will serve as key evidence for the vaccine's safety and efficacy for years to come.

Subjects in a Phase 3 trial are randomly divided into one of two groups: the *trial group*, which receives the test vaccine over a specified period of time, and the *control group*, which receives a placebo (dummy) or some other compound (see the detailed explanation in the next section). Throughout the study period, researchers monitor trial participants' health and collect information that will be used to evaluate the vaccine's efficacy and safety. The large quantity of subjects, as well as their separation into trial and control groups, affords a deeper probe into the vaccine's safety and its potential side effects, including those that occur relatively infrequently (i.e. one case in hundreds or thousands of subjects).

Successful completion of a Phase 3 trial paves the way for the long-awaited approval for commercial production and marketing of the new vaccine. However, even after the vaccine has been in general use for a while, additional trials are sometimes called for.

These "post-marketing" trials may be required to investigate unexpected adverse events reported after licensing or negative effects that have emerged in a specific population segment. This type of trial is called a *Phase 4 Clinical Trial*.

As mentioned above, after the vaccine successfully passes Phase 3 trials, the doors open for commercial use. However, for new vaccines, receiving approval from the authorizing body is not sufficient. The product must also receive the approval of the authority responsible for distribution of vaccines. In the US, the FDA is in charge of licensing new vaccines, while the Centers for Disease Control and Prevention (CDC) is responsible for making recommendations for their actual use, including who should receive them (their ages and health status), the timing and number of doses to be received, and which vaccines can be given concurrently. The final step in the long process of marketing a new vaccine is its integration into the national vaccine programs of the US and other countries around the globe. Adding a vaccine to the American schedule recommended by the CDC instantly guarantees sales of millions of units per year in the US alone, thus assuring its manufacturer a handsome return on its initial investment.[3]

The Randomized Controlled Trial (RCT)

In a "simple" vaccine clinical trial (one without a control group, as is the case for trials in Phases 1 and 2), researchers face an inherent difficulty in determining whether a specific condition reported during the trial period is actually caused by the experimental compound or not. If a trial subject experiences a severe and immediate phenomenon following the receipt of the test vaccine, such as fainting or cardiac arrest, it could be reasonably assumed that the recently consumed vaccine was the culprit. When the side effect is less pronounced, or appears days or weeks following vaccine administration, however, the researchers' decision is less obvious. For example, if the subject's temperature rises to 103°F less than 48 hours after administration of the test vaccine, the researchers do not have enough information to decide whether this is a true side effect or merely an unfortunate coincidence. One option is to have every participant who experiences a health-related condition during the trial undergo a series of in-depth medical examinations in order to uncover possible links to the experimental vaccine. This strategy is not feasible or economical, however, if only because the vaccine is new and its specific effect on the human body is virtually unknown. Consequently, such an investigation could prove lengthy, costly, and unlikely to yield conclusive results.

A better option is to conduct an "enhanced" clinical trial – a controlled, randomized, and blinded trial (also known as a *randomized controlled trial* – RCT). In an RCT, subjects are divided into two groups:[c] the *trial group*, receiving the test compound, and a *control group*, receiving a dummy or existing compound (whose efficacy and safety profile is well known). Subjects are randomly assigned to the two groups prior to the start of the trial to ensure that the groups are virtually alike in every relevant characteristic (age, gender, area of residence, demographic status, and so on). The term *blinded* (or *blinding*), means that the trial subjects do not know which group they are in and thus do not know whether they received the test or dummy compound. In a *double blind* trial, the researchers also do not know which subjects belong to which group. Thus, prior knowledge of which compound a participant received is not likely to influence either subjects or researchers and skew the results of the trial. In a non-blinded trial, subjects who receive the test compound, rather than the dummy one, may complain more about side effects, since they expect them to occur.[d] Similarly, a researcher who knows a particular subject belongs to the control group also knows that any reported side effects are not

---

[c] Sometimes the experiment may include three groups, or more. For example, a trial might consist of two trial groups and a control group.

[d] In clinical trials with infant subjects, as many vaccine trials are, biased reporting from participants is impossible. However, if parents are aware of their child's grouping (trial or control), reporting bias is plausible.

due to the vaccine and may inadvertently (subconsciously) underreport medical conditions occurring during the trial period. Only when the trial is over, after all relevant information has been collected, is the specific compound administered to each of the study subjects revealed, and the researchers, with the complete data in hand, can begin the post-clinical data analysis.

When it comes to pre-licensure testing of drugs, vaccines, and other medical products, RCTs are widely considered the industry's "gold standard". The random distribution of subjects to trial and control groups, as well as the minimization of potential biases through the use of double-blinding, facilitates a reliable and meaningful comparison of trial and control group data.[4] As an example, in a vaccine trial in which the control group is receiving a dummy compound, one can measure the level of antibodies produced in trial group subjects and compare it to that of the control group, thus getting a measure of vaccine efficacy. Similarly, a researcher could compare the incidence of adverse events following vaccination in the two groups, thus getting an estimation of vaccine safety. The larger the number of trial participants and the better the researchers adhere to RCT standard practices, the more reliable and comprehensive the trial results will be.

Due to the high quality and reliability of RCTs, they are the method designated by regulatory agencies (and accepted by the pharmaceutical industry) for evaluating efficacy and safety of vaccines in Phase 3 clinical trials.[5]

The Control Group in a Clinical Trial

As we have seen, the use of a control group in a clinical trial allows researchers to examine the therapeutic effect of the compound (efficacy) and the rate of adverse events it causes (safety) by comparing outcomes in the trial group with those of the control group. This comparative statistical analysis, then, will be influenced by the nature of the compound the researchers give to the control group.

As a general rule, when deciding upon the type of compound given to the control group in an RCT, there are two options. For a trial of a completely new drug or vaccine, i.e. one which does not have an approved equivalent, the control group should receive an inert compound (*placebo*)[6] that does not affect the parameters measured in the trial.[e] However, if a proven treatment already exists, it may be unethical to prevent control group participants from receiving it. For example, in trials of new cancer drugs, it is considered unethical to prevent the control group's subjects from receiving an existing drug for their illness. In this scenario, then, the control group would receive the current approved treatment. This practice is also the norm for vaccines even though vaccines are used preventatively (not treatment for an existing condition) and are given to healthy individuals.[7]

If we apply the above guidelines to the clinical trials for the two generations of the Prevnar vaccine,[f] then the original Prevnar, a new vaccine that had no therapeutic alternative at the time it was developed, should have been tested in an RCT in which the control group received an inert injection as a placebo. In the trials of Prevnar-13, the next-generation vaccine, the control group should have received the (original) Prevnar vaccine, assuming that it would be unethical to deprive that group's subjects of the current Prevnar vaccine's protection, whose efficacy is already proven.

So how do researchers determine the incidence of adverse events associated with the new compound being tested in a controlled clinical trial? By comparing the rate of adverse events observed in the trial group to that of the control group. For example, if in a new vaccine's trial group of 1,000 infants there were 20 cases of high fever, and in the control group (which has

---

[e] In vaccine trials, the conventional placebo is usually a saline (salt water) injection that is widely accepted as having no side effects (except those related to the physical act of injection).

[f] A vaccine for preventing infection caused by the pneumococcal bacteria.

the same number of subjects) there were only 10 such cases registered, the results would imply the risk of high fever in the vaccinated is twice as high as in the unvaccinated. In absolute terms, the data shows that the vaccine increases the risk of high fever occurrence from 1 in every 100 infants to 1 in 50.[g]

When the control group's subjects are given a placebo, an inert substance not known to cause high fever, it is assumed that the incidence of high fever recorded for the group represents the *background rate* (or *baseline rate*) of the phenomenon. In other words, the background rate is the number of subjects who would experience high fever naturally, regardless of any trial intervention. In our example above, we would assume that 1 in 100 control group subjects developed high fever due to random causes (unrelated to the trial). Since the trial group would likely experience a similar background rate of high fever (1 in 100), any significant deviation from this level should be attributed to the experimental vaccine. It follows, then, that an RCT in which the control group receives an *inert placebo* is designed to answer the critical question of *How many adverse events does the new vaccine cause?* Of course, we should keep in mind that trial results are no more than a good estimation. If or when the vaccine is released to the market, the actual reported adverse event rate might deviate significantly from that observed in the clinical trial. Still, the results of RCTs are the best estimate of safety available to science during the vaccine approval process, and in many cases, throughout its lifetime.

In a trial in which the control group receives a different vaccine (as in the trial of Prevnar-13 vs. Prevnar, its predecessor), the results obtained are always relative, answering the question *How many more (or less) adverse events does the new vaccine cause compared to the current vaccine?* For example, if (out of 1,000

---

[g] The above calculation is intentionally simplistic and is intended to demonstrate the basic principle applied in analyzing the results of an RCT, which is the comparison of different quantitative parameters between trial and control groups. In practice, researchers apply complex mathematical calculations that utilize various statistical functions and parameters.

subjects) 24 cases of high fever were observed in the trial group, while 20 such cases were reported in the control group, the new vaccine would appear to increase the odds of high fever by 20% (relative to the current vaccine). That is an important piece of information as it reveals how the new-generation vaccine's safety fares against that of its predecessor. However, it is impossible to calculate from a trial such as this one the absolute rate of adverse events caused by the experimental vaccine – that is, the rate of adverse events from vaccinating compared to not vaccinating. The absolute rate could not be calculated because the control group received a compound (the current vaccine) which is not inert (neutral), but rather has side effects of its own. In the above example, 24 cases of high fever were observed in recipients of the new vaccine, and 20 cases in current vaccine recipients. But how many cases would have been reported in trial subjects given a true placebo? This trial cannot answer that question; therefore, the absolute rate of adverse events caused by the new vaccine cannot be calculated from trial data. The new vaccine could be said to cause 24 cases of high fever per 1,000 subjects, but this number would not represent a reliable estimate[h] as it does not take into account the background rate of the phenomenon, which was not measured in the trial.

In order to determine the true rate of adverse events of a new generation vaccine, a *three-arm trial* must be conducted, combining the two methods described above. In this kind of trial, subjects would be randomly allocated into three groups, one trial and two controls: The trial group would receive the new generation vaccine, the first control group would receive the current vaccine, and the second control group would receive an inert placebo. This trial design is considered to be of excellent quality, as it measures both the *absolute* rate of adverse events (comparing the new vaccine to the placebo) and the *relative* rate (comparing the new vaccine to the current vaccine).[8] From a

---

[h] The 24 per 1,000 rate represents a "ceiling" of the phenomenon, as was observed in the trial. The "floor" is, of course, zero.

public health perspective, the three-arm trial answers two important questions: (1) *How many adverse events does the new vaccine cause when compared to not vaccinating?* and (2) *How many adverse events does the new vaccine cause when compared to the existing vaccine?*[i] Continuing with our Prevnar example, if the placebo-receiving control group reported, say, 8 high fever cases per 1,000 subjects, then the study would indicate that the new vaccine – which, as we recall, had 24 cases of high fever per 1,000 subjects – increased the risk of high fever by a factor of three (or, put differently, caused 16 more cases per 1,000 subjects), compared to not vaccinating.

Another scenario in which a three-arm trial would be appropriate is re-establishing the safety of a legacy vaccine that was originally tested many years ago. The environment into which today's infants are born may differ significantly in crucial health-related aspects from the environment in which a first-generation vaccine was tested decades ago. For example, the current measles-mumps-rubella-varicella (MMRV) vaccine (ProQuad) is the "grandchild" of the original MMR vaccine, which was tested in the late 1960s. Back then, the vaccine schedule consisted of only the diphtheria-pertussis-tetanus (DPT) and polio vaccines, with the first dose administered at age two months. If ProQuad were clinically tested against the original MMR and proved to have a similar safety profile, could we assume it is safe just because its grandparent vaccine was deemed safe 50 years ago? MMR vaccines are typically administered in the second year of life, after most of the infant vaccine schedule has already been delivered. If, hypothetically, the MMR's risk of harmful side effects were related to the load of previously administered vaccines, then we could not automatically accept the present safety of the original

---

[i] In order to overcome ethical objections to a three-arm trial, administration of the existing vaccine to placebo group participants could be delayed for several months, so as not to prevent them from getting the protection it is supposed to provide. Alternatively, the trial could be carried out in a country where the existing vaccine was not routinely provided, so the control group would not be deprived of a treatment the subjects would otherwise receive.

MMR. Remember that the MMR was first tested when the vaccine schedule consisted of only two other vaccines. If it were tested today, with many more vaccines on the schedule, some of which are given to pregnant mothers, others to newborns and infants one month of age, would it still be proven safe? And the changing vaccine program is just one aspect of the environment that may affect the safety of a given vaccine. Other factors, such as chemical exposure, changing diets, air pollution, radiation, etc., could also play a role. Therefore, a clinical trial comparing ProQuad to MMR alone is deficient, as it would rely on the presumed safety of a vaccine (MMR) that might no longer be safe. Once more, a third group receiving a placebo is the proper solution to the problem.[j]

To summarize, in a clinical trial of an (entirely) new vaccine, the control group should receive a placebo so that the absolute rate of the vaccine's adverse events can be determined. This design does not pose an ethical problem, since the vaccine has no existing alternative. In a trial of a new-generation vaccine, one control group should receive the current vaccine and another should receive a placebo (a three-arm trial).

External Control Group

Another important point to consider is that an RCT control group cannot be replaced with data from another trial, or any other externally calculated background rate. In other words, it is not scientifically valid to draw conclusions by comparing the observed rate of any phenomenon in a randomized controlled trial to the rate reported in another trial or to a rate observed in

---

[j] One might claim that safety issues with a vaccine that has been in use for many years would have been discovered earlier by other surveillance means such as adverse event reporting systems and epidemiological studies. However, as will be discussed in chapters 3, 4, and 5, these measures are far less reliable than RCTs.

the general population.[k] For example, if in a particular vaccine trial the reported incidence of sudden infant death syndrome (SIDS or "crib death")[l] in the trial group were 0.5% (1 in 200), researchers could not then compare this rate to the background rate of the phenomenon in the population (say 0.8%), thus determining that the vaccine lowered the risk of SIDS. This is because trial participants comprise a subgroup which could possess specific characteristics, known or unknown, which are not representative of the entire population. This could potentially yield trial results that are not comparable to rates in the general population.[9] For example, the proportion of infants participating in a trial whose parents smoke may be much lower than the background rate in the entire population, skewing the incidence of crib death in trial participants in a downward direction. Of course, skewing in the opposite direction is equally possible.

Similarly, there is little scientific merit in comparing results from different clinical trials. For example, no significant insights could be derived from comparing the results of a Prevnar-13 trial carried out in infants from the New York area in 2010 with those of a Prevnar trial conducted in Philadelphia in 2005. This is due to the randomization principle of the Randomized Controlled Trial (RCT), which requires that the trial participants be randomly divided between the trial group and the control group. Obviously, groups whose members were selected at different times and places would not satisfy this requirement. In the above examples, any differences in trial results could be entirely due to dissimilarities between the groups, such as different socioeconomic status, environmental exposures, or behavioral characteristics.

The principle described above is well known to the pharma-

---

[k] Except in very specific and limited cases that are not relevant to this discussion.

[l] Crib death, formally named sudden infant death syndrome (SIDS), is the term used when an infant dies for no discernible reason.

ceutical industry and it appears in numerous vaccine manufacturers' leaflets. For example, the package insert for Glaxo-Smith-
Kline's (GSK) hepatitis A vaccine (Havrix) reads: "Because
clinical trials are conducted under widely varying conditions,
adverse reaction rates observed in the clinical trials of a vaccine
cannot be directly compared to rates in the clinical trials of
another vaccine, and may not reflect the rates observed in
practice."[10]

Clinical Trials in Children

Throughout most of the 20th century, the prevailing opinion in
the world of medicine was that due to the relative fragility of
children (compared to adults), they should be protected from the
perils of medical research. The result was a distinct lack of
scientific knowledge about the effects of medical interventions
(such as medication) on children. Administering medication to
children, therefore, was largely a wide-ranging experiment
conducted on the public. Circumstances began to change in 1977
when the American Academy of Pediatrics (AAP) published new
guidelines regulating the participation of children in clinical
trials. In the new guidelines, the AAP said that drugs and vaccines should be tested on the population for which they are
intended – in this case, children – and that this requirement is
not only ethical, but essential to their health as well.[11]

Over the following decades, various international medical
organizations have formulated ethical rules governing the participation of children in clinical trials of drugs and vaccines.
According to these rules, children may only be included in
experiments intended to achieve an important scientific or
public health objective directly related to the health and well-
being of children. Children should not participate in studies that
do not promote such goals, such as studies designed merely to
confirm the results of other studies or studies designed to advance scientific knowledge that does not concern children.[12]

In addition, the medical code of ethics states that all parties involved in a trial must carefully weigh the potential benefit to child participants against the potential dangers involved. If the study's participants cannot be expected to benefit from the given intervention, then the intervention's inherent risk must be "minimal", especially if the subject has not consented to participate in the trial (as is the case with infants). For example, if children assigned to the control group of a drug trial were to receive a dummy medication (placebo) and a blood test, then both the medication and the blood draw must present no more than "minimal" risk. Also, the potential benefit must be substantial enough to justify the intervention's risk.[13] For example, in a trial of a children's cough syrup, the risk associated with the new drug should be relatively low as the potential benefit would be relatively low, while the potential benefit in a trial of a child cancer medication would be significantly higher, thus the risk posed by the drug could be proportionately higher as well.

A more lenient approach holds that even if a trial procedure has no expected benefit, a "minor increase over minimal risk" is allowed if the experiment has the potential for gaining knowledge about the subjects' disorder that is considered to be of "vital importance". However, even with this approach, the risk associated with the intervention must not exceed the risk a healthy child would face in everyday life and should not cause permanent or irreparable damage. In any case, there must be prior knowledge of the level of risk inherent in the procedure. If the risk is unknown, it cannot be determined to be "a minor increase over minimal risk".[14] It is important to note that the above discussion holds equally true for both the trial and control groups of an experiment.

Now that we are familiar with the different clinical phases of the vaccine approval process, the purpose of control groups in randomized controlled trials, and the ethical limitations imposed on children's participation in medical research, we can better examine the deliberately flawed procedure the industry uses to conduct vaccine clinical trials.

A Problem and a Solution

Let's take a moment to examine a hypothetical scenario: A major pharmaceutical company has developed a new drug against a particular medical problem. Following its preliminary trials, the company realizes that the drug is associated with a relatively high incidence of serious side effects that may negatively affect its chances to win FDA approval. Let us suppose that, since the company spent hundreds of millions of dollars developing the drug and the target market segment is worth billions of dollars in sales per year, the company decides to move forward with the licensing process and start a Phase 3 clinical trial. Given all of the above, what are the company's options, legal and illegal, for ensuring that the trial demonstrates a positive safety profile, thus clearing the way for the drug's approval?

One option is to artificially lower the incidence of adverse events reported in the trial group (the group receiving the new drug), by withholding or modifying data for specific cases. The difficulty with this technique is that for the duration of the trial, because of the enforced double-blinding, researchers do not know which subjects belong to which trial group. Thus, one cannot suppress or dilute reports for a specific group (the trial group, in this case) while leaving those of the other intact. Randomly suppressing reports would not be likely to accomplish the desired effect as the ratio of adverse events in each of the two groups would probably not change much.

Another theoretical option would be to modify the results following the conclusion of the clinical stage of the trial, at which point the blinding is removed and the data becomes fully available to the researchers.[m] The difficulty with this approach is that falsifying trial data is a criminal offense, which can lead to grave consequences for the company and the researchers them-

---

[m] Triple-blind RCT studies prevent this kind of possibility by hiding the group identity even in the analysis stage. Studies of this type are rare and not usually part of vaccine pre-licensure trials.

selves, making this an unattractive option.

Another option would be to use various statistical techniques (which will be discussed later in the book), to build a false safety profile for the drug being tested. The difficulty with this approach is that the RCT study design greatly reduces researchers' ability to affect the results since they gain access to the full data set at a time when the data can no longer be altered. With limited ability to control the data, it can be quite difficult to eliminate undesired signals by statistical manipulation while at the same time successfully covering one's tracks.

The last option available to the company wishing to hide their product's undesirable side effects is to design a trial in which the reported rate of adverse events in the control group would likely be very similar to that of the trial group. As described previously, the RCT's control group represents the baseline rate to which the trial group is compared. A similar proportion between the two groups would indicate that the adverse events reported in the trial group were the result of "background noise" only and not caused by the experimental drug. This technique has three distinct advantages: (1) It is 100% legal, (2) it is very effective, and, as it turns out, (3) it has the full approval of licensing authorities around the world. As we shall shortly see, this method is exactly the one vaccine manufacturers employ to deliberately obscure the real incidence of vaccine adverse events.

The entire vaccine program is founded upon this deception.

Fake Placebo

It is virtually impossible to state the bottom line of the analysis presented above mildly, so here goes: **Vaccine trials in general, and childhood vaccine trials specifically, are purposely designed to obscure the true incidence of adverse events of the vaccine being tested.**

How do they do this? By using a two-step scheme: First, a new vaccine (one which does not have a predecessor), is always tested in a Phase 3 RCT in which the control group receives another vaccine (or a compound very similar to the experimental vaccine, see explanation below). A new pediatric vaccine is never tested during its formal approval process against a neutral solution (placebo). Comparing a trial group to a control group that was given a compound that is likely to cause a similar rate of adverse events facilitates the formation of a false safety profile. The rate of adverse events of the tested vaccine is said to be similar to the "background rate", hence it is considered safe. The researchers, and the vaccine manufacturer they work for, seem to "forget" that the compound they administered to the control group is a bioactive substance, carrying its own risks and side effects, and hardly represents the baseline or background rate that is essential to an RCT for a new vaccine.

Thus, the vaccine is approved and added to national vaccine programs throughout the world. Then, when the "next genera-tion" vaccine comes along, its pre-licensing clinical trials will always compare the new vaccine to the current vaccine and never to a placebo. Thus, all parties involved ensure that the true rate of vaccine adverse events is never discovered – for either the original or upgraded vaccine – and that rate is never shared with the public, or even the medical world.

The practice of giving a different vaccine to the control group in an RCT of an entirely new vaccine and calling it "placebo" is a deliberate misrepresentation of the term. As explained previous-ly, a placebo is a compound (or procedure) that does not affect the parameters measured in the trial. When testing the efficacy of a new vaccine, researchers measure the level of disease anti-bodies in both study groups, so the substance given to the control group must not affect that antibody level, or the compar-ison becomes meaningless. For example, in a hypothetical new hepatitis C vaccine trial, it would not make scientific sense to inject the control group subjects with a compound that could increase (or decrease) the subjects' hepatitis C antibodies. Doing so would preclude a valid assessment of the effect of the vaccine on the antibody level, as the substance taken by the controls could have distorted the comparison.[n]

The above analysis holds true for safety testing as well. If the compound given to the control group has its own significant side effects, it cannot be regarded as a true placebo. If the rates of adverse events observed in the trial and control groups appear similar, is it because the experimental vaccine is safe or because the control compound is just as unsafe as the vaccine? It would be impossible to know. Giving the control group an active substance in an RCT intended to test safety would be a bad design decision, then. Yet this is exactly how new vaccine Phase 3 trials are performed: Instead of a placebo, the control group receives a different vaccine, which is certain to cause its own adverse events and can in no way be deemed a neutral substance.

This practice of administering a different vaccine to the control group in a new-vaccine trial has no bearing on efficacy testing: It is highly likely that the control vaccine, which usually targets a different disease, would have no effect on the antibody level of the disease targeted by the test vaccine. Thus, using our hepatitis C example, if the control group subjects in the vaccine trial were given the Prevnar vaccine, no change in their hepatitis C antibody level would be expected; thus, the true efficacy of the test vaccine could be determined. But this lack of effect is not the case when it comes to safety: Because the Prevnar vaccine has its own side effects, it cannot be considered neutral in this context. Therefore, the true rate of adverse events for the experimental hepatitis C vaccine cannot be determined by comparing it to the rate in the group that received Prevnar since the controls did not receive a neutral compound.

This deliberate distortion of the placebo concept in clinical trials of new vaccines is so prevalent that researchers and vaccine

---

[n] Thus, a positive effect (a significantly higher level of antibodies in the trial group) could be the result of the control group's compound *lowering* the antibody level rather than the vaccine *raising* it. The opposite would hold true for a negative effect: The vaccine could have done a decent job raising the antibody level, but the control substance, for some unknown reason, was almost as effective, thereby diminishing the vaccine's positive effect.

package inserts frequently refer to the bioactive compound given to a control group as "placebo", even when it's clear it is another vaccine or a similar bioactive compound, which in itself is not safety-neutral.[15] Falsely using the term "placebo" allows researchers to conclude that the new compound "was proven safe" because its rate of adverse events was similar to that of placebo – even though the substance the control group received was decidedly not a placebo. For example, in one of the DTaP° vaccine trials, the rate of hospital admissions in the trial group was almost 1 in every 22 subjects. The researchers did not consider this statistic alarming, however, because in the control groups that received different DTP vaccines,[p] the hospitalization rate was similar.[16] Was such a high hospitalization rate in trial participants unrelated to the vaccines used, or were they the main culprit? Only the use of a true placebo control group could answer that question.[17]

No logical explanation can be found for the ubiquitous practice of administering bioactive compounds to control groups in trials of new vaccines other than a desire to conceal the true rate of adverse events of the vaccine. Testing a new vaccine against a placebo in an RCT is the simplest, safest, cheapest and most reliable option. Saline (sterilized salt water), for example, is a safe, reliable, widely available, and inexpensive compound – certainly when compared to a vaccine. Because it does not cause significant adverse events, nor does it produce disease-specific antibodies, it provides a reliable baseline for both safety and efficacy testing and is therefore ideal for control group usage. Calculation of the true rate of adverse events of the test vaccine becomes straightforward and simple. Despite its clear benefits as a placebo, vaccine makers prefer not to use saline in vaccine trials, and the reason for this should be obvious by now.

° A vaccine against diphtheria, tetanus, and pertussis that contains an acellular pertussis component.

[p] The older version of the DTaP vaccine that contains a whole-cell pertussis component.

How Were Vaccines on the Schedule Tested?

Now that the groundwork has been laid, it's time to consider the vaccines on the CDC's recommended childhood vaccine schedule: How were they tested for safety before getting marketing approval? Were the clinical trials of these vaccines "cooked" in the manner described above? Were they tested against (real) placebos? Is their true rate of adverse events known?

According to the current CDC vaccination program,[18] all children routinely receive vaccines against 13 different diseases by the age of two years.[q] Let's examine each of these vaccines.

Diphtheria-Tetanus-acellular-Pertussis Vaccines (DTaP): The DTaP vaccine is administered in various combinations – with or without inactivated polio, Hib, and hepatitis B components – and is manufactured by two companies: GlaxoSmithKline (GSK) and Sanofi Pasteur.

GSK's Pediarix vaccine protects against five diseases: diphtheria, tetanus, pertussis, hepatitis B, and polio. The safety section of the vaccine's package insert mentions 14 clinical trials involving 8,088 subjects. In the largest of the trials, conducted in Germany, the trial group received the Pediarix vaccine and a Hib vaccine, while the control group received Infanrix (DTaP vaccine, see below), Hib, and oral polio vaccines. In another trial explicitly mentioned in the leaflet, Pediarix was tested against a control group receiving Infanrix, hepatitis B, and inactivated polio vaccines. The leaflet does not describe the compounds given to the control groups in the remaining 12 safety studies, other than indicating that all of them received "comparator vaccines".[19]

GSK also manufactures a 4-in-1 vaccine called Kinrix, which is identical to the above Pediarix, minus the hepatitis B component. In the vaccine's largest clinical trial, the control group received Infanrix and IPOL (polio) vaccines. All trial participants were also concomitantly administered a dose of the MMR vac-

---

[q] As of April 2020. Not counting the annual influenza vaccine.

cine. The leaflet does not mention any trial involving a placebo control group.[20]

And how was the aforementioned Infanrix vaccine itself tested? The vaccine, which includes diphtheria, tetanus, and acellular pertussis components, was tested for safety in one clinical trial against a control group that received the DTP vaccine (the older, whole-cell pertussis, version), and in another that had no control group.[21]

What about the older generation DTP vaccine? What safety testing did it undergo? Although this vaccine is known to have caused serious side effects in infants (and was therefore replaced by the newer DTaP vaccine in the late 1990s),[22] it was never tested in a modern clinical trial in which the control group received a true placebo.[23] The vaccine, which was developed in the first half of 20th century, underwent a series of trials in the 1930s and 1940s at a time when the concept of the randomized controlled trial was still in its infancy. Hence, in most of these trials, there was no randomized control group, and the researchers devoted little effort to gathering information on the side effects of the tested vaccine.[24]

In addition to the above, a search of the *clinicaltrials.gov* web-site, a repository of clinical trials conducted since the year 2000, yields dozens of results for GSK's Infanrix vaccine family. None of them specifies an RCT with a placebo control group.[25]

To summarize, the safety of GSK's 5-in-1 and 4-in-1 vaccines was tested against the triple vaccine (DTaP), which was tested against the older generation vaccine (DTP), whose safety was never tested in an RCT with a placebo control group. A turtle standing on the back of a turtle, standing on the back of yet another turtle – all the way down.

In addition to GSK's diphtheria-tetanus-pertussis family of vaccines reviewed above, Sanofi Pasteur's DTaP line of vaccines is also approved for use in the US. The Pentacel vaccine (DTaP, polio and Hib) was tested in four clinical trials during its licensing process. In three of the trials, the control group participants received an assortment of different vaccines.[26] The fourth trial appears to have had a control group that received no vaccines. However, the clinical review document submitted to the FDA reveals that the trial actually had no control group.[27]

Sanofi's Quadracel 4-in-1 vaccine (DTaP and polio) was tested for safety in one large clinical trial. The control group received Sanofi's 3-in-1 (Daptacel) and polio vaccines.[28]

Daptacel, Sanofi's triple DTaP vaccine, underwent four clinical trials during its licensing process. All of the trials were randomized and controlled, and in all of them, the control group received different combinations of DTaP or DTP vaccines, sometimes concurrently with other vaccines as well.[29]

The rates of adverse events in the trials reviewed above were always compared with rates observed in control groups whose participants also received vaccines. For example, a major study conducted in Sweden in the early 1990s compared four different DTP-related vaccines and found that serious adverse events – seizures, life-threatening events, onset of chronic illness, and more – occurred in approximately 1 in 200 vaccinees. Adverse events classified as "prohibiting future vaccination" were reported for 1 in every 100 vaccinees, and about 1 in 22 subjects were admitted to a hospital.[30] However, since the rates for the new-generation-vaccine (DTaP) groups were similar to that of the old-generation-vaccine (DTP) groups, the new vaccines received the green light.

The bottom line is that none of the many products in either of the DTaP vaccine family lines routinely administered in the US has been tested for safety in a clinical trial with a placebo-controlled group.

Haemophilus Influenzae Type B (Hib) Vaccine: The vaccine protects against infection caused by the Haemophilus influenzae type b bacterium. It can be administered as a component of the 5-in-1 Pentacel vaccine, discussed above, or as a separate vaccine. At present, there are three standalone Hib vaccine brands approved for use in the United States.

Hiberix is produced by GSK. Its package insert reports a single RCT in which the vaccine was administered concomitantly with several other vaccines (DTaP, polio, hepatitis B, and others). The two control groups received a different Hib vaccine or a DTaP-polio-Hib vaccine, along with several other vaccines. Seven other trials mentioned in the leaflet were not blinded ("open label") and apparently had no control groups.[31]

ActHIB, manufactured by Sanofi Pasteur, was clinically tested for safety in three RCTs. In the first, the vaccine was simultaneously administered with the DTP vaccine, while the control group received the DTP vaccine alone. In the other two trials, the trial groups received a combination vaccine with ActHIB as one of its components, while the control groups received the same combination vaccine (without the ActHIB component), and a separate ActHIB vaccine.[32]

PedvaxHIB, by Merck, was tested in Native American infants. The package insert states that the control group received a placebo; however, all trial participants were also given the DTP and OPV vaccines concomitantly.[33]

Polio Vaccine (IPV): Similar to the Hib vaccine, the inactivated polio vaccine is administered as either a component of DTaP combination vaccines (discussed previously) or as a standalone vaccine. The IPOL vaccine, by Sanofi Pasteur, is the only brand currently licensed and used in the United States. Its package insert does not mention any pre-licensure RCTs that were performed for the vaccine.[34] Wasn't the vaccine clinically tested before it was introduced into the US schedule in the early 1990s?

Well, no. According to a document released by the FDA in 2018 following a Freedom of Information Act (FOIA) request, the vaccine underwent two clinical trials. However, these trials did not meet the current requirements for a Phase 3 randomized controlled trial. The first trial, which was conducted in 1980-1983, consisted of only 371 subjects in the IPOL trial group and about the same number in the control group, which (and this shouldn't be surprising by now) received the oral polio vaccine (OPV). The OPV, manufactured by Lederle, was the only polio vaccine licensed in the US at the time. In addition, all trial participants received the DPT vaccine. The trial was controlled, randomized, and possibly blinded (though the licensing documents do not state this explicitly), but obviously not placebo bound. The second study, conducted in Buffalo, New York, in the late 1980s, enrolled 114 children who underwent a series of three vaccinations with either IPOL, OPV, or a combination of both. Most of the children received the DPT vaccine as well. This trial was not controlled, randomized, or blinded.[35]

So, the inactivated polio vaccine (IPV) "safety turtle" – established in two small trials, only one of them an RCT with any sort of control group – stands on the back of Lederle's oral polio vaccine (OPV) safety turtle. And what lies below that turtle's feet? Only thin air, apparently. The Lederle vaccine, introduced in the US in the early 1960s, has no public documentation of any clinical trials performed pre-licensure, or thereafter.

Prevnar Vaccine: The Prevnar vaccine brand protects against multiple strains of the pneumococcus bacterium that can cause pneumonia. The Prevnar-13 vaccine protects against 13 bacterial strains and has been in routine use in the US since 2010.[r] The vaccine replaced the older-generation vaccine called Prevnar, which was introduced in 2000 and protected against 7 bacterial strains.

How was Prevnar-13's safety tested before approval? Browsing the vaccine's package insert reveals that it was tested against its predecessor, Prevnar.[36] In these trials, severe adverse events were reported in 1 in 12 infants receiving Prevnar-13 (8.2% of subjects) and slightly less often in Prevnar subjects (7.2%).[37] But how many babies who participated in the trial would have experienced severe medical events if not vaccinated at all? That question cannot be answered because the Prevnar-13 trials did not include a placebo control group. Unsurprisingly, the rate of

---

[r] The Prevnar-13 vaccine is routinely given to infants at ages 2, 4, 6, and 12 months.

adverse events in the Prevnar-13 was generally similar to, albeit slightly higher than, the rate of its predecessor; thus, the vaccine was declared "safe" and approved for use by the FDA.

The Prevnar-13 turtle stands on the back of the Prevnar turtle. And what is the Prevnar turtle standing on? The answer: On the back of another turtle, which is standing on nothing but thin air, as we shall immediately see.

Prior to its approval, the Prevnar vaccine underwent a major clinical trial in the United States. In this trial approximately 17,000 infants received Prevnar and a similar number of controls received a vaccine against the meningococcus bacterium.[38] A review of the scientific paper reporting the results of the trial reveals that about 1,000 subjects in total were hospitalized (about 1 in every 35 infants), and about 1 in 16 had emergency room (ER) visits within 30 days of receiving the vaccine.[39] In addition to the Prevnar or meningococcal vaccine, all trial subjects received concurrent DTP or DTaP vaccines. (Note that administering the trial and control vaccines concurrently with other vaccines further obscures the results, as it impossible to determine which adverse events are due to which vaccine(s).)

And what about that meningococcal vaccine received by the control group subjects? In 1998, the year its trial took place, there was no existing alternative to the Prevnar vaccine. Thus, there were no ethical reasons not to give the control group an inert saline injection. Yet the manufacturer chose to give the control group the meningococcal vaccine instead, despite the fact that it had not yet been approved by the FDA and was still "experimental".[40] Why would the manufacturer, as well as FDA and other licensing approval bodies, prefer using an experimental vaccine over the safe, economical, practical, and ethical alternative of a saline placebo? There can be only one answer: to hide the true rate of Prevnar's adverse events.

Hepatitis B Vaccine: Engerix-B is a hepatitis B vaccine manufactured by GSK, which is routinely given to US infants.[s] How was it tested for safety? The vaccine package insert provides an exceptionally brief description: "The incidence of local and systemic reactions was comparable to those of plasma derived hepatitis B vaccines."[41] The package insert mentions another safety study, carried out in children aged 11 to 15 years, where both trial and control groups received the Engerix-B vaccine, though different dosing regimens were applied.[42]

Twinrix, also made by GSK, is a combined hepatitis A and B vaccine. This vaccine was tested in clinical trials against a control group receiving the company's single hepatitis A and B vaccines (Havrix and Engerix-B, respectively).[43]

Recombivax-HB is a hepatitis B vaccine produced by Merck. Surprisingly, its package insert does not mention any safety RCT in infants that was performed for this vaccine.[44]

In summary, the safety of the three hepatitis B vaccines routinely given to newborns has not been tested in a single randomized controlled clinical trial in which a control group received a placebo. As should be all too familiar by now, it's "turtles all the way down" again.

Hepatitis A Vaccine: Two hepatitis A vaccines are routinely used in the United States:[t] the GSK Havrix vaccine and Merck's Vaqta vaccine.

In a large-scale trial in Thailand with over 40,000 participants, GSK's Havrix was compared with a control group which received Engerix-B, the company's hepatitis B vaccine. In three other clinical studies, the trial groups received the Havrix vaccine concurrently with another vaccine and the control groups received several other vaccines (MMR, varicella, and more).[45]

The safety testing of Merck's vaccine, Vaqta, was not much different. According to FDA licensing documents, the vaccine

---

[s] Hepatitis B vaccine is typically given on the day of birth, and at the ages of 1 month and 6 months.

[t] Hepatitis A vaccine is given twice in the second year of life.

was tested in two clinical trials:[46] The first one ("Monroe") had no control group, while the second, in addition to having no control group, administered Vaqta along with two other vaccines.[u] Vaqta's package insert mentions several additional studies but none with a control group that received a placebo. It is interesting to note that contrary to the FDA licensing document, the package insert states that there was a control group in the "Monroe" study and that it received a placebo. A closer look reveals that the "placebo" used contained the vaccine's aluminum adjuvant,[v] [47] and further examination reveals that it also contained the preservative thimerosal (a mercury-based substance removed from most vaccines in the early 2000s).[48] As mercury is a potent neurotoxin and aluminum adjuvants are used because they stimulate a strong immune reaction, both of these substances are a far cry from being inert and safety-neutral.

Measles, Mumps, Rubella, and Varicella (Chickenpox) Vaccine: Merck manufactures a single-dose varicella vaccine called Varivax. The safety section of its package insert mentions a "double-blind, placebo-controlled study" of 914 healthy children and adolescents, in which only two mild symptoms, pain and redness at the injection site, "occurred at a significantly greater rate in vaccine recipients than in placebo recipients."[49] Does that mean a real placebo was used in this trial? Definitely not. The paper describing the study reveals that the so-called placebo given to the control group was actually the test vaccine from which the viral component was removed.[50] No wonder the rates of adverse events were similar between the trial and control groups.[51] Another controlled study compared the safety of two different formulations of the Varivax vaccine. According to the leaflet, the

---

[u] The observed adverse events in the second trial were compared to a "historical" control group, that is, to the results of another, and different, vaccine trial. As explained previously in this chapter, this technique is not scientifically valid because it conflicts with the principle of randomization, which is one of the pillars of an RCT study.

[v] Adjuvant is an immune system stimulant that is present in some vaccines.

safety profiles of the two formulations were comparable.

The two measles-mumps-rubella vaccines licensed for use in the US[w] are a 3-in-1 vaccine called MMR II, and a 4-in-1 vaccine (measles-mumps-rubella and varicella) called ProQuad. Both are manufactured by Merck.

ProQuad's safety was tested in several randomized clinical trials, most of which were not blinded ("open label" studies). The largest RCT compared ProQuad to a control group that received the older-generation MMR II and the Varivax vaccine at the same time. Another study in children 4-6 years old divided the subjects into three groups: The first received ProQuad and "placebo"; the second, MMR II and "placebo"; and the third, MMR II and Varivax. In the open label studies, the participants of both trial and control groups received additional vaccines.[52]

The package insert for MMR II does not mention any safety trials.[53] As with the polio vaccine (IPOL) described earlier, a FOIA request revealed that the vaccine was tested in the mid-1970s in eight small clinical trials.[54] The control groups in all of the trials received either the predecessor vaccine (MMR), a measles-rubella (MR) vaccine, or a single-dose of the rubella vaccine. A total of approximately 850 children received MMR II. Some of the trials seem to have been randomized, but none were blinded. These trials, considered either singly or in combination, do not meet the current requirement of a Phase 3 randomized controlled trial, which might explain their complete absence from the package insert.

Finally, let's examine how the original MMR vaccine, licensed in 1971, was tested before getting the nod from the regulator. Will we find a placebo-receiving control group in this legacy vaccine's trials? Well, almost. Similar to MMR II, the original MMR was tested in a few small-to-medium trials wherein the newer vaccine was given to a total of more than 1,000 infants and children. The control groups' subjects totaled about

---

[w] The MMR and MMRV vaccines are administered at the age of 12–15 months and again between the ages of 4 and 6.

one tenth that number, and most of them were siblings of the vaccinated children (which violates the randomization principle). The control group participants received no injection at all, which means the studies were not blinded; everyone knew who got the vaccine and who didn't. As with MMR II, the MMR trials fail to meet the Phase 3 RCT bar.[55]

Evidently, the safety of the MMR line of vaccines, like the rest of the vaccines in the US childhood vaccination program, was tested according to the de facto industry rule of "turtles all the way down".

Mere Coincidence or Deliberately Flawed Design?

As we've clearly illustrated in the preceding sections, not one of the vaccines the CDC recommends all American children receive was tested for safety in a Phase 3 clinical trial where the control group received an inert placebo. All the vaccines reviewed in the preceding pages – of which tens of millions of doses are administered to infants and toddlers in the US every year – were tested in trials which did not include any control group at all, or ones in which the so-called control group received at least one other vaccine.

Is it just coincidence that none of these vaccines has been tested against a true placebo, despite the fact that in many cases doing so would have been easier, cheaper, and yielded more valid results than the testing that was done? Is it just an accident of fate that the accepted methodology of all childhood vaccine trials obscures the real rate of adverse events of the new vaccine? That seems highly improbable.

As explained at the start of this discussion, testing the safety of a next-generation vaccine against its predecessor is justifiable on ethical grounds: Withholding an existing and proven treatment from control group subjects would be immoral. However, there is no justification for conducting a chain of trials (turtle upon turtle upon turtle) that ultimately stands on nothing but air. Moreover, what possible rationale could justify trials for new vaccines wherein the control groups receive other (sometimes experimental) vaccines? Would a safety trial for a new cigarette have any credibility at all if the "control" group consisted of subjects who smoked a different kind of cigarette?

Whether or not you believe this trial methodology is ethical, its consequence remains the same: The true rate of adverse events of routine childhood vaccines is virtually unknown; therefore, there is no scientific basis for claiming they're safe.

The fact that we don't know how often childhood vaccines hurt the children who receive them casts a dark shadow over the legitimacy of vaccine programs the world over. But that is not all. Even worse, as we shall shortly see, safety trials conducted for some childhood vaccines blatantly and seriously violate the medical code of ethics. In any vaccine clinical trial, a balance must be struck between the vaccine's potential benefits (disease protection) and potential risks (adverse events). When control subjects in vaccine trials receive another type of vaccine, even if it's done in order to obfuscate the real rate of adverse events of the vaccine being tested, the compound they receive is at least of some potential benefit to them. However, in the rotavirus vaccine trials this imperative ethical risk-to-benefit balance was blatantly violated.

The Clinical Trials of the Rotavirus Vaccines

Designing clinical trials for the RotaTeq and Rotarix vaccines was particularly challenging for their manufacturers, Merck and GSK, respectively. To begin with, the first rotavirus vaccine brand (RotaShield) was recalled from the market[56] after it was found to significantly increase the risk of intussusception, a highly dangerous condition in infants.[x] This meant that clinical

---

[x] Intussusception is a condition in which part of the intestine folds into the section immediately ahead of it. This, in turn, could cause bowel obstruction and even require surgical intervention. If left untreated, intussusception can result in death.

trials for the new rotavirus vaccines had to adhere to higher safety standards. In addition, the companies faced an equally serious problem: With RotaShield off the market, there was no suitable vaccine to give to control group subjects.

A rotavirus vaccine dose, a few drops of an opaque liquid, is consumed orally.[y] Hence, the control group in its clinical trials could not receive a vaccine administered via injection as it would violate the RCT blinding principle. If the trial group were vaccinated orally, while the control group was injected, it would be easy to tell the two groups apart. At the time the rotavirus vaccine trials began, there was no other orally ingested vaccine licensed for use. The use of the live polio vaccine (OPV), also consumed by mouth, was terminated in Western countries several years earlier.[z] As a result, there was no oral vaccine available to compare with rotavirus vaccines in clinical trials.

Another option would be to give the control group a few drops of a neutral liquid, such as a solution of sugar or salt water. These compounds are safe, inexpensive and convenient to use – ideal for the purpose of testing the vaccine's efficacy and safety. Because these were entirely new vaccines, which had no alternative, there were no ethical objections to using such a solution.

So, on the one hand, rotavirus vaccine manufacturers did not have a ready-made vaccine available for use in the control group, and on the other, there was no impediment to using a cheap, available and effective substance, such as sugar water. How, then, did they choose to conduct their Phase 3 clinical trials? A preliminary examination of the clinical trial record of the rotavirus vaccine shows that the control groups in the RotaTeq and Rotarix trials received... a placebo![57] Was this, then, the industry's first breach of the sacred tradition that vaccines never be tested against a true placebo? Were the rotavirus vaccine trials

---

[y] The rotavirus vaccine is routinely administered to babies at the age of 2, 4, and 6 months.

[z] This occurred after it was discovered that the vaccine could cause paralysis in a small proportion of vaccinees.

the first to provide reliable and relevant information about the rate of adverse events of a childhood vaccine?

The answer to these questions is, unfortunately, "no and no".

Examining one of the licensing documents submitted to the FDA by GSK[58] indicates that the placebo received by the control group in the main Rotarix trial (which included approximately 63,000 infants) is nothing but the tested vaccine without its antigenic component.[aa] This compound, the vaccine-sans-antigen (*sans* means *without*), is well suited for testing the efficacy of the vaccine as it does not produce rotavirus antibodies. However, when it comes to safety, it's a whole different ballgame: The vaccine-sans-antigen is a potentially potent compound whose side effects are likely to be quite similar to those of the vaccine being tested.

And what was the placebo in Merck's RotaTeq vaccine trial? That's difficult to say because Merck deleted its description from the licensing document submitted to the FDA.[59] It appears that the trial's placebo is a trade secret, which implies its contents were very similar to the vaccine's. Further examination of RotaTeq documents supports this hypothesis: In another RotaTeq clinical trial, the control group received the vaccine-sans-antigen, similar to the compound control group subjects received in the Rotarix trial.[60]

The bioactivity of the compounds given to the control groups in rotavirus vaccine trials was seemingly apparent in the rate of adverse events reported in the trials. In the Rotarix trial, about 1 in 30 control group subjects experienced a "severe" medical event (a rate which was even slightly higher than that of the trial group), and a similar proportion of participants was hospitalized. In addition, 16 infants suffered intussusception and 43 died.[61] In the RotaTeq trial, similar rates were recorded in the control group: Serious adverse events were reported in 1 of every

---

[aa] The antigen in the vaccine is the substance that stimulates the desired immune response. It is usually composed of attenuated or killed particles of virus or bacteria.

40 subjects, 15 suffered intussusception, and 20 infants died.[62]

Using the word placebo to describe the vaccine-sans-antigen leaves the false impression that it is a safe compound that has no side effects of its own. Formal documents, which reference the rotavirus vaccine trials, rely on the supposed biological neutrality of that "placebo". One example is the Rotarix vaccine package insert, which states in the clause discussing the rate of intussusception reported in pre-licensure trials: "No increased risk of intussusception was observed in this clinical trial following administration of ROTARIX when compared with placebo."[63] (The trial in question is the same trial referenced above. There are plenty of other examples, too).[64] Nowhere is there any reference to the actual contents of that "placebo".

The rotavirus vaccine makers were evidently able to find a creative solution to the challenge they faced. They gave their trials' control groups compounds that were very similar to their vaccines, and – as was, no doubt, expected – the resultant rates of adverse events were not significantly different from those observed in the trial groups. In future trials of next-generation rotavirus vaccines, GSK and Merck will be able to give their control groups the standard "placebo" – the currently licensed vaccine – whose safety "was already proven" in its pre-licensure trials.

But there's a fly in this sticky ointment.

Unethical Trials

As previously discussed, the ethical standards for using children as subjects in clinical trials are exceptionally high. Clinical trial designers must ensure that planned procedures are balanced with respect to the expected benefit and risk to the participating infant or child. If a child subject is likely to receive no benefit, the potential harm must be "minimal" or only "slightly above the minimum", and by no means permanent or irreparable. In addition, the risks associated with any procedures must be well-known in advance.[65]

In stark contrast to the standards above, tens of thousands of infants in the control groups of the rotavirus vaccine trials received compounds that could provide no potential benefit to the recipient yet carried significant risk. Neither GSK's nor Merck's vaccine-sans-antigen could possibly prevent rotavirus as they did not contain the antigenic particles that evoke immune reactions to the virus. On the other hand, these compounds had significant potential to cause harm, as demonstrated in the trials. (Remember, 1 in every 30 or 40 control group subjects experienced a serious adverse event). In addition, the safety profiles for the vaccines-sans-antigens were unknown (and, for all we know, still are) as they were new compounds specifically formulated for the rotavirus trials with no documentation of past safety studies. Hence, the health risks associated with administering them to infants was undetermined.

To sum up, tens of thousands of infants were given an utterly useless compound whose safety was unknown and whose side effects could be (and probably were in some cases) severe and permanent. Thus, the Phase 3 clinical trials of the rotavirus vaccine constitute blatant violations of the medical code of ethics.

This ruthless breach of ethics and morality is highlighted by the fact that there was no scientific justification for giving the vaccine-sans-antigen to the control group other than a malicious intention to conceal the experimental vaccine's true rate of adverse events. Using a real placebo that posed no health risk – a few drops of sugar or salt water – would have cost less and led to more scientifically valid conclusions by enabling straightforward calculations of the true adverse event rates as well as vaccine efficacy.

The manner in which the rotavirus vaccine trials were conducted raises grave questions which should not be directed solely toward the vaccines' manufacturers. The FDA supervises the vaccine approval process, and it is the FDA that approved these trials.[bb] The vaccine also received CDC approval and that of other health authorities around the world, even though its pre-licensure trials unnecessarily endangered tens of thousands of children and may have caused serious harm to hundreds, as well as dozens of needless deaths.

The Declaration of Helsinki is the ethical code governing the conduct of human medical experimentation. The Declaration was formulated for the medical-scientific community by the World Medical Association and is considered the ethical corner-stone of the medical research field. It leaves no doubt as to the ethical violations perpetrated in the rotavirus trials:

> *Physicians may not be involved in a research study involving human subjects unless they are confident that the risks have been adequately assessed and can be satisfactorily managed. When the risks are found to outweigh the potential benefits [...] physicians must assess whether to continue, modify or immediately stop the study.*
>
> *... [A] potential research subject who is incapable of giving informed consent [...] must not be included in a research study that has no likelihood of benefit for them unless [...] the research entails only minimal risk and minimal burden.*[66]

The *Nuremberg Code*, the medical code of ethics established in the late 1940s to bring Nazi doctors to justice, constitutes the basis of the Declaration of Helsinki. It too underlines the immorality of the rotavirus vaccine trials: "[An] experiment should be so conducted as to avoid all unnecessary physical and mental suffering and injury."[67] A similar conclusion was also reached by a World Health Organization (WHO) committee that recently examined placebo use in clinical trials.[68]

Ponder it as you will, you won't find a satisfactory explana-

---

[bb] A similar, though not identical, design was employed in the pre-licensure trials of the human papillomavirus (HPV) vaccine Gardasil.

tion for the way the rotavirus vaccine trials were conducted other than the malicious desire to assist the manufacturers in obscuring and concealing the vaccines' true adverse event rates. This demonstrates that the public health establishment is willing to go to great lengths to maintain the pretense of vaccine safety, casting aside medical ethics and even fundamental principles of morality in the process.

Childhood Vaccine Clinical Trials: A Summary

The table below summarizes the safety testing performed in Phase 3 clinical trials for the vaccines included in the CDC-recommended childhood vaccination program.

Table 1: The control group in Phase 3 clinical trials of CDC's routine childhood vaccines

Disease	Vaccine	The Control Group in Phase III Clinical Trials
Diphtheria-Tetanus-Pertussis (with and without Polio, Hepatitis B and Hib)	Pediarix *(Diphtheria-Tetanus-Acellular Pertussis-Hepatitis B-Polio)*	Control groups in the trials received either the Infanrix vaccine along with hepatitis B, Hib, and polio vaccines, or other, unspecified vaccines. No control group received a placebo.
	Kinrix *(Diphtheria-Tetanus-Acellular Pertussis-Polio)*	In the only trial specifically described in the package insert the control group received the Infanrix and polio vaccines. The package insert doesn't mention any trial involving a placebo control group.
	Infanrix *(Diphtheria-Tetanus-Acellular Pertussis)*	Tested against a control group that received the DTP vaccine or no control group.
	DTP *(Diphtheria-Tetanus-Pertussis)*	The vaccine was developed in the 1930s and has never been tested in an RCT against a control group receiving a real placebo.

	Pentacel *(Diphtheria-Tetanus-Acellular Pertussis-Polio-Hib)*	The control groups in 3 of the 4 trials received an assortment of different vaccines. The 4th trial's control group may have received no vaccines; however, its safety data is not presented in the package insert.
	Quadracel *(Diphtheria-Tetanus-Acellular Pertussis-Polio)*	The control group in the trial received the Daptacel and polio vaccines.
	Daptacel *(Diphtheria-Tetanus-Acellular Pertussis)*	The control groups in the trials received other vaccines.
Haemophilus Influenzae Type B	Hiberix	The only blinded RCT had two control groups receiving another Hib vaccine or a DTaP-polio-Hib, along with several other vaccines.
	ActHIB	Control groups received either the DTP vaccine or other combination DTaP-based vaccines.
	PedvaxHIB	Most of the control group subjects received DTP and OPV vaccines along with a "placebo" whose ingredients were not specified.
Polio	IPOL	The package insert does not mention any RCT performed for the vaccine.
Pneumococcal Disease	Prevnar-13	Tested against a control group receiving Prevnar (older-generation vaccine).
	Prevnar	Tested against a control group that received an experimental meningo-coccal vaccine.
Hepatitis B	Engerix	Its side effect rate was compared to that of a previous generation product (plasma vaccine).
	Twinrix	Tested in clinical trials against a control group that received separate hepatitis A and B vaccines.

	Recombivax HB	The package insert does not mention any safety RCT performed in infants.
Hepatitis A	Havrix	The control group in the main trial received the hepatitis B vaccine. In three other trials, the control group received several other vaccines (MMR, varicella vaccine, and more).
	Vaqta	In one trial, there was no control group (according to another document, the control group received a compound that included aluminum and thimerosal), and in the second trial the vaccine was given concurrently with other vaccines and without a control group.
Measles, Mumps, Rubella, Varicella (Chickenpox)	ProQuad *(Measles, Mumps, Rubella, Varicella)*	Safety was tested in several randomized clinical trials, most of which were not blinded. None of the trials contained a control group receiving only a placebo.
	MMR II *(Measles, Mumps, Rubella)*	Tested in eight small unblinded clinical trials. All of the trials had one or more control groups receiving either the predecessor MMR vaccine, a measles-rubella (MR) vaccine, or a single-dose of the rubella vaccine.
	MMR *(Measles, Mumps, Rubella)*	Tested in several small to medium unblinded and partially randomized trials. The control groups totaled about 1/10 the number of subjects in the trial groups and received no injection.
	Varivax *(Varicella)*	In one RCT the "placebo" given to the control group was actually the test vaccine from which the viral component was removed. Another trial compared two different formulations of the vaccine.

| Rotavirus | RotaTeq | The control group in the trial probably received the vaccine-sans-antigen compound (the description of the control compound was intentionally deleted from FDA licensing documents). |
| | Rotarix | The control group in the trial received the vaccine-sans-antigen compound. |

Counter Arguments

As summarized in the table above, the manufacturers' package inserts and FDA licensing documents indicate that none of the US routine childhood vaccines has been tested against a true placebo. It is very unlikely that new documents which attest to the opposite will suddenly appear. It is also highly improbable that a new technique for calculating the true rate of vaccine adverse events in an RCT by comparing it to population background rates or to a non-placebo control group will miraculously emerge. A moral justification for giving control group infants a compound that could seriously harm them, while providing them with no potential benefit, will also not be forthcoming anytime soon.

However, because the arguments made in this chapter undermine the very foundations of the childhood vaccine program, devout believers in the "vaccines are safe and effective" mantra try hard to refute them. Their popular arguments and suggested responses are presented below.

Important Note: When addressing alleged refutations to the content of this chapter, the first response should be to politely request scientific references backing them up. When facing the inevitable and grave consequences of the material presented in this chapter, vaccine proponents sometimes resort to baseless, even borderline imaginary, claims. In many cases, asking for a valid scientific reference that backs up a claim will quickly put the argument to rest.

"A placebo in vaccine clinical trials is only used for the purpose of testing vaccine efficacy." – This is a bizarre claim which has no scientific basis (just ask for a scientific reference – you won't get one). A (real) placebo given to the control group in a vaccine clinical trial provides a "background rate" for both efficacy and safety. Therefore, in a trial which has a placebo group, both vaccine efficacy and the incidence of adverse events could be easily calculated by comparing results in trial vs. control groups.

"It is unethical not to give the control group another vaccine." – The practice of always testing vaccines against other vaccines gives rise to the "turtles all the way down" scenario, where the true rate of adverse events of any childhood vaccine is never determined. In fact, the opposite is true: It is unethical not to conduct at least one trial from which one can reliably estimate the rate of adverse events before a vaccine is licensed and widely used.

As reviewed in this chapter, medical ethics guidelines permit the administration of a placebo to a control group in a clinical trial of a completely new vaccine and to a control group in a three-arm trial of a next-generation vaccine.

"When testing a next-generation vaccine, it is unethical not to give the control group the current vaccine." – This argument is similar to the previous one, but focuses specifically on the next-generation vaccines. It certainly makes sense to test the safety of a next-generation vaccine against the current one, but if the current vaccine has never been previously tested against a placebo, it is "turtles all the way down" again; that is, the data collected from the vaccine's clinical trials is inadequate for establishing a true safety profile.

The solution to the above is straightforward: Conduct a three-arm trial with next-generation vaccine, current vaccine, and placebo groups. This allows the comparison of the safety of the new vaccine to the existing one, as well as obtaining an estimation of the absolute rate of the new vaccine's adverse events (by comparing it to placebo). A trial of this kind has never been conducted for any of the routine childhood vaccines.

"It is sufficient to test a new vaccine against another vaccine whose rate of adverse events was determined in a previous trial (or measured for a country/region/city population)." – As explained in the chapter, the results of one randomized controlled trial (RCT) cannot be compared to that of another RCT, nor to population "background rates" (even if those are known, which is uncommon) because it violates randomization. Known or unknown differences may exist between the studies' populations that could potentially skew the results significantly. Vaccine package inserts, which are published by the manufacturers and approved by health authorities, state this explicitly.

"It is sufficient to test a next-generation vaccine against the current vaccine, as the current vaccine has already been given to millions over many years and proven safe." – The argument implies that if we know that a certain current vaccine is safe and a control group in a next-generation vaccine trial is given that vaccine, then if adverse events are comparable between the groups, it can be concluded that the new vaccine is also safe for use.

First, this presupposes that the current vaccine is safe. But we cannot make that assumption if the current vaccine itself was tested in clinical trials designed to obfuscate its true rate of adverse events. That is, the industry's "gold standard", the RCT, was "cooked" (as was the case in this chapter's examples) in order to hide the health risks of the tested vaccine. Instead, we must base our judgment of its safety on inferior studies[cc] performed only after the vaccine has been on the market for several years.

Secondly, without a placebo control group there is no way to

[cc] See chapter 4 for a review of types of epidemiological studies.

prove that the vaccine being tested is actually safe. For example, in one of the DTaP vaccine trials, 1 in every 22 subjects in the trial group was admitted to the hospital. A similar hospitalization rate was also reported in the control group (which received the older-generation DTP vaccine).[69] Is this a normal background rate? Would nearly 5% of all infants really end up in the hospital if they didn't receive these vaccines? Should we regard both these vaccines, which appear to cause an alarmingly high rate of hospitalizations, as "safe" simply because they have similar hospitalization rates? Or is the reality that neither of them are safe? Definitive answers to these questions could only be obtained by adding a placebo group to the trial. Only then could we calculate a meaningful baseline hospitalization rate that could be put to good use in evaluating the vaccine's safety.

In any case, the above claim is irrelevant for trials of entirely new vaccines for which there are no valid reasons not to use a real placebo control.

"The safety of the [xyz] vaccine was extensively studied after it was approved for wide use and was found to be excellent." – Statistical (epidemiological) studies, which are typically conducted only after a vaccine has been in wide use, are considered inferior to RCT studies. The RCT is the industry's "gold standard", and every new vaccine must undergo such a trial before it is approved for use. It would not be acceptable or reasonable to approve a vaccine for use without adequate clinical studies, and then, after it was administered to millions of babies, retroactively endorse it based on methodologically inferior studies.

"The assertion that vaccines are never tested against a placebo is false. Here are some references to vaccine clinical trials in which the control group received a real placebo."[70] – The claim made in this chapter is not that vaccines in general are never tested against placebo in their pre-licensure process. Rather, it is childhood vaccines recommended by the CDC that were never tested against a placebo. The references provided to support the above statement do not refute this claim, as they link to trials of adult vaccines, or vaccines that are not used in the United States. In fact, these references reinforce this chapter's arguments, as they demonstrate that using a placebo control group in a vaccine RCT is valid, feasible, methodologically sound, and ethical.

"Contrary to your claim, a placebo is not mandatory in a vaccine clinical trial. Instead, the control group could be given nothing (i.e., no intervention)." – In a double-blinded randomized controlled trial (RCT), the control group must receive a compound that looks the same and is administered in the same way as the tested compound. This eliminates potential reporting bias. For example, subjects who know they received the experimental vaccine are more likely to report adverse events than control group participants who received no intervention. This rule also applies to trials with infant subjects even though it is generally believed they are not affected by this bias, because their parents, who are usually present at the time of vaccination, can certainly be affected.

In any case, there are no current childhood vaccines that were tested in clinical trials that included a no-intervention control group, which renders the above claim irrelevant.

"The vaccine-sans-antigen that was given to the control group in the rotavirus trials is a safe compound since it is made of a mixture of ingredients, each of which is generally considered to be safe." – This is yet another baseless claim that has no scientific or factual basis. Even if we presuppose that the individual ingredients in the compound given to the control group in the rotavirus trials were harmless, we cannot assume their specific mixture was harmless, too. This is a fundamental tenet of drug and vaccine testing methodology: A compound's safety is not the sum of the safety of its parts. Thus, we cannot presume its safety based on a theoretical calculation of the aggregated safety of its ingredients. It must be clinically tested before it is approved for wide use (even more so, if given to babies).

Additionally, in the case of the rotavirus vaccine trials, neither the manufacturers nor the licensing bodies claimed that the vaccine-sans-antigen that was given to the control group was considered, or proven to be, safe or that its safety profile was known. If anyone claims the opposite, they must provide the scientific references to back it up.

"Giving the control group the vaccine-sans-antigen is the proper way to test the vaccine's antigen efficacy and safety." – Once again, this is a baseless claim that has no scientific merit. A clinical trial in which the trial group receives the test vaccine and the control group the vaccine-sans-antigen compares two experimental compounds whose safety profiles are unknown. Therefore, such a trial design precludes calculation of the true rate of adverse events of the test vaccine. For a valid determination, the control group should receive a placebo, which is a compound whose rate of adverse events is known and is very close to zero. In clinical trials using vaccine-sans-antigen compounds in the control group (for example, the rotavirus vaccine trials), researchers reasoned that "no significant difference in the rate of adverse events was observed in trial and placebo groups." However, this claim is critically flawed, since the "placebo" given to the control group was not neutral (i.e., one which had zero side effects), but rather a bioactive compound whose rate of side effects was unknown.

In addition, the safety of the vaccine antigen is irrelevant as it is not administered by itself, but rather in combination with all the vaccine's other ingredients. It's the safety of the vaccine as a whole that matters, and that is not best tested by comparing it to the vaccine-sans-antigen.

In any event, the above discussion should only be considered theoretical, since administering a potentially harmful substance with no potential benefit to infants in a clinical trial violates the medical code of ethics as well as fundamental moral principles.

"It is inconceivable that every doctor and researcher in the entire

world would approve, or retroactively approve, of a flawed methodology for testing vaccines' safety before they are licensed. Are all of them taking part in a huge conspiracy?" – Providing a complete and comprehensive answer to this claim goes beyond the scope of this chapter. In short, the vast majority of physicians and researchers are completely unaware of the manner in which vaccine safety trials are designed and conducted and the methodological flaws inherent in that process.

Regardless, this claim is essentially irrelevant, as it does not directly answer the arguments presented in the chapter and therefore cannot refute them. A doctor or researcher who has studied vaccine safety and maintains there are no flaws in their licensing process should respond directly to the arguments made in this chapter instead of asking the public to blindly agree based on professional authority alone.

Summary

Vaccines, as opposed to drugs, are given to healthy babies and thus must meet a particularly high safety standard. Clinical trials of new vaccines must be impeccably designed and performed, thereby providing high-quality, reliable data about the products' efficacy, and more importantly, about their safety. Anything less is socially and morally unacceptable.

Vaccine manufacturers and health authorities worldwide frequently assure us, the public, that vaccines are tested at the highest possible level and that the rigorous series of clinical trials they undergo as part of the licensing process ensures that vaccines are truly safe and effective.

These assurances, however, are meaningless at best and deliberately misleading at worst.

As we have seen in this chapter, vaccine trials are designed and performed in such a way as to ensure that the true extent of adverse events is hidden from the public. There is not a single vaccine in the US routine childhood vaccination program whose true rate of adverse events is known. The assertion that vaccines cause serious side effects in "one in a million" vaccinees contradicts the results of numerous clinical trials in which serious adverse events were reported in 1 in 40, 30, or even as few as 20 vaccinated infants. After becoming acquainted with the finer details of vaccine safety trials, hearing the familiar tune of "a similar rate of adverse events was reported in the control group" (which received another vaccine or similar compound) comes off as ludicrous, cynical, and patently immoral.

Current vaccine clinical trial methodology completely invalidates the claims that vaccines are safe and that they are thoroughly and rigorously tested. And pulling out that bogus card completely topples the childhood vaccine program's house of cards, as officials' assurances of vaccine safety rely primarily on deliberately flawed, industry-sponsored clinical trials.

Furthermore, some of the clinical trials that have been conducted for routine childhood vaccines, which were approved by relevant health authorities, blatantly violated the medical code of ethics (the Declaration of Helsinki) and fundamental principles of morality. In these trials, infants in the control groups were given completely useless compounds (an antigen-free vaccine) whose safety was unknown and which had the potential to cause serious and irreversible damage to health, including death.

Any reader looking for a quick and definitive understanding of the truth about vaccine safety – well, you can put this book down right now. You have your answer: The entire vaccine program is based on a deliberate cover-up of true vaccine adverse event rates. This seemingly mighty fortress, carefully constructed over many decades and fortified by countless officials, researchers, and physicians – actually stands on nothing but turtles all the way down.

Ask your doctor:

• Was the vaccine that you are recommending tested in a pre-licensure clinical trial with a (real) placebo control group? If not, how do you (or anyone else, for that matter) calculate its true rate of adverse events?

• Is it morally acceptable to conduct a clinical trial in infants for a new vaccine, where the "control group" receives an untested compound, i.e., the vaccine-sans-antigen, which is likely to cause irreversible side effects and has no potential benefit?

Share this chapter with colleagues, friends and family (free PDF):

https://tinyurl.com/TurtlesBookChap1Eng

2

THE SCIENCE OF VACCINE ADVERSE EVENTS: A MISSING LINK AND AN EMPTY TOOLBOX

Isaac's Story

Isaac,[a] his parents' only child, came into the world in a normal, uneventful birth. Although his head was smaller than average (a condition known as microcephaly),[b] he developed normally in the first few weeks of life. At the age of two months, Isaac's mother took him to the pediatrician's office for his first "well-baby visit" and first round of vaccinations.[c] The doctor, noticing

---

[a] Though the story is real, the child's name was changed for privacy and the timing was modified slightly to reflect the US vaccine schedule.

[b] Microcephaly is a rare neurological syndrome wherein a child's head circumference is significantly smaller than average. The phenomenon is linked to a number of environmental and genetic factors that delay the development of the fetal brain. A baby with microcephaly may experience developmental problems (motor, speech), intellectual disability, seizures, hyperactivity, and more. Nevertheless, some children affected by the syndrome develop normally.

[c] According to the US recommended vaccination schedule, a two-month-old baby should receive DTaP (diphtheria, tetanus, and pertussis), rotavirus, Prevnar-13, Hib, and polio vaccines.

that Isaac's head circumference was smaller than average, was hesitant. She consulted with a colleague and eventually decided to administer only the pentavalent DTaP-IPV-Hib vaccine, which protects against five different diseases.[d]

In the days following his well-baby visit, Isaac cried for hours and hours. In addition, behavioral patterns that his parents had not observed before began to emerge. At times, his gaze got "stuck" to one side for several seconds. His mouth occasionally "locked", and he insisted on breastfeeding from one side only (as his mother realized later, these were signs that Isaac was having mild convulsions). Two weeks later, after crying constantly for hours, Isaac lost consciousness and stopped breathing. His grandfather, who arrived on the scene before the ambulance arrived, resuscitated him, saving his life.

At the hospital, the doctors suspected Isaac was suffering from congenital epilepsy and wanted to begin drug treatment. His mother, however, insisted they perform an electroencephalogram (EEG) to verify their conjecture. The EEG was negative. The neurologist who examined him believed that Isaac's seizures were caused by the pertussis component of the pentavalent vaccine. He recommended that Isaac not be vaccinated further with that vaccine and that he skip the MMR vaccination at 12 months as well.

Following this recommendation, at four months Isaac was given only a monovalent polio vaccine instead of the multiple vaccines that were normally given at this age. Shortly thereafter, the seizures reappeared and lasted for about three weeks. Similar symptoms appeared after Isaac's next dose of the polio vaccine at age six months, after which the neurologist instructed his mother to stop vaccinating him altogether.

Sadly, the doctors didn't stop vaccinating soon enough for Isaac and his family. Isaac, now four years old, was badly injured and permanently disabled. He is unable to sit up by himself or

---

[d] Those are diphtheria, tetanus, pertussis, polio, and haemophilus influenzae type b.

stand without assistance and cannot hold objects with his hands.

Apart from the devastation wreaked upon one child and his family, Isaac's sad story highlights the failure of the healthcare system to prevent serious harm to infants by screening out those who would be susceptible to vaccine injury. Although his doctor recognized Isaac's microcephaly as a potential susceptibility, due to a lack of relevant medical expertise and diagnostic tools, she was unable to make an informed medical decision regarding his vaccinations. After witnessing the first signs of injury following the pentavalent vaccine Isaac received, the neurologist mistakenly assumed that the pertussis component alone caused Isaac's seizures. This arbitrary and erroneous assumption led to Isaac receiving two more doses of the monovalent polio vaccine, which resulted in further, apparently irreversible, deterioration in his health.

David's Story

David was also born with microcephaly. Unlike Isaac, David's pediatrician detected his potential susceptibility to vaccine injury before he received his first round of vaccines. His doctor ordered a series of specialized genetic, immunological, and neurological diagnostic tests. Following the results of the tests, and after consulting a specialist, the doctor gave David a personalized vaccination schedule tailored to his specific medical profile. As recommended in his individualized plan, David began receiving vaccinations at age 12 months and subsequently received only a handful of vaccines which were determined to pose only a low risk to him. In addition, he was administered only one vaccine at a time, and only if he had been healthy in the preceding three weeks.

David's personalized vaccine program achieved its goal: He received all of his prescribed vaccines without suffering significant side effects. In his case, the innovative array of vaccine susceptibility testing implemented in the US healthcare system in recent years made a big difference. This progress in medical practice, which David's doctor exploited so effectively, was based on research from thousands of scientists from around the world. These researchers laid the theoretical groundwork required to understand the biological mechanisms that underlie vaccine adverse events and helped develop practical tools for preventing most of them. These tools include screening for genetic suscepti-bilities, assessing potential adverse consequences of vaccinating during or shortly after an illness, testing for sensitivities to specific vaccine components, and modeling the potential cross-reactions of multiple vaccines administered simultaneously.

Sounds impressive, right? Unfortunately, while Isaac's story is a genuine and painful reminder of the medical establishment's impotence when it comes to preventing vaccine injury, David's story is entirely... imaginary. A "science fiction" story, if you will.

Fictional Science

It is widely agreed that vaccines are the linchpin of public health and that they have played a major role in decreasing mortality and morbidity from infectious disease for the past 150 years. Hundreds of millions of vaccine doses are administered yearly in the United States alone, and many more worldwide. Given the primary importance of vaccination, it could reasonably be ex-pected that, as depicted above in David's fictional case, vaccine safety would be, and always had been, thoroughly and diligently investigated by scientists and doctors worldwide, and that a vast body of theoretical and practical knowledge had accumulated in this field.

The reality, it turns out, is quite different. At present, official-ly sanctioned medical science knows very little about the harmful effects of vaccines. It cannot, and does not, anticipate which children will be injured by vaccination, in what manner, or to what extent.

What's worse is this lack of knowledge is not accidental. It is the inevitable consequence of more than sixty years of deliberate inaction.

Sixty Years of Non-Research

The first vaccine that was introduced in a nationwide campaign in any country in the modern era was Jonas Salk's polio vaccine.[e] This groundbreaking vaccine was given to US children beginning in 1955 and was soon adopted by many countries around the world.

More than sixty years have passed since the cornerstone of the modern vaccine program was laid. Since then, dozens of vaccines for numerous diseases have been developed and marketed, and tens of billions of vaccine doses have been administered to billions of people worldwide, most of them infants and children. Over the last several decades, countless studies have been conducted in the field of vaccinology and related medical fields. However, only a tiny fraction of those have sought to improve our fundamental understanding of the biological mechanisms that underlie vaccine side effects. As will be shown below, sixty years of modern vaccine research has provided precious little theoretical or practical insight into exactly how vaccines hurt people like Isaac. As of today, fundamental questions pertaining to this topic remain largely unanswered: How can one recognize and diagnose vaccine adverse events? What are their possible causes? Which individuals are at increased risk of vaccine injury? What factors affect the severity of a vaccine injury? How can we treat vaccine-related health conditions effectively? Remaining unanswered, these critical questions highlight the regrettable fact that medical

---

[e] Vaccines that preceded the Salk vaccine were based on pre-modern methods of prophylaxis (e.g., Edward Jenner's smallpox vaccine or Louis Pasteur's rabies vaccine), or were not widely distributed until the late 1940s (e.g., diphtheria, pertussis, and tetanus vaccines).

science has failed to develop biological models that explain the mechanisms underlying the majority of vaccination injuries, as well as effective protocols for treating them.

A bold claim such as this one obviously requires compelling evidence. In order to compile such evidence, a comprehensive review of the relevant scientific literature must be performed. One must browse through thousands, or possibly tens of thousands, of scientific papers, identify those that actually deal with the subject, examine their methodology, tabulate their findings, analyze the resulting data, and finally, formulate conclusions. Fortunately, an intrepid organization took on this Herculean task for us: the US Institute of Medicine.

The IOM 2011 Report

Part of the American National Academy of Sciences, the Institute of Medicine (IOM)[f] is a nonprofit, non-governmental organization that serves as an advisory body to the nation on medical and health issues. Its role is to provide objective and reliable information and advice to policymakers, the medical profession, and the public. The organization is made up of volunteer health professionals from various healthcare sectors who are nominated based on their expertise and past accomplishments. The IOM initiates most of its investigations following formal requests coming from the federal government and its agencies. A small share of the research is done at the request of the business sector.

The IOM has published a number of vaccine-related reports over the last 20 years. These reports have dealt with topics such as the link between the MMR vaccine and autism (2001),[1] the association between thimerosal-containing vaccines and neurological disorders (2001),[2] vaccines and sudden infant death syndrome (2003),[3] vaccines and autism (2004),[4] the safety of the

---

[f] In 2015, the IOM changed its name to the National Academy of Medicine (NAM).

US national vaccine program (2013),[5] and more. Evidently, these reports have tackled the "hottest" topics in the field, issues that were, and still are, the focus of intense debate between vaccine advocates and their critics. The conclusions of these IOM reports, as well as other IOM vaccine-related reports, have been overwhelmingly and unequivocally supportive of the federal agencies that govern the US vaccination program[g] and the policies they implement.

In 2011, in response to a request submitted by the US Department of Health in 2009, the IOM issued a special report on vaccine adverse effects.[6] The IOM was asked to convene an expert committee "to review the epidemiological, clinical, and biological evidence regarding adverse health events associated with specific vaccines covered by the [vaccine program]" and to state its opinion on "the evidence bearing on causality, and the evidence regarding the biological mechanisms that underlie specific theories for how a specific vaccine is related to a specific adverse event."[7] In short, it was asked to examine whether vaccines are causally linked to certain adverse events. In order to fulfill its mission, the IOM expert committee had to conduct a comprehensive and thorough examination of the scientific literature. The committee browsed thousands of scientific articles, the most relevant of which it rated according to quality. Then, it weighted the results and summarized them in a specialized model developed specifically for the purpose of this task.

It took the committee two full years of demanding work to complete the report, during which it carried out a thorough investigation into the available evidence, including epidemiological (statistical), clinical (medical studies in humans), and biological (animal and *in vitro*) studies. The committee's conclusion was that there were only a handful of adverse events of specific vaccines for which a causal link between the event and the vaccine had been established. Of the 158 adverse event and

---

[g] The CDC, the FDA, and the US Department of Health and Human Services.

vaccine combinations examined by the committee,[8] [h] a causal link was confirmed for only 14 of them and suggested for 4 others ("the evidence favors acceptance").[9] The committee rejected a causal link for only 5 adverse event and vaccine pairs. For the remaining 135 pairs, it concluded that the evidence was insufficient to either prove or refute a causal link.[10]

Further examination of the cases where a causal link was established between the side effect and the vaccination that preceded it raises an interesting point: For the vast majority of them, the causal link between the adverse event and the vaccine is virtually self-evident. Almost half, 6 of the 14, were labeled "anaphylaxis", an acute, immediate, and often life-threatening allergic reaction, which the committee associated with 6 different vaccines. Four other causally related pairs involved immunocompromised vaccine recipients suffering symptoms of the diseases they were vaccinated for. Those were attributed to the attenuated viruses contained in the vaccines. Two other events, shoulder inflammation following an injection and fainting shortly after vaccine administration, were linked to the act of injection itself rather than to any specific vaccine.[11] Thus, the link between vaccination and outcome was virtually irrefutable for 12 of the 14 adverse events that the committee confirmed were causally linked to vaccination.

Despite the indisputable nature of the links the IOM confirmed, the report's authors took pains to soften any potential blow to vaccines' image by making it clear that these causally linked adverse events were not a source of public concern. They were, the committee noted, typically either very rare, mild, or transient, or they were caused by the physical act of injection and were not, therefore, specific to vaccination.[12]

---

[h] The committee examined 158 pairs of adverse-events/vaccines. Some of the adverse events were investigated with relation to several vaccines. Thirty different adverse events were examined for the MMR vaccine; 15 for varicella; 27 for influenza; 8 for hepatitis A; 27 for hepatitis B; 13 for human papillomavirus; 26 for tetanus, diphtheria, and pertussis; 9 for meningococcal; and 3 related to the act of injection itself.

The conclusions of the report, which were widely publicized by the media as further proof of vaccine safety and yet another refutation of the alleged link between vaccines and some publicly attributed illnesses and conditions,[13] came as no surprise. The IOM, as indicated by its past publications, has always been committed to scientific consensus. As a longtime partner of the government and federal agencies, it couldn't be reasonably expected to publish radical conclusions that could undermine the public's trust in the vaccine program.[14] The committee made its stance clear by expressing its unequivocal support for the vaccine program in the report's introductory chapter, stating: "The overwhelming safety and effectiveness of vaccines in current use in preventing serious disease has allowed them to gain their preeminent role in the routine protection of health."[15]

Regardless of any potential bias that may have affected the committee's work and conclusions, the published report makes a decisive contribution to the issue at hand. The report, possibly inadvertently, publicly exposed the current sorry state of scientific knowledge about vaccine safety. In this regard, the report's significance lies not with the causal links it was able to establish or refute (23 out of 158), but rather with the numerous potential links it was unable to prove or disprove. In more than 85% of the adverse events the committee examined (135 out of 158), it found no adequate scientific studies that could corroborate or refute a causal link to the vaccine. Practically, this means that the medical world has no body of scientific knowledge to rely on when determining whether these 135 health conditions are caused by vaccines or not.[i]

According to the committee's findings, the dearth of studies examining vaccine side effects is evident in both the epidemiological (statistical) and biomedical (mechanistic) research

---

[i] Also, keep in mind that the committee investigated only a small fraction of adverse events reported following vaccinations. Thus, the report didn't include any adverse events for several vaccines routinely administered in the US (Prevnar, rotavirus, Hib, and polio vaccines). Nor did it include all reported events for vaccines they did consider (e.g., the human papillomavirus vaccine).

categories. The lack of high-quality mechanistic studies, those that look at the underlying "mechanics" of vaccine injury, is particularly noteworthy because they, and they alone, are capable of proving a causal link, as the committee points out.[16] For most of the adverse events considered, only a handful of mechanistic studies were found in the scientific literature, nearly all of them "case studies", that is, descriptions of individual patients with various health issues that began following vaccination. Most of these case studies did not mention the performance of any specialized medical tests that might have shed light on the event's specific circumstances. Consequently, these studies were largely deemed "low quality" by the committee as they did not provide supplemental medical information linking the vaccine to the adverse event beyond the fact that the condition first appeared shortly after vaccination.[17]

For example, a review of the medical literature on ADEM[j] following the administration of the hepatitis B vaccine found eight such reports. Six of the eight studies were disqualified by the committee as they had merely reported the proximity in time between vaccination and disease commencement while not providing additional medical information. While the remaining two articles did provide supplemental medical findings in the vaccinees, which were consistent with ADEM's clinical picture, the committee concluded that in the absence of a proven biological mechanism linking the disease to the vaccine, "the evidence is inadequate to accept or reject" a causal link.[18] The committee similarly dismissed a causal link between the MMR vaccine and transverse myelitis.[k] The five case studies in the medical literature did not provide any evidence to suggest the existence of a biological mechanism linking the vaccine and disease.[19]

So the majority of the scientific literature regarding disease

---

[j] ADEM, acute disseminated encephalomyelitis, is an autoimmune disease similar to multiple sclerosis.

[k] Transverse myelitis is a neurological disease in which inflammation of the spinal cord leads to loss of the myelin sheath of the nerves, and subsequently to organ numbness and loss of motor function.

mechanisms consisted of superficial case studies, and the committee determined that only a handful of papers met the criteria of basic scientific research – studies that looked for causal links between vaccines and medical conditions through in-depth investigation of biological mechanisms. It is no wonder, then, that the committee could not confirm or deny a causal link to vaccination for over 85% of the adverse events examined.

Scientific research into the mechanisms underlying side effects of vaccines should investigate, among other things, (1) the effects that vaccine ingredients (like aluminum adjuvants) have on the body; (2) the biochemical interactions between vaccine components; (3) the biochemical interactions among multiple vaccines administered at the same time; (4) genetic characteristics that may increase vulnerability to vaccine injury; and (5) permanent or transient health conditions that may increase susceptibility to injury. In addition, investigation of potentially susceptible subpopulations, such as infants and pregnant women, should be made a priority. The absence of basic research in this field is particularly alarming because current medical science cannot even identify the source of most of the serious diseases and syndromes reported post-vaccination, much less cure them. Such is the case for ADEM,[20] optic neuritis,[21] Guillain-Barré syndrome,[22] transverse myelitis,[23] lupus,[24] vasculits,[25] juvenile diabetes (type 1),[26] autism, ADHD, and many other conditions.

The shortage of applicable scientific research on adverse events documented in its own report should have prompted the IOM committee to sound a long and loud alarm. The report's finding that biomedical aspects of post-vaccination conditions are rarely investigated contrasts starkly with the constant assurances from medical authorities that vaccine safety is thoroughly investigated. Yet, instead of sounding the warranted alarm, the committee chose to give the "all-clear". The report's conclusions don't convey any sense of urgency, nor does the report call for health authorities to take any immediate action. While the report does not state it explicitly, news articles following the report's publication conveyed the committee chairperson's implicit message that *All is fine*: Only a handful of adverse events have been proven to be linked to vaccines, and even those are mild and rare.

The IOM committee members knew that "the absence of evidence is not evidence of absence"[27] but went ahead and acquitted vaccines anyway based on a lack-of-evidence argument. Oddly, the committee seems content with the current paucity of scientific evidence, while expressing the wholly unjustified expectation "that more can and will be known about vaccine safety in the future."[28]

Until that day comes, however, we ought to consider the serious practical and theoretical consequences of the gaping holes in vaccine safety science that were exposed in the IOM report.

The Missing Causal Link

As hauntingly illustrated by the story of little Isaac at the beginning of this chapter, the lack of solid science on vaccines' potential side effects has grave and often tragic consequences. With no scientific foundation to work from, there is no practical way to establish a causal link between vaccines and the myriad adverse health events that often follow. This, in turn, means that even the idea of a causal link is excluded from the conversation about vaccines, greatly reducing the likelihood that such a link would ever be suspected, investigated, or diagnosed.

The absence of the causal link from the safety conversation begins with the pre-licensing approval process. Regulatory bodies do not require manufacturers to perform biomedical research investigating possible associations between their experimental products and any side effects reported in the trials.[1] Although considered the industry's gold standard, a randomized controlled trial (RCT) is actually a sort of medical compromise. Since trial researchers cannot rely on existing medical science to assist them when deciding whether an adverse event is causally

---

[1] See section "Vaccine Approval Process" in Chapter 1.

linked to the test vaccine, they must settle for a statistical comparison of rates between the trial and control groups. Unfortunately, in comparison with the (regrettably theoretical) alternative of performing medical tests on trial participants to identify adverse effects of the test vaccine, such a statistical analysis can yield only limited and superficial information.

Consider a vaccine clinical trial in which 10 cases of ADEM were reported in the trial group, while the placebo control group had 5 such cases. The comparison of these two numbers amounts to no more than a rough estimation that the vaccine doubles the risk of ADEM. That is just a fraction of the information we want. It cannot help answer medically essential questions such as (1) Does the vaccine cause ADEM? (2) Who is at high risk of developing ADEM following vaccination? (3) How could we reduce the risk of ADEM following vaccination? (4) How could we effectively treat post-vaccination ADEM patients? Only a thorough biomedical investigation of ADEM cases in the trial could generate information that could answer these questions.

The lack of solid science illuminating the mechanics of vaccination side effects has another important downside: It allows researchers conducting clinical trials to arbitrarily decide whether a particular adverse event observed in the trial is related to the vaccine or not.[29] Thus, with the stroke of a pen, researchers can eliminate whole categories of adverse events potentially caused by the trial vaccine. There are many examples of clinical trials in which researchers have casually dismissed, usually without any explanation, potential links between the trial vaccine and serious side effects observed in trial subjects. Here's one typical example: "Of 55 SAEs [serious adverse events] reported during the active phase of the protocol, and 12 reported during the 180 day extended safety follow-up, none were considered to be vaccine related."[30] No government or formal medical body challenges these offhand dismissals of possible associations between the test vaccine and subsequent adverse events.

Discussion of potential causal links to adverse events continues to be absent from the conversation even after the vaccine is approved for use. The manufacturer's package insert, for example, will hardly ever use language that suggests a causal link. Statements such as "the vaccine is known to cause (health condition) X", or "X is likely caused by the vaccine" rarely appear in these leaflets. Instead, manufacturers prefer noncommittal language such as "condition X was reported following use of the vaccine" and emphasize that "a causal association could not be established" between the reported adverse event and the vaccine.[31] Naturally, there is never any mention of the fact that no attempt was made to establish whether or not a causal link exists.

Once the vaccine is on the market and widely used, the absence of any documented causal link on the package insert allows healthcare professionals – doctors, nurses, and officials – to categorically dismiss any link between vaccines and most reported serious side effects.

The Empty Toolbox

As is evident from Isaac's case, doctors do not have any diagnostic tools at their disposal that allow them to reliably associate a particular medical condition to the vaccine or vaccines that preceded it.[m] With the exception of a handful of allergy tests for some vaccine components – even those aren't particularly reliable and results should be interpreted cautiously[32] – their toolbox is empty.

The IOM report reviewed above corroborates this indirectly: In the absence of biomedical studies investigating the link between vaccines and their side effects, the healthcare system cannot be expected to come up with appropriate diagnostic or

---

[m] Unconventional ("functional medicine") doctors use a number of tests to treat side effects of vaccines (for example, testing for the presence of metals in the body or various tests of the digestive system). These tests are generally not recommended by health agencies or mainstream medical associations as means for diagnosing vaccine damage.

therapeutic tools.[n] These tools can only be built on top of solid scientific and medical models. In other words, without a scientific foundation explaining the mechanisms by which vaccines (adversely) affect the human body, one cannot develop appropriate medical tests or effective therapies for vaccine-injured individuals.

Since their diagnostic toolbox is empty, doctors must settle for the accepted medical wisdom regarding vaccination, which is currently based almost entirely on large-scale statistical studies. These studies look for a statistical correlation between two phenomena in a population, receipt of the pertussis vaccine and seizures in infants under the age of 12 months, for example. The study can confirm or reject a correlation in the studied population, but its conclusions are not automatically applicable to individuals. That is, physicians cannot confirm or rule out anything in specific patients based on the results of a large-scale statistical study (more about this in chapter 4). Thus, when only a few vague "rules of thumb" are available for linking vaccines to subsequent health events, a physician's judgment on whether or not the two are related amounts to mere speculation, or, at best, an informed guess.[33]

The large gaps in medical knowledge of vaccine side effects make the daily practice of medicine far more difficult, which can have dire consequences for patients like Isaac. For example, pediatricians cannot predict whether a particular infant will be adversely affected by one vaccine or another, nor the degree of the injury. They cannot make educated decisions about future vaccinations for infants who were previously injured by one or more vaccines. They cannot test an infant's sensitivity to most vaccine ingredients. Nor can they recommend a particular brand of vaccine over another, a safer vaccination schedule, or specific combinations to avoid.

---

[n] A few basic precautions are observed in special cases such as preventing a person who is on immunosuppressive medications because of a transplant from receiving live-virus vaccines.

The empty toolbox also boosts conformity with the recommended vaccine schedule. Since the milieu in which medical professionals operate values high vaccination rates while emphasizing the rarity of serious adverse events, the average physician is unlikely to deviate from the formal schedule. With no practical medical tools available to anticipate or confirm vaccine injury, doctors are left to their own devices should they recognize or acknowledge one. Similarly, they are not very likely to report any injuries they witness to medical authorities (more about this in the next chapter).

Perhaps the most tragic consequence of the missing knowledge regarding mechanisms of injury from vaccination is that doctors have no effective therapies to offer those who "took one for the team" and were harmed, often permanently, by something they were told would protect them. Understanding the mechanism that underlies an injury is imperative when devising effective treatments to reverse or ameliorate it. It is not surprising, then, that effective medical treatments for many serious health conditions attributed to vaccines don't exist.

And the last, but certainly not least, consequence of the lack of research that allows the medical establishment to pretend that all is well in the land of vaccines, is that it precludes any system-wide effort to improve vaccine safety. You have to have a good grasp of how something is causing harm in order to make it safer. In other words, the absence of basic vaccine safety science means that nothing will get better, and children like Isaac will continue to get hurt.

Counter Arguments

"Statistical studies are the only/best/correct way to confirm or rule out a causal link between a vaccine and a side effect." – Not true. Statistical (epidemiological) studies can only corroborate, or fail to corroborate, a correlation (of any degree) between two phenomena. Correlation alone, as we know, does not imply causation. In addition, a statistical correlation tells us nothing about an individual's susceptibility to injury. There is extended discussion of this topic in chapter 4.

"Statistical studies could prove causation." – As mentioned above, statistical studies can only find a correlation and cannot prove a causal link. That is because such studies cannot explain how phenomenon A may cause phenomenon B, but only estimate the frequency with which B follows A. More on this topic is presented in chapter 4.

"It is impossible to deduce a causal link between a vaccine and an adverse event from a single case and even a series of reported cases." – True, but any such case deserves thorough investigation into the medical circumstances and any plausible biological models that could illuminate a link between the vaccine and the adverse event. This is frequently done for medication side effects. As the IOM 2011 report attests, this has hardly been the norm in the field of vaccines.

"The side effects of vaccines are very rare. Therefore it is not a priority to investigate them biologically." – First, this is an example of circular thinking. Which came first, the chicken or the egg? Vaccine side effects are only considered "very rare" because they are not recognized or documented as such in the medical literature, or even in patients' medical records. This lack of recognition is itself due to the lack of a solid scientific foundation linking adverse events to vaccines. So, vaccine injury is rarely reported because the basic research is missing. In fact, as long as this research is missing, the claim that vaccine side effects are "rare" is scientifically unfounded.

Second, in recent years, there have been many parental reports of post-vaccination adverse events, and the public is increasingly linking those to vaccines. This, in itself, is a very compelling reason for funding biomedical research on the subject, since the scarcity of meaningful research significantly impairs public confidence in vaccine safety.

Third, when a society expects all its members to be vaccinated for the "good of the herd," it has a moral obligation to do everything in its power to prevent harm to those who are vaccinated and to provide the vaccine-injured (no matter how few there are) with the best medical therapy possible.

"Biomedical research in the field of vaccine side effects is constantly being done. However, these studies haven't found any links so far." – This claim contrasts starkly with the findings of the IOM 2011 report, which details only a small number of high-quality biomedical studies devoted to the investigation of potential side effects of vaccines. Consequently, the report could not rule out causal links between most of the vaccines and adverse events examined. The glaring lack of scientific research is also evident in medical science's failure to prevent and treat many diseases and conditions reported after vaccination and in the "empty toolbox" of the physician concerned about vaccination risks.

"The 2011 IOM report claims vaccines are safe!" – The IOM 2011 report is not concerned with the question of whether vaccines are safe or not but rather with the possible links between specific vaccines and specific side effects reported following their administration. The opinion of the IOM authors, expressed in a single written sentence[34] and in additional media interviews, is not factually supported by the report. What is important for this discussion's purpose is the evidence the report provides, which clearly indicates that most serious side effects reported after vaccination have not been investigated with high-quality biomedical studies.

Summary

Although modern vaccines have been in widespread use for over 60 years, science and medicine have failed to lay the scientific foundation required to properly assess the associations between vaccines and their reported side effects. The theoretical knowledge base on this issue is very limited and covers only a few of the myriad serious adverse events that have been reported post-vaccination, mainly those for which the connection to the preceding vaccine is obvious. Accordingly, there is also an acute lack of diagnostic and therapeutic tools available for use by medical professionals. As far as vaccines and their adverse events are concerned, the doctor's toolbox is practically empty.

It's no accident that there is so little scientific research on the side effects of vaccines, a state of affairs that has persisted for decades. Hundreds, possibly thousands, of studies in the field of vaccinology are being conducted every year, and many of them are publicly funded. It seems that health authorities in charge of budgeting these studies, however, are not too keen on committing resources to biomedical research on vaccine side effects, nor do they require manufacturers to perform such studies. They seem content with the fact that nearly all vaccine safety research being done, from pre-licensure and onwards, is purposely superficial and ineffectual. Instead of conducting studies that seek to gain a thorough understanding of the underlying biological mechanisms, vaccine safety research settles for mere statistical correlations that provide little theoretical or practical knowledge that can be used to develop tools for prevention, diagnosis, and treatment of vaccine injury.

Yes, scientific research that could provide a thorough understanding of vaccine side effects would require significant financial investment. However, since vaccines are given to healthy people and pressed upon the entire population, most of whom are infants and children, the safety bar should be set particularly high. Health authorities that urge everyone to be vaccinated have a moral obligation to do everything within their power to minimize the harm vaccines can do and to provide effective therapeutic measures for those who are injured. The persistent and severe lack of meaningful research has serious social and economic consequences. Because of the medical establishment's inability to anticipate who will be hurt by vaccines, its inability to associate a specific side effect with the specific vaccine(s) that caused it, and its inability to make adjustments in vaccination parameters to account for individuals' genetic makeup and specific health conditions, catastrophic vaccine injury cannot be prevented.

Investigating the underlying scientific foundation of vaccine side effects could potentially result in significantly safer vaccines, the development of effective treatment options for adverse events, and improved accuracy in cost-to-benefit analysis. This becomes ever more important as each new vaccine is added to the vaccine schedule.

The findings of the IOM 2011 committee report, which reveal a critical shortage in basic scientific research on vaccine side effects, clearly contradict health authorities' claim that vaccine safety has been thoroughly researched. These authorities ignore the fact that vaccine safety research, for the most part, is based on a statistical methodology with limited practical benefit and does not even attempt to contribute biomedical information that could lead to the development of diagnostic and therapeutic tools. Medical science's ongoing failure to provide practical answers is even more glaring in light of its inability to identify causes or provide cures for many of the serious conditions reported after vaccination that have become increasingly common in recent decades.

Ask your doctor:

• If our child experienced a health problem following vaccination, what medical tests are at your disposal to decide whether the condition was actually caused by the vaccine?

• We fear that our child could be adversely affected by a particular vaccine. What medical tests can you perform in order to determine whether or not she is at high risk of being injured by that vaccine?

3

DEFICIENT BY DESIGN: VACCINE ADVERSE EVENT REPORTING SYSTEMS

Once a vaccine has successfully passed through the lengthy licensing process and received the coveted regulatory approval, it is typically integrated into national vaccination programs in the US and other countries. From that point on, it will be routinely administered to tens of millions of people every year, many times more than the thousands, or tens of thousands, of subjects who received it in pre-licensure clinical trials.

Experience of the past few decades demonstrates that when new vaccines or drugs are widely distributed, health events that were not identified in clinical trials often emerge.[1] A clinical trial involving 5,000 subjects, for example, is not large enough to detect adverse events occurring at a rate of 1 in 5,001 vaccinees.[a] The large number of individuals vaccinated in the general population brings a greater human diversity that can affect vaccination outcomes in unexpected ways. Personal characteristics such as genetic makeup, current health status, dietary habits,

---

[a] Even more common adverse events, 1 in every 1,000 for example, may not occur in significant numbers during clinical trials. Yet on a population level, such rare events can affect a large number of people: A rate of 1 in 1,000 adds up to a total of 4,000 affected infants in the US alone every year.

medication use, and socioeconomic status may vary much more than those of the relatively narrow slice of the population in a controlled clinical trial environment. Thus, new types of adverse events may emerge, triggered by a synergy of specific personal traits and health conditions that did not occur in the trials. For example, one child might prove to be allergic to a vaccine component, or a vaccine might cross-react with a medication taken by another. In addition, adverse events that were reported at low rates in clinical trials could prove to be more common in the general population or in specific subpopulations.[2] Accordingly, all parties involved in vaccine development, licensing, and distribution agree that safety should be closely monitored after new vaccines are released to the market.[b]

Health agencies carry out post-licensure vaccine safety monitoring through two main avenues. The first is by collecting reports of adverse events in a specialized database and periodically analyzing the collected data to identify patterns. The second is performance of statistical studies which explore any association between the vaccine and specific adverse health events. The use of these two tools, health authorities say, ensures comprehensive, reliable, and continuous monitoring of vaccine safety. Any anomaly is, supposedly, quickly detected, promptly investigated, and handled appropriately.

On first glance, authorities do indeed seem to be covering all the necessary bases to ensure that vaccine safety is maintained even after vaccines are put on the market. However, closer examination of the design and operation of vaccine adverse event reporting systems paints a radically different picture. This chapter, therefore, describes vaccine adverse event reporting systems and examines to what extent, if any, they achieve their stated objectives.[c]

---

[b] The same practice is applied in the pharmaceutical drug field, too.
[c] The topic of epidemiological studies will be addressed in the next chapter.

VAERS

Vaccine adverse event reporting systems around the world have similar modes of operation and functionality. Therefore, we will focus on the world's leading system: the US Vaccine Adverse Event Reporting System commonly referred to as VAERS.

The VAERS system, jointly managed by the CDC and FDA, was established under the National Childhood Vaccine Injury Act of 1986 and began operation in 1990.[3] VAERS's stated objectives are the following:

a) Identification of new or uncommon adverse events of vaccines (i.e., those not found in clinical trials).

b) Detection of unexpected upsurges in the incidence of known adverse events.

c) Identification of risk factors for specific adverse events.

d) Identification of "hot" vaccine batches.

e) Evaluation of the safety profile of new vaccines.[4]

In its 30 years of operation, VAERS has accumulated over half a million reports. In the last decade, 20,000 to 30,000 new case records have been added yearly.

VAERS receives reports from three main sources: vaccine manufacturers, healthcare professionals, and the general public. Only the manufacturers are required by law to report vaccination adverse events.[d] Reports filed in the system are usually crude case descriptions that do not include analysis or interpretation and rarely, if ever, seek to establish a causal association between the vaccine and the ensuing adverse event. CDC personnel are supposed to monitor VAERS and analyze its data to look for any "signal" which might indicate a safety issue. The system is accessible through a website that allows members of the public to file reports of vaccine adverse events and search the database for information.[5]

So, on the surface, VAERS appears to be well suited to perform its formal tasks and meet its stated objectives. Now let's

---

[d] With a slight reservation, as will be explained later in the chapter.

take a "look under the hood" at VAERS's inner workings to see if it is truly delivering on its promises.

Underreporting Bias

Similar to its counterparts in other countries, VAERS is a passive reporting system. This means that reports are not solicited by VAERS personnel; they are initiated by the reporting parties themselves. Vaccinated individuals, parents of vaccinated children, and medical professionals who vaccinate or treat post-vaccination health events can all file VAERS reports if they wish to. But no one from the VAERS team, or any other state or government health agency, will ever proactively contact them to collect information on post-vaccination events.[6] Solicitation of such information is called "active reporting", and such reporting is used to monitor the safety and efficacy of vaccines in clinical trials. As one might expect, passive reporting systems have universally lower reporting rates when compared with those of active reporting systems.[7]

Another important feature of VAERS is that reporting is generally voluntary, not mandatory. Only the vaccine manufacturers themselves are required to report all adverse events that come to their attention – and even they are not held to any reporting quality standards, as we shall see shortly. Healthcare professionals, on the other hand, are required to report only a handful of adverse reactions that are acknowledged by the federal "Vaccine Court"[e] to be caused by vaccines. This means they are not required to report the majority of health events that occur in close proximity to vaccination, even if they are severe or disabling.[8]

Reporting vaccine adverse events is hardly likely to be beneficial to either a pediatrician's business or peace of mind. Firstly,

---

[e] The Vaccine Injury Compensation Program (VICP) is a federal program intended to compensate people who are injured by vaccines on the childhood immunization schedule. It is known colloquially as "Vaccine Court."

US pediatricians who routinely administer vaccines have no financial motivation to report potential vaccine adverse events. Detailed and accurate reporting can take a significant amount of work, and medical personnel are not compensated for that time.[9] Furthermore, if doctors reported adverse events of vaccines they administered, that could be construed by others as an implicit admission, however informal, of responsibility for any resulting harm. Obviously, neither doctors in private practice nor those working in clinic or hospital settings would have any interest in paving the way for patients or their parents to sue for damages. In addition, doctors, like the rest of us humans, may not be too keen to admit, even to themselves, that medical procedures they recommended and performed might have caused serious harm to their patients.

The public is also not required to report vaccine adverse events. In fact, most parents are completely unaware that they can report their child's post-vaccination adverse health event directly. Even among the parents who are aware, most lack the professional expertise required to provide a detailed and comprehensive record of their child's injury.

Since medical professionals are not obliged to report post-vaccination events, only a tiny fraction of adverse events is actually reported to VAERS. The exact rate of underreporting is unknown, as stated in an official document outlining the VAERS system: "Thus, when the product leaves the controlled study environment of clinical trials and is put into general clinical use by practitioners, the ability to determine the actual incidence of adverse events is questionable."[10] Different estimations put this number anywhere between 1 and 10 percent, which means that only one-tenth, or even one-hundredth, of actual vaccine reactions is ever reported to VAERS.[11] In fact, these estimates, too, are merely educated guesses, as a reliable scientific method for calculating the underreporting rate has yet to be devised.

To estimate the rate of reported adverse events for any vaccine, one must count the number of adverse events reported – the numerator – and divide it by the number of vaccine doses administered (or the number of people vaccinated) – the denominator.[f] Thus, one can determine that for every X vaccine doses administered (or Y people vaccinated) there will be one report of a specific adverse event for a specific vaccine. Since the number of adverse events reported is much lower than the number that actually occur (the numerator), and since the denominator is the number of doses distributed rather than the number actually administered,[12] any rate calculated from VAERS data will inevitably be significantly lower than the true rate, probably by at least one order of a magnitude. As should be apparent, if a calculated rate is only a tenth or a hundredth of the actual rate, that rate cannot be considered a reliable indicator of a vaccine's safety.[13] For example, assuming a particular health event was reported to VAERS following a particular vaccine 100 times in one year, and assuming the vaccine was given to the entire birth cohort of 4 million infants that year, then the calculated rate would be about 1 in 40,000 infants per year. This may seem a relatively low rate for a health phenomenon that is not considered "severe". However, if we account for VAERS underreporting, then the actual rate could be anywhere from 10 times higher (1 in 4,000 infants) up to 100 times higher (1 in 400), and those are not insignificant numbers.

Another noteworthy weakness of VAERS is the fact that most reports are not verified by system operators after they are filed.[14] Many turn out to be inaccurate, implausible, or lacking critical details, which makes them scientifically unusable. Thus, these records are typically omitted from statistical analyses performed on VAERS data, artificially lowering calculated

---

[f] Currently, there is no feasible way to get an accurate number for vaccine doses that were actually administered. Therefore, the denominator most often used in calculating adverse-event rates is the number of doses distributed, which is provided by the manufacturer. This number is always higher than doses administered due to inevitable wastage built into the distribution system. Using this inflated denominator artificially lowers any adverse event rates calculated from VAERS. However, in order to simplify our discussion, calculations in the text will ignore this point.

adverse event rates (which, as we have seen, are already biased downward due to severe underreporting) even further. Reports submitted by manufacturers are particularly likely to be incomplete or inaccurate. For obvious reasons, manufacturers have no motivation to document vaccine adverse events properly. Because they are legally required to pass on any reports they receive, their lack of motivation often manifests in poor reporting quality: missing or incorrect information, vague and inaccurate wording, and the like. Thus, a big question mark hovers over the credibility of at least the 37% of VAERS reports which originate from vaccine manufacturers.[15]

Meaningless Analysis

How, then, do US health authorities utilize VAERS to monitor vaccine safety? Although information collected in the system is meant to enable thorough investigation of alleged vaccine injuries – researchers could potentially contact the sufferers and their families, consult their doctors, ask for further tests to be performed, and so on – this is virtually never done. In practice, VAERS information is only used to produce infrequent statistical analyses that look for patterns that may represent safety signals.

Recall that VAERS's formal objectives include identification of upsurges in vaccine adverse event rates, risk factors for adverse events, and susceptible subpopulations. Statistical analysis is the appropriate tool for achieving these objectives, but as we've seen statistical comparisons using rates calculated from VAERS reports are invalid. The high and virtually unknown rate of underreporting in VAERS renders quantitative comparison of its data to that of other systems scientifically meaningless. Thus, even if the background rate of a specific phenomenon, such as seizures in infants, were known, it wouldn't make sense to compare that rate to the rate reported to VAERS, since that figure could be only a tenth, a hundredth, or even a thousandth of the number of actual cases. For example, if 1 in every 1,000 infants experienced seizures every year and the rate calculated from VAERS for the same age group was also 1 in every 1,000 recipients of all vaccines,[g] one could not argue that vaccines do not appear to increase the risk of seizures, as the real rate of seizures following vaccination could be 10 or 100 times the VAERS rate. Similarly, VAERS data cannot be used to reliably identify susceptible subpopulations, that is, groups who are more susceptible to vaccine injury, such as preterm babies. In this case, too, the absence of reliable and accurate data means that no valid insights can be gained by comparing VAERS data with that of other systems.

Consequently, the flaws inherent to VAERS design and operation, which are typical of many, if not all, of the world's vaccine adverse event reporting systems, render it almost scientifically useless for vaccine safety monitoring. To illustrate this point further, the next section spotlights a VAERS study of the safety of Gardasil, a human papillomavirus (HPV) vaccine, which was published by CDC researchers.

Slade 2009: A VAERS HPV Vaccine Safety Study

On June 8, 2006, following an abridged licensing process, the FDA approved Merck's human papillomavirus vaccine, Gardasil, for commercial use in the United States. A few weeks later, the CDC's Advisory Committee on Immunization Practices (ACIP) met and recommended that the vaccine be given to all girls 11 to 12 years old and that "catch-up programs" be implemented for girls and women aged 13 to 26 years.[16] Shortly thereafter, disturbing reports of serious illnesses following HPV vaccination began to emerge. Testimonials of girls and young women experiencing neurological damage, autoimmune diseases, chronic pain, paralysis, and even death began to accumulate in VAERS and to pop up in media news stories and internet websites.

---

[g] The discussion heavily simplifies the statistical analysis that should be performed in this case. For example, the number of 1,000 should be adjusted to a one-year period.

In 2009, in response to widespread publicity detailing serious adverse events attributed to the vaccine, the FDA and CDC initiated a study to examine Gardasil's safety profile based on VAERS case reports. The lead researcher was Dr. Barbara Slade from the CDC Vaccine Safety Office; her research colleagues also came from CDC and FDA ranks.[17]

The study, published in August 2009, analyzed all VAERS reports filed since Gardasil's mid-2006 approval through the end of 2008, a period of two and a half years. The researchers found that over two-thirds (68%) of reports were submitted by representatives of Merck, the vaccine's manufacturer. As we already know, manufacturers are required to report any adverse events that come to their attention but have little motivation to do so. As would be expected, Merck's Gardasil reports were largely incomplete or inaccurate. With regard to Gardasil, Slade and her colleagues discovered that about 90% of Merck's reports lacked information essential for conducting medical assessments. Since more than two-thirds of the reports were filed by Merck, we can see that a majority, over 60 percent, of Gardasil reports recorded in the study period were critically flawed.[18]

In addition to the low quality of the majority of reports, the study authors also note the unreliability of VAERS rates. As a passive reporting system, they write, VAERS suffers from "underreporting",[19] and, worse, the rate of this underreporting is "unknown",[20] On top of this, they add, "vaccine distribution data do not [...] provide the numbers of doses actually administered",[21] which means that not only is the numerator used in rate calculations inaccurate and uncertain, the denominator is as well.

Although Slade and her colleagues acknowledge that they cannot even estimate relevant rates, let alone accurately calculate them, they do specify a rate of 53.9 VAERS reports per 100,000 vaccine doses distributed in the United States.[22] We know that this number is scientifically meaningless as the true rate of injury may be 10 or 100 times higher (or any other figure, for that matter), and the actual number of doses administered is unknown.

The authors go on to assert that Gardasil's "post-licensure safety profile" as calculated from VAERS data is "broadly consistent" with safety data collected in its clinical trials.[23] This claim, for which no supporting evidence is provided, is inconsistent with the fact that the researchers relied on flawed and underreported data which could not validly be compared with Gardasil clinical trial data. The data presented in the article, in contrast to the authors' illogical conclusion, actually highlight the large apparent difference between the rate of adverse events recorded in clinical trials and in VAERS. For example, the researchers found only 51 VAERS reports of autoimmune diseases following vaccination with Gardasil. Since several million women and girls were vaccinated during the study period, this number roughly translates to a rate of about 1 in 100,000 recipients of the vaccine,[h] while Gardasil's primary clinical trial documented new autoimmune diseases in 1 in 43 young women in the trial group (250 cases out of ~11,000 participants).[24] This huge difference underscores the senselessness of comparing VAERS and clinical trial rates.

The researchers also compared the proportion of VAERS reports for selected adverse events (e.g., death) between Gardasil and other vaccines.[25] This comparison is even more senseless than the comparison with clinical trial results since both numbers in this comparison come from VAERS, and as such are subject to unknown, and probably different, rates of underreporting.[26] The study authors do not provide any evidence to support their assumption that VAERS reporting rates are similar, or similarly distributed, among different vaccines.[i]

---

[h] The researchers used Merck's self-reported 23 million doses of Gardasil distributed in the US during the study period.

[i] There is no reason to assume that the rate of VAERS (under)reporting for various vaccines is similar or evenly distributed. The researchers themselves mention in the article that Gardasil reports to VAERS may be biased due to

Although the authors admit that VAERS does not provide reliable data to realistically assess safety, they willfully leap all methodological obstacles and conclude that Gardasil's safety profile was generally similar to that of other vaccines.[27] This is certainly a noteworthy achievement, especially when one considers that they stated at the outset that "the VAERS reporting rate for [Gardasil] is triple the rate for all other vaccines combined."[28] Did VAERS data and the research techniques at the authors' disposal enable them to come up with a reasonable explanation for the abnormally high rate of reported adverse events for Gardasil? The answer seems to be no. The paper does not contain an evidence-based explanation, merely the speculation that the high reporting rate might simply "reflect greater public attention to HPV" that was purportedly "stimulated" by "widespread media coverage".[29]

Despite Slade and company's acknowledgment of the inherent limitations of VAERS – "underreporting, inconsistency in the quality and completeness of reported data, stimulated reporting due to extensive news coverage, and reporting biases" – and despite their own warning that "VAERS data need to be interpreted with caution,"[30] the authors illogically conclude that Gardasil is at least as safe as other vaccines.[31] This ringing endorsement was amplified when news stories about the Slade 2009 study started appearing in mainstream media shortly after it was published. In these news stories, the caveats and question marks brought out in the paper, the methodological limitations, and the call for caution in interpreting VAERS data all vanished as if they had never existed. All that remained was the decisive *The vaccine is safe!* message promulgated by the lead researcher, Dr. Slade.[32] Later, prominent health organizations, including the CDC and WHO, repeated this *nothing to see here, all is well* message while citing the Slade study as conclusive evidence of

---

"extensive news coverage" or because it was a new vaccine. Those are two examples of unknown variables that may affect the reporting rate and distribution.

Gardasil's safety.[33]

Slade 2009 is a classic example of the way US and international health authorities, assisted by the media, use flawed and incomplete VAERS data to construct a soothing façade of vaccine safety. CDC researchers, well aware that VAERS data cannot provide a valid assessment of vaccine safety, nonetheless concoct a supportive study that media outlets and health authorities then disingenuously cite to lull the public into a false sense of "evidence-based" vaccine safety.

Deficient by Design

As you may recall, the three pillars of vaccine safety are pre-licensure clinical trials, adverse event reporting systems, and post-marketing epidemiological studies. Now that we have familiarized ourselves with the way VAERS operates as well as its limitations and deficiencies, it is time to look at how reporting systems fit in the overall scheme and to evaluate their true contribution to vaccine safety.

Vaccine adverse event reporting systems are designed on the (false) premise that a vaccine's basic safety is established during pre-licensure clinical trials. According to this line of thinking, there is no need to spend extra funds to build a robust reporting system that captures comprehensive data regarding vaccine adverse events. Instead, a more limited system that gathers only a fraction of actual reports and generates alerts for exceptional scenarios is sufficient. Thus, passive systems, like VAERS, that do not mandate reporting from healthcare professionals are designed with built-in flaws. Such systems always suffer from underreporting and, as a result, cannot provide reliable information on the true magnitude of vaccine adverse events.[34]

As we saw in chapter 1, vaccine clinical trials are deliberately designed to conceal the real and high rate of adverse events. Recall that the rate of adverse events recorded in the vaccine group in a clinical trial is "balanced out" by the rate of events in the control group, which also received a vaccine or similarly active compound. Thus, if the rate of serious adverse events in the trial group is a whopping 1 in every 15 subjects, and a similar rate is recorded in the control group, the vaccine is declared "safe".[j] By contrast, if a reporting system such as VAERS collected all adverse health events following vaccination with a particular vaccine and serious adverse events were reported for 1 in 15 or 1 in 20 infants who received it, it would be much more difficult to convince the public that the vaccine was indeed safe. Unlike a clinical trial, VAERS does not have a control group and thus cannot "balance out" high rates of adverse events. However, such high rates can be "watered down" by using a voluntary reporting system, which all but guarantees that a mere fraction of events will be reported. Such a system would not pose a threat to the official vaccine safety message, as it could not expose the true magnitude of adverse events. Whether by design or by accident, the reality is that studies using data from adverse event reporting systems are inherently too weak to contradict vaccine safety dogma or undermine its stability.

Another important point worth considering: High underreporting rates make it extremely difficult to use passive reporting systems to identify rare or unusual adverse events. This is due to the lack of a common numerical basis that would permit meaningful comparisons to population background rates or rates observed in clinical trials. Also, since there is no guarantee that reports are submitted randomly and there is no control group, it is also not particularly useful to compare reporting rates for different vaccines.

While VAERS, with its grossly underreported, incomplete, non-randomized, and uncontrolled data, cannot contribute meaningfully to vaccine safety, it is ideal for those who might wish to obscure any links between vaccines and adverse events.

---

[j] Recall from chapter 1 that in the Prevnar-13 vaccine trial 1 in 12 infants (8.2%) experienced a serious health event in the vaccine group, whereas the control group, which received the older Prevnar vaccine, had a serious health event rate of 1 in 14 (7.2%).

On the one hand, it is conveniently ill-suited to provide meaningful estimates of the actual adverse-event rates[k] or prove causal links between vaccines and subsequent adverse events. On the other hand, the information stored in the system is good enough for health authorities to produce ostensibly respectable scientific studies which reinforce the apparent safety of the vaccine program and relieve public concern.

The methodological flaws inherent in vaccine adverse event reporting systems, as presented above, are well recognized by relevant members of the scientific community. The Slade 2009 authors, for example, explicitly refer to VAERS's limitations several times and emphasize the difficulty of evaluating vaccine safety based on its data. However, despite the authors' numerous reservations as to the validity of their findings, a reputable medical journal published the article, and its conclusion that "the vaccine is safe" received favorable media coverage and has been widely cited in scientific literature since.[1]

Keep in mind that the underreporting typical of vaccine adverse event reporting systems is an artificial limitation due entirely to the fact that reports are neither solicited nor required from medical personnel. In contrast, health agencies around the world implemented similar systems decades ago for reporting and monitoring infectious diseases. In the US, reporting began as early as the late 19th century.[35] Since healthcare professionals are required to report cases of "notifiable" infectious diseases, the reporting rate is extremely high. In addition, when the CDC receives a report of an infectious disease outbreak in a particular area, they immediately send a special team to investigate,[36] an action that is almost never carried out for suspected vaccine-

---

[k] It should be noted that the rate of underreporting in VAERS and similar systems is generally unknown, which further muddies the waters around the true magnitude of vaccine adverse events. Had this rate been known, the true rate of adverse events could have been estimated by simple multiplication. However, recent studies shed light on the subject. See later in the chapter.

[l] As of May 2020, the Slade 2009 article was cited 289 times in the scientific literature.

related events. Therefore, the inherent deficiencies in vaccine adverse event reporting systems that necessitate a "cautious interpretation of their data", as noted by Slade and colleagues, are a direct consequence of health authorities' deliberate choice not to require medical personnel to report vaccine adverse events and to refrain from taking active measures to improve the rate and quality of reports.

This suggests that VAERS and similar systems were intentionally designed to serve as "window dressing", that is, to provide a mere semblance of vaccine safety monitoring rather than the real thing. In practice, these reporting systems constitute another link in a chain, which began in clinical trials, aimed at preventing the truth about the alarming rate of vaccine adverse events from gaining public attention.

Stop Calling Us, Lazarus

The CDC's unwillingness to improve its vaccine adverse event reporting process was inadvertently exposed by a researcher named Ross Lazarus in 2010. Lazarus and his team were awarded a research grant by the US Agency for Healthcare Research and Quality (AHRQ).[37] The purpose of their research was "to create a generalizable system to facilitate detection and clinician reporting of vaccine adverse events, in order to improve the safety of national vaccination programs."[38] Such a system, they write, "has the potential to speed the identification of problems with new drugs [i.e., vaccines] and more careful quantification of the risks of older drugs."[39]

The software designed by Lazarus and his team was intended to extend the capabilities of an existing software package already used by several US healthcare providers for reporting cases of notifiable diseases to public health authorities.[40] Lazarus and his team developed algorithms to identify potential vaccine adverse events, both "expected and unexpected", and to facilitate accurate reporting. The software automatically tracked every vaccinee for a period of 30 days following vaccination and detected and analyzed relevant medical events – hospitalization, laboratory tests, and new drug prescriptions – that could indicate a vaccine reaction had occurred. When such a pattern was identified, the system automatically sent an electronic message to the patient's physician, attaching case details and information about the patient's medical history. The doctor would then decide whether to report the case as a vaccine adverse event, and, if so, the report was sent directly to VAERS in an electronically secure message.[41]

In order to test the new system, Lazarus and colleagues planned to collaborate with the CDC on a joint randomized trial comparing the quantity and quality of reports produced by their software with corresponding reports in VAERS. The trial design, as well as the full research proposal, was distributed among relevant CDC units, which promptly sent their comments back to Lazarus's team.[42]

One might expect that the CDC, the governmental body charged with monitoring vaccine safety, would have seized upon this golden opportunity to upgrade their obviously deficient vaccine adverse event reporting by fully collaborating with Lazarus and his team. The team's system was specifically designed to alleviate VAERS's main deficiencies: severe underreporting by healthcare professionals and poor information quality. Thus, it had the potential to dramatically improve vaccine adverse event reporting, which in turn should lead to better vaccine safety.

As it turned out, however, the CDC had its own considerations. According to Lazarus and colleagues, they completed initial development of the new system, but repeated attempts to proceed with testing were blocked by the CDC; the relevant CDC officials stopped responding to their inquiries.[43] "Due to restructuring at CDC and consequent delays in terms of decision making, it became impossible to move forward with discussions regarding the evaluation of [the system's] performance in a randomized trial, and compare [its] performance to existing VAERS [...] data," the researchers concluded with academic courtesy.[44]

The CDC did not bother to share its reasons for cutting off contact with the research team. However, it would not be unreasonable to infer that the CDC's decision was heavily influenced by the fact that preliminary data from the new system suggested an adverse event rate of roughly 1 in 10 vaccinees, several orders of magnitude higher than the VAERS reported rate.[m] [45] Regardless, if it were only "structural changes" that hindered the new system's implementation, the CDC, the federal agency responsible for monitoring vaccine safety, could have resumed its efforts at any time in the intervening years.

As you may have already guessed, that hasn't happened.

Counter Arguments

"The mission of the VAERS system is to continually monitor vaccine adverse events after they are widely distributed. Because it is a voluntary and uncontrolled system, its sole function is to raise a warning signal when a potential vaccine adverse event is identified, which it does." – That is a partially correct claim. Indeed, VAERS was not intended to provide real data on the rate of vaccine adverse events or to prove causality. However, its inherent deficiencies do not allow the system to effectively fulfill its stated mission and provide true alerts about vaccine adverse events. This is due to the high rate of underreporting, which makes any comparison to population background rates or clinical trial results meaningless. To identify a vaccine safety signal, one needs to compare the rate of reported adverse events to some other "base rate". However, if rates aren't comparable, which is the case for passive reporting systems like VAERS, the comparison isn't scientifically valid.

---

[m] Analysis of information collected on about 1.4 million vaccine doses in 376,452 vaccinees found 35,570 potential adverse events, which roughly amounted to 1 in 39 doses or 1 in 10 vaccinees. This is far higher than rates calculated from VAERS data, which are based on 20,000 to 30,000 yearly reported cases.

"VAERS's goal is to compare its reporting rate to population background rates. For instance, if VAERS receives reports of people fainting in the two weeks following vaccination, it could be compared to the occurrences of fainting in the population to determine whether they are higher, lower, or similar." – As explained in this chapter, because VAERS data is heavily underreported, non-randomized, and uncontrolled, it cannot be meaningfully compared to population background rates or rates observed in vaccine clinical trials.

"Anomalies of an irregular magnitude for a particular vaccine can be identified in VAERS by comparing the rate recorded for a specific vaccine with that of rates of other vaccines recorded in the system." – The VAERS reporting rate for any vaccine is influenced by many factors, at least some of which are unknown. The impact of these factors cannot be quantified or even roughly assessed. The assumption that VAERS reporting rates for different vaccines is identical, or even similar, has no scientific basis. There is also no scientific method to estimate the difference in VAERS reporting rates for different vaccines. Consequently, comparing VAERS reporting rates between different vaccines is not scientifically valid.

"The cases documented in VAERS are mostly health conditions occurring following vaccination that were reported by laypeople who are inexperienced in diagnosing medical and physiological phenomena. As a result, the vast majority of cases reported to VAERS are unrelated to vaccines." – This is a partially correct claim. About a third of VAERS reports come from medical personnel who are, or should be, experienced in diagnosing and reporting medical events. This is indeed a relatively low rate, but it stems directly from the decision of the US health authorities not to require medical personnel to report vaccine adverse events (unlike notifiable infectious diseases). Secondly, it is impossible to ascertain whether a VAERS case was caused by a vaccine without a thorough examination of the case details, including the patient's medical record, and potentially performing additional medical tests. This is almost never done by VAERS personnel or anyone else. Also, recall from chapter 2 that medical science has yet to develop a theoretical framework for reliable diagnosis of vaccine adverse events. In any case, VAERS's shortcomings only serve to emphasize its inability to perform its stated mission of monitoring vaccine safety.

"VAERS is considered to be a very unreliable tool. One can easily file false reports in the system." – That's correct and begs the question, why did US health authorities create such a deficient and unreliable reporting system? Why aren't healthcare professionals required to report? Why aren't reports verified? Why did the CDC block the government-funded project that demonstrated that the system could be improved significantly? Could it be that a deficient and unreliable vaccine adverse event reporting system actually serves US health authorities' interests?

"According to the CDC, the rate of VAERS reporting for serious adverse events is higher than that of minor symptoms, and so for serious symptoms, the VAERS rate is similar to the actual rate, and that's what matters." – Indeed, the VAERS website claims that serious adverse events after vaccination are reported to VAERS at a higher rate compared to mild symptoms.[46] However, this claim is not backed up by any scientific reference or evidence.

"VAERS is not the only US vaccine monitoring system for adverse events. There is also the Vaccine Safety Datalink (VSD) system, which is similar to VAERS but does not suffer from the same drawbacks." – The VSD system is not an adverse event reporting system and is therefore not covered in this chapter. It is a CDC-run information network that pools data from several major US healthcare providers' computerized records. These providers have agreed to make available their clients' data to CDC researchers for the purpose of vaccine adverse event analysis and monitoring (as well as some other uses).[47] VSD analysis reports are not fundamentally different from epidemiological studies performed by researchers using data stored in other healthcare information systems. Epidemiological studies will be discussed in chapters 4 and 5.

The CDC's Vaccine Safety Office manages the VSD system.[n] [48] It is inaccessible to outside researchers, healthcare professionals, and the general public. Researchers who wish to analyze VSD data must submit a formal request to the CDC detailing their research proposal and intentions. Only CDC-approved research- ers gain access to the system.[49] In this way, as an Institute of Medicine special committee explained, the CDC ensures that only researchers within its circle of trust have access to infor- mation in the VSD.[50] Thus, data on the true magnitude of vaccine adverse events can continue to be concealed from the public indefinitely.

Summary

Vaccine adverse event reporting systems are an essential element of the official testing and monitoring process intended to ensure vaccine safety. Vaccine pre-licensure clinical trials are relatively limited in scope and cannot identify uncommon adverse health events or susceptible population subgroups. As a result, comput- erized reporting systems were developed in the US and other countries for the collection of adverse event reports from healthcare professionals, pharmaceutical companies, and the general public. These systems are supposed to identify unusual patterns and warn against potential safety issues of widely used vaccines.

Unfortunately, the promise of vaccine adverse event report- ing systems has not been realized because these systems are

---

[n] At the time of writing, Dr. Frank DeStefano is the head the CDC Vaccine Safety Office. Remember that name for reference later in the book.

intentionally designed to be unable to fulfill their stated mission. Since healthcare professionals are not required to report, and system operators are not soliciting reports (passive reporting), the reporting rate for the system is very low, estimated to be between 1 and 10 percent of the actual rate. In addition, reports are not verified for content or followed up by system personnel. Consequently, the system cannot provide reliable estimations of the true magnitude of vaccine adverse events. In addition, since system rates cannot be meaningfully compared to population background rates or rates observed in vaccine clinical trials, it cannot produce reliable warnings about unusual adverse events of specific vaccines.

The flaws inherent in vaccine adverse events reporting systems are well known to the agencies that operate them and to the researchers who analyze their data. However, neither seems to be bothered by it. On the contrary, health authorities appear quite comfortable with deficient and unreliable-by-design reporting systems, whose data cannot be used to challenge their *Vaccines are safe!* message, as exemplified by the CDC inexplicably blocking a government-funded project to improve VAERS. Nevertheless, these agencies try to have it both ways by exploiting VAERS's unreliable and underreported data to concoct deceptive, scientifically shaky studies that bolster their claim that adverse events are extremely rare. Health authorities' decision to create and maintain deficient-by-design vaccine adverse event reporting systems is even more jarring when one considers that the very same agencies have been operating high-quality mandatory reporting systems for infectious diseases for decades.

Evidently there is a common thread running through vaccine clinical trials, the lack of basic scientific research into vaccine adverse events, and vaccine adverse event reporting systems. In the next two chapters, we will look into epidemiological studies, yet another component of the vaccine safety testing and monitoring process, and examine how they fit into this picture.

Ask your doctor:

• Are you familiar with the VAERS system? Have you ever filed a case with VAERS?

• If your patient experiences an adverse health event following vaccination, do you check VAERS for reports of similar symptoms before deciding how to proceed with the case? Do you report it to VAERS?

• Do you think healthcare professionals should be required by law to report adverse health events following vaccination, similar to their obligation to report cases of notifiable infectious diseases?

4

EPIDEMIOLOGY 101

Epidemiology[a] is a branch of medical science that studies disease at the population level rather than the individual level. Epidemiological research collects data about diseases in a specific population or subpopulation and analyzes it with statistical tools to try to gain insight into their causes, patterns, and effects. For example, an epidemiological study of the effect a particular vaccine had on a particular country may compare the number of disease cases before and after the vaccine was introduced, correlate vaccine coverage (the percentage of people vaccinated) with disease levels over time, and check for unusual morbidity patterns. Thus, researchers can estimate the impact the vaccine had on disease incidence: Did morbidity decline following vaccine introduction? Is there a correlation between disease incidence and vaccine coverage?[b] Did the severity of illness change following vaccine introduction? and other relevant questions.

Epidemiologists, for the most part, rely on collecting health-

---

[a] Literally, the word comes from Greek, meaning "the study of what occurs in populations".

[b] Vaccine coverage: the percentage of vaccinated persons in a population or a relevant subpopulation.

related data from computer systems and processing it using statistical analysis software. Thus, epidemiologists work with computers, not patients. They rarely, if ever, perform physical examinations of study subjects. In fact, in most epidemiological studies the researchers never meet the study subjects or even know their names.

In contrast to epidemiological research, biomedical research (also known as "experimental" research) studies the human body, its systems, components, and mechanisms. Biomedical researchers typically perform laboratory and/or medical procedures using specialized tools and devices. In addition to measuring various physiological parameters, researchers conduct experiments, or trials – in test tubes, laboratory animals, or humans – and analyze the results.

In short, epidemiology views the individual as a "black box" and studies disease characteristics at the "box" population level, while biomedical research investigates the inner workings of the "black box".

With the ever-increasing use of computers to keep track of medical data in the modern era, the relative importance of epidemiology to the study of disease in general, and vaccination in particular, has also increased. How a vaccine affects the individual is the domain of the biological sciences – immunology, virology, etc. But public health officials have to consider the effect vaccines have at the population level, and that is where epidemiology comes in. Consequently, it is crucial to understand the role epidemiology plays in determining vaccine policy and how the health establishment uses it to reinforce the claim that vaccines are safe and effective. To do so, we must familiarize ourselves with epidemiological tools and techniques – their strengths and weaknesses, and their advantages and disadvantages.

Even laypeople who devote considerable time to studying the science of vaccination often avoid delving into epidemiological research. This is due to the arcane technical terms, research methods, and statistical tools of the field. This chapter, therefore, will provide a quick introductory course in epidemiology. We will explain the basic terms in simple, understandable language, helping the reader to grasp both the strengths and limitations of epidemiological research. This understanding will enable readers to spot the weaknesses of vaccine safety epidemiological studies presented in the next chapter and later in the book.

For this crash course in epidemiology we will use a classic historical example of epidemiologic research in action: the discovery of the association between cigarette smoking and lung cancer.

Cigarette Smoking and Lung Cancer

Lung cancer was very rare in the 19th century, so rare, in fact, that when medical professors encountered a patient with the disease they told their students to pay close attention as they might never see another case in their lifetimes.[1] That began to change in the early 20th century as reports of a steady increase in lung cancer, mainly in men, began to emerge. These reports came from three distinct sources: death registration repositories, autopsy reports from pathologists, and doctors who treated cancer patients. In the 1920s, about 1.5 percent of men in the UK were already dying of lung cancer. By 1947, that number had risen 13-fold, to nearly 20 percent. Similar numbers were reported in the US, Australia, Switzerland, and Denmark.[2]

The beginning of the 20th century also marked the point when cigarette consumption began to rise. Until that time, cigarettes were rolled by hand, which made them relatively expensive and, as a result, not very popular. The invention of cigarette-making machines pushed down the price of cigarettes, significantly increasing their popularity. Cigarette consumption in the US rose 80-fold between 1900 and 1960, from about 50 cigarettes a year per person to 3,900, while consumption of cigars and pipe tobacco decreased.[3]

The rapid, sustained rise in lung cancer that began in the early 20th century naturally attracted the attention of doctors, researchers, and public health officials. The common assumption was that such a rapid rise was likely caused by changes in living conditions, that is, by "environmental factors". Suggested potential causes included cigarette smoking, air pollution from car exhaust and factory smokestacks, toxic tar vapors coming off newly built asphalt roads, and aftereffects of influenza or tuberculosis. A minority opinion was that the apparent increase in lung cancer incidence was not a true increase but rather due to better diagnosis or an indirect result of a rise in life expectancy.[4]

As time passed, however, the theory that cigarette smoking was primarily responsible for the huge increase in lung cancer gained dominance. Experts began voicing the opinion that cigarette smoking was causing lung cancer in the early 20th century. These voices multiplied in the 1930s and 1940s with the publication of initial epidemiological studies that demonstrated a statistical association between smoking and lung cancer. Then, in 1950, two large-scale studies found a strong correlation between smoking and lung cancer.[5] These studies, the first American and the second British, were heavily criticized in scientific circles. One argument was that the studies did not demonstrate a causal association between cigarette smoking and lung cancer but a mere statistical correlation. In addition, some scientists highlighted the weaknesses of the research method used and its inherent biases.[c] Another critique stressed the facts that some lung cancer patients hadn't smoked a day in their lives and no cancer-causing substance had yet been found in cigarettes. The harsh criticism directed at these studies stemmed in part from academic disagreement but also from the fact that that by then cigarettes were very lucrative products promoted by a rich and powerful industry.[6]

In response to the criticism, two larger, improved epidemiological studies were designed and performed in the early 1950s and published in 1954. These studies, which analyzed data from tens of thousands of people, found a clear statistical association

---

[c] A retrospective case-control study. See explanation later in the chapter.

between cigarette smoking and lung cancer. In addition, they found that cancer rates increased as subjects smoked more and were higher for cigarette smokers than pipe smokers, and the death rate in subjects who had quit was lower than in those who hadn't.[7] However, even these studies were not sufficient to convince the entire scientific establishment. Prominent statisticians (Berkson, Fisher) still refused to acknowledge a causal link between cigarette smoking and lung cancer, stating that such a link would be proven only if convincing biological evidence was found. They based their criticism on methodological weaknesses of the studies and some seemingly contradictory results.[8]

Of course, scientists were looking for physiological evidence as well. They studied the components of cigarettes hoping to identify any carcinogens. Attempts to trigger cancer in laboratory animals were only partially successful. Smearing cigarette smoke-derived substances on the skin of laboratory animals produced cancer,[9] but attempts to generate lung cancer through inhalation of cigarette smoke failed. These mixed results meant that experimental research had not yet conclusively linked cigarette smoking to the development of lung cancer.[10] (It should be noted, however, that cigarette manufacturers had ample scientific evidence for this connection in their possession as early as the 1950s[11] but chose to hide this information from the public and deny the damage done by cigarettes for decades to come.)

Despite the lack of decisive physiological proof, the accumulation of further high-quality epidemiological evidence finally tipped the scales. In 1957, the British Medical Research Council (MRC) determined that smoking, and particularly cigarette smoking, was a major cause of lung cancer. A few years later, the US Surgeon General also determined that cigarette smoking was the main cause of lung cancer.[12] From then on, the causal link between cigarette smoking and lung cancer was indisputable in scientific circles, and in time, became common knowledge.[d]

Correlation and Causal Link

Interpreting the results of epidemiological studies is always tricky due to the inherent limitations of statistical analysis. Demonstrating that a statistical correlation exists between two phenomena cannot shed any light on the biological mechanism that may underlie the association. In other words, while an epidemiological study may discover a correlation between two phenomena, A and B, it cannot explain why B occurs following A. As we have seen with smoking and lung cancer, the lack of a proven biological mechanism for the development of lung cancer delayed acceptance of the causal link by scientists for many years. The scientific world could not make up its collective mind whether the correlation repeatedly found in epidemiological studies represented a causal association or not.

What is, then, the difference between statistical correlation and causal association? A correlation between two phenomena exists if an increase in the incidence of one is accompanied by an increase in the other.[e] [13] A correlation is established by statistical calculation alone. To demonstrate correlation, one does not have to explain, theorize about, or even speculate as to a mechanism that may link the two phenomena.

In contrast, determination of causation relies on an experimentally demonstrated mechanism by which one phenomenon can lead to the other. The relationship between smoking and shortness of breath, for example, is explained by the fact that cigarette smoke damages lung tissue, impairing its ability to perform the crucial exchange of oxygen and carbon dioxide.[14] A causal link in medicine is proven through physiological (biologi-

---

[d] Some aspects of this controversy, especially those relating to the tobacco companies' attempts to hide the connection through buying science and scientists, nicknamed "tobacco science", were exposed many years later.

[e] Or, in the case of a negative correlation, an increase in the rate of one phenomenon is accompanied by a decrease in the other.

cal, biomedical) research. Epidemiologic studies may provide supportive or contrary evidence of a causal link, but they cannot prove or disprove it (more on this later).

As mentioned above, epidemiological studies can only confirm or refute the existence of a statistical correlation. An epidemiological study investigating the association between cigarette smoking and lung cancer could potentially find no correlation between the two (similar rates of lung cancer in smokers and nonsmokers), a positive correlation (lung cancer is more common in smokers than nonsmokers), or a negative correlation (lung cancer is less common among smokers, implying that smoking protects against lung cancer). A correlation also has a strength qualifier. For example, a study may find that smokers of a single pack per day may be five times more likely then nonsmokers to get lung cancer, a strong correlation, while two-pack-a-day smokers may be eight times more likely to get lung cancer (an even stronger correlation).

It is important to remember that a chance correlation between two phenomena is not rare. There are many examples of a phenomenon whose incidence increases or decreases in accordance with that of another despite no causal association between them. In the early 20th century, for example, along with the rise in lung cancer and cigarette consumption in the US, there were corresponding rapid increases in candy consumption, agricultural pesticide use, and paving of asphalt roads (and probably many other measurable phenomena). By using statistical tools and techniques, epidemiologists can usually distinguish meaningful correlations from those that are due to chance alone. For example, the correlation between the increase in lung cancer incidence and the acceleration of asphalt paving led some researchers to speculate that there might be a connection between the two. According to this hypothesis, inhalation of toxic fumes from freshly paved roads was the main culprit behind lung cancer. This hypothesis could be tested using epidemiological tools. For instance, the correlation between lung cancer and the number of paved roads in different geographical areas could be examined. In addition, the population could be stratified by level of exposure to asphalt roads – with those who live or work in high-traffic areas at the top and farmers living miles from any paved roads at the bottom – and the correlation to lung cancer for each of the groups could be calculated.

However, in the end, even the best epidemiological studies cannot prove or disprove a causal link between two phenomena.[15] In the absence of an evidence-based explanation of how phenomenon A is related to phenomenon B, one cannot rule out the possibility that the observed correlation between the two is coincidental or due to a third phenomenon not yet considered (more on that later). In order to unequivocally prove the existence of a link between two phenomena, such as cigarette smoking and lung cancer or a vaccine and a subsequent adverse health event, biomedical studies must be conducted that illuminate an underlying physiological mechanism.

Therefore, a statistical correlation established by an epidemiological study, no matter how strong, is considered less conclusive than a causal link demonstrated in physiological studies, since it represents a lower level of certainty. If we know nothing about how one thing leads to the other, we cannot rule out the possibility that the correlation between them is mere coincidence and does not represent a true cause-and-effect relationship.

Determination of Causal Links in Medicine

As noted above, despite the accumulation of epidemiological studies in the 1940s and 1950s that indicated a correlation between cigarette smoking and lung cancer, the scientific world was slow to acknowledge the reality of a causal link between the two. This hesitation was in part due to the fact that determining causation in medicine is inherently uncertain and inconclusive. Scientists had to evaluate the supportive evidence, while at the same time considering contradictory study results. Though epidemiologic research repeatedly found a correlation, there were plenty of counterexamples: people who had smoked several packs a day for decades and never got cancer and people who had never smoked and got lung cancer anyway. The second fact is easily explained: Lung cancer could have multiple causes, including secondhand smoke as well as other, non-smoking-related, exposures. But how could smoking be said to cause lung cancer when so many heavy smokers never develop lung cancer?

The answer is that the term *causal link* has a different meaning in medicine than in exact sciences like chemistry and physics. When physicists knock billiard balls into other billiard balls, they can predict how the collision will affect the direction and speed of each of the balls, and exactly where they will come to a halt on the table. All the factors involved in the event – from the number and size of the balls to the friction produced by the felt surface – are knowable, as are the laws of physics that govern their motion. In this scenario, scientists can easily describe the movement of the balls in terms of causal relationships: The stick hits the white ball and causes it to roll in a certain direction and at a certain speed; the white ball hits the red ball at a certain angle and speed and makes it change direction and speed; the red ball hits the blue ball, and so on. Whenever we arrange the balls in the same formation and move the white ball toward them in the exact same direction with the exact same speed, an identical result will occur: The balls will stop at exactly the same positions on the billiard table.

In medicine, however, the situation is radically different. Such certainty doesn't exist. The human body, infinitely more complex than a billiard table, is made up of countless "moving parts" that interact with each other and are simultaneously influenced by many external factors. In fact, the human body is so complex that science currently understands only a small fraction of its workings. It is nearly impossible for biologists to predict all the downstream effects of a single change in a particular human body. Myriad biological processes affect other processes, any of which could be affected in multiple ways, directly or indirectly. Thus, lung cancer could develop in a person who smoked a pack a day since he was 20 years old and not in his classmate, who started at the same age and smoked two packs a day. To date, science has no definitive answers as to why one gets cancer while the other does not.

If scientists cannot accurately predict which smokers will develop lung cancer, why, then, do they maintain there is a causal link between the two? In other words, why do we say that cigarette smoking causes lung cancer? The answer is that smoking increases the risk of developing lung cancer. While smoking does not cause lung cancer in every individual, it certainly increases an individual's likelihood of developing lung cancer.[16]

Similarly, if a vaccine increased the risk of a certain side effect, the vaccine would be considered a cause of the side effect, even if it did not occur in every vaccinee. In this case, too, there are many factors, too many to accurately evaluate, operating simultaneously in the vaccine recipient's body, shaping the end result. Thus, a vaccine could cause paralysis in a particular person while not harming any of the other 999 individuals vaccinated on the same day. Moreover, the same vaccine, administered a day earlier or a day later, might not have caused paralysis even in the affected person. Even though so many people received the vaccine with no ill effects, an epidemiological study could still find a solid correlation between the vaccine and paralysis, and a physiological study could explain how the vaccine caused paralysis in that specific individual.

It is important to remember that, despite the tremendous advances made by medicine in the modern age and the vast knowledge we have accumulated about the human body, many present-day medical policies and recommendations are based on statistical correlations alone. In the absence of scientific evidence solidly linking two phenomena, it is quite common for formal medical bodies to base policy recommendations on nothing more than a statistical association between them. A typical example is the "Back to Sleep" campaign, begun in 1994, which recommended laying infants on their backs, as opposed to their stomachs or sides, in order to reduce the risk of "crib death"

(SIDS). This recommendation is made despite the fact that medical science still does not know exactly why back sleeping appears to be safer for babies.[17]

Characteristics of Epidemiological Studies

In chapter 1 we introduced the concept of a clinical trial. That discussion briefly touched on some of the features of epidemiological research. You may recall that the RCT, the form of clinical trial which is considered the industry's "gold standard", is controlled (includes trial and control groups), randomized (subjects are randomly assigned to a group), and double-blinded (subjects and researchers are not aware of who is in which group).

RCTs are *interventional* studies, studies in which participants are asked to behave in a particular manner at the researchers' request. Subjects could be asked to consume a specific medical product, such as a drug or vaccine, or perform some activity periodically, such as exercise for 15 minutes a day or drink a glass of red wine at dinner every night.

In contrast to interventional studies, an *observational* study does not interfere with subjects' daily lives; researchers simply collect and analyze relevant health information. Nowadays, most observational studies are conducted by analyzing data that is stored in computerized data banks. Thus, observational studies are generally easier, quicker to perform, and less costly than interventional studies. In addition, they facilitate analysis of much larger volumes of data. On the other hand, however, observational studies are more prone to bias. Thus, their results are considered lower quality than those of clinical trials.

Another important feature of epidemiological research relates to the time perspective of the study. In a *prospective* study (looking ahead), the researchers select a group of subjects, monitor them for a certain period of time and document changes in relevant health parameters (such as the number of subjects diagnosed with lung cancer during the study period). At the end of the study, the researchers analyze the data collected, summarize the results, and formulate their conclusions.[18] In a *retrospective* study (looking back), the researchers select a group of subjects and examine relevant personal data that already exists, usually in one or more computerized systems.[19]

Prospective studies generally produce higher quality results than retrospective studies as they are less prone to bias. Because recruitment is complete before any of the studied events occur, the risk that the results would be skewed by a biased sample of subjects is reduced. In addition, the information collected by researchers is generally more complete and accurate, since much of it is recorded in real time. Retrospective studies, on the other hand, similar to observational studies, are faster, simpler, and cheaper to perform. They also allow for much larger study groups, enabling the investigation of relatively rare phenomena.

How do the two features of epidemiological research described above fit together? An interventional study (a trial) is always prospective, since the data the researchers seek does not yet exist (or they wouldn't need the trial). An observational study may be prospective or retrospective. An observational prospective study might, for example, monitor smokers of varying levels for several years and look at how the incidence of lung cancer changes over time. An observational retrospective study might, instead, use existing patient records in a health provider's computer system to answer the same questions.

Types of Observational Studies

Observational studies are usually divided into four main categories:[20]

Cross-section: a study that examines data at a specific point in time in different populations. The raw data is evaluated at the population level (as opposed to the individual person level).

Example: Comparing lung cancer rates in various countries around the world and looking for factors that could explain any differences, such as the country's level of industrialization.

Ecological: a study that looks for a correlation between two phenomena in a population. Similar to the cross-section, the ecological study also compares data at the population level and not at the individual level.

Example: A study examining the correlation between air pollution levels and the incidence of lung cancer in various US cities.

Cohort: a study investigating a group of individuals who share relevant characteristics but were variously exposed to the factor whose impact is to be examined.

Example: Evaluating the correlation between the quantity of cigarettes consumed per day and lung cancer incidence in urban men aged 50 to 60.

Case-control: a study comparing individuals who suffer from a common condition (e.g., type 1 diabetes) to a control group consisting of people without that condition. Control group subjects are deliberately chosen to closely match potentially relevant characteristics of subjects in the trial group. Each subject in the trial group is matched with one or more controls with similar characteristics, such as age, gender, and area of residence. The researchers try to identify risk factors by comparing the two groups.

Example: A study matching lung cancer patients with healthy controls who share similar demographic characteristics in order to find differences between the two groups that might hint at the cause for the disease (such as differences in smoking habits).

If you're a little confused and having trouble remembering the distinctions between different types of observational studies, don't worry. They're all quite similar. The bottom line is this: Different types of observational studies use different statistical methods to look for correlations between phenomena in a population.

Sources of Error: Biases and Confounders

The quality of epidemiological research is determined, first and foremost, by the quality of the data on which it is based. It is next to impossible to draw valid conclusions from partial or inaccurate data. There are two main sources of bias, or error, which can potentially impair research quality: *selection bias* and *information bias*.[21]

Selection bias occurs when researchers, consciously or unconsciously, select a group of subjects (or a data set) that does not accurately represent the research population or does not suit the study's research questions well. Including inappropriate subjects or excluding appropriate ones can skew a study's results. For example, in our hypothetical ecological study investigating the correlation between air pollution and lung cancer cases in various US cities, including only a small number of cities could potentially bias the results in one direction or another if those cities are not representative of the nation as a whole.

Information bias occurs when researchers fail to gather accurate or complete data on subjects. For example, a study that examined the effects of cigarette smoke exposure could suffer from information bias if researchers collected information on the subjects' smoking habits but didn't consider other potential smoke exposures such as a spouse's smoking. In addition, the smoking data itself could be inaccurate if it was obtained from a database that suffered from incomplete or unreliable reporting.

Data collection is followed by data analysis, which comes with its own potential sources of error. Researchers weed out bad data, apply statistical "corrections" to the data or parts of it, compute correlations, and the like. Naturally, the analysis techniques themselves could be flawed or not appropriate for the study. In addition, the conclusions drawn could be erroneous. The professional literature usually mentions one major potential source of error in data analysis: the *confounder*.

A statistical correlation between two phenomena, however robust, could be an optical illusion if there's a confounder. A confounder is a separate variable, not included in the initial analysis, which is associated with the two phenomena examined. For example, several epidemiological studies found a positive correlation between alcohol consumption and lung cancer. This correlation suggested that alcohol consumption could be a significant risk factor for lung cancer. However, subsequent physiological studies that searched for biological proof for the alcohol-lung cancer connection could not find much supporting evidence. This failure led many in the scientific community to suspect that the correlation between alcohol consumption and lung cancer was artificial and did not represent a causal association. Indeed, further epidemiological studies found that the apparent link between the two stems from the fact that heavy drinkers are more likely to smoke, and smoking, as we already know, increases the risk of lung cancer. Supporting evidence for this assertion was found when researchers separated alcohol-drinking subjects into smokers and non-smokers. The lung cancer rate among alcohol-drinking smokers was very high, and it was close to average in alcohol-drinking non-smokers.[22] Thus, when investigating the connection between alcohol consumption and lung cancer, cigarette smoking played a confounding role, since it, rather than alcohol consumption, is the true risk factor for lung cancer. The above example also demonstrates how statistical techniques in epidemiological research can reveal confounders and highlight their impact.

Bias and confounders are considered the main pitfalls of epidemiological research, but that presupposes that researchers behave honestly and objectively, in line with the scientific ideal. In practice, however, as we shall see in the next chapter, when researchers choose not to abide by ethical research guidelines, there are numerous techniques they can use to skew study results.

Capabilities and Challenges

As was mentioned previously, epidemiology's various kinds of observational studies are quite similar in nature. In all of them, a group of "subjects", whether persons or populations, is selected and stratified according to various criteria. Then, researchers do statistical analysis, seeking correlations between group characteristics and one or more health outcomes.

Epidemiological studies can provide a good estimate of the incidence of a particular health condition in a population. They are also capable of generating, rather quickly, warning signals regarding emerging illnesses in a population, even when science can tell us nothing else about them. In addition, they can point to promising future research directions. Physiological research is less suited for studying all of the above.

On the other hand, since epidemiological studies can only determine statistical correlations, rather than causal links, they produce relatively low certainty. It's difficult, therefore, to use the results of these studies to devise diagnostic or therapeutic tools or to make decisions regarding an individual patient's care. Physiological research, as already discussed in chapter 2, can potentially provide assistance with all of those. For example, a study identifying the carcinogenic substances in cigarettes could lead directly to the production of safer cigarettes.

Despite its intensive use of statistical tools and methods, epidemiology is not considered a pure technical science. Some even describe it as a form of "art".[23] To conduct a high-quality study, researchers must formulate good research questions, select an appropriate study type, select a suitable group of subjects, collect comprehensive and reliable data, apply fitting statistical methods, neutralize biases, and identify confounders. There is no fixed blueprint to follow. The researchers are free to choose their tools and techniques and must use this freedom wisely if they wish to produce valuable and meaningful results. Even a small methodological misstep can significantly tarnish the quality of the research and the scientific merit of the results.[24]

Individual, Group, and Population

Epidemiological research is highly suitable for assessing the incidence of phenomena and discovering correlations at the population level but, as we've seen, its findings are not applicable to individuals. For example, epidemiological studies can find a correlation between smoking and lung cancer, but they cannot determine whether a specific smoker will ever develop lung cancer.[25] Physiological research, however, because it investigates the biological mechanism that links two phenomena, could potentially shed light on an individual's medical condition.[26] Epidemiological studies may also fail to detect risks that are relatively rare, or those that are expressed in only a small population subgroup.[27]

So what happens when epidemiological and physiological studies contradict each other? In this case, physiological research has the upper hand. In the somewhat technical wording of the 2011 IOM report (discussed in chapter 2): "Epidemiologic evidence [...] can support [...] a causal association or can support the absence of [...] a causal association in the general population and in various subgroups that can be identified and investigated, unless or until supportive mechanistic evidence is discovered [...]."[28] The reason for this, as mentioned previously, is the higher level of certainty inherent in physiological (mechanistic) research.

It is important to understand – and this point will come up again later in the book – that epidemiological studies, no matter how well done, cannot rule out a causal link between two phenomena (such as a vaccine and a new autoimmune condition) for an individual. In addition, sound physiological research that demonstrates a causal association in a specific person or group of people, cannot be refuted by epidemiological studies. This, too, is true for vaccines and adverse events as noted in the IOM 2011 report: "Even in the presence of a convincing protective effect of [a] vaccine in epidemiology, studies may not rule out the possibility that the [adverse] reaction is caused by [the] vaccine in a subset of individuals."[29] In other words, even if a correlation between a vaccine and an adverse event was not found in a large statistical study, that would not preclude the possibility that the vaccine did cause the adverse event in a specific person or group of people.

Summary

Epidemiology is a field of medicine that investigates disease on a population level through the use of statistical tools. Epidemiological research looks for statistical correlations between different phenomena in an attempt to elucidate a relationship between them. While such a study can demonstrate a statistical correlation, it cannot provide insight into a physiological mechanism by which A causes B (causal link). In order to prove a causal association in science, physiological (biomedical, mechanistic) studies must be performed.

In medicine, a causal link between two phenomena is often ambiguous and difficult to identify. A certain condition may be caused by several co-factors operating synergistically, each required for its development, but none causing it on its own. That is, a risk factor present in a particular person, heavy and prolonged smoking, for instance, might not necessarily cause the disease, lung cancer, in that individual. The difficulty in identifying relevant risk factors – including their roles, relative importance, and interrelationships – makes it challenging for modern medicine to explain the origins of many diseases. It is quite common, therefore, for medical bodies to make recommendations without a thorough understanding of the mechanism underlying a specific health condition. One such recommendation is the advice to parents to lay babies on their backs to prevent "crib death", which is based entirely on epidemiological data.

Epidemiological studies come in several varieties. In an interventional study (trial), subjects are asked by researchers to take specific actions (e.g., take a drug), while in an observational study, researchers only gather information about the subjects. A prospective study tracks a group of people for a specific period of time and collects relevant data about them. A retrospective study analyzes existing data. Interventional studies are more expensive to perform than observational studies, but their results are generally of higher quality. Prospective studies are more expensive and take longer than retrospective studies, but they suffer less from selection and information bias, which makes their results more reliable.

Epidemiological studies cannot predict whether a particular individual will get a certain disease, nor can they prove that a particular factor was, or wasn't, the cause for that individual's disease. Since they only deal with statistical correlations, they cannot refute the results of physiological studies. The fields of epidemiological and physiological research complement each other. Each has its own advantages, disadvantages, and uses.

Despite the fact that formal techniques and statistical tools are used in epidemiological research, there are no fixed recipes to follow when designing studies. Researchers must carefully select the research method, collect complete and reliable data, neutralize any bias, and apply correct analytical methods. Producing high-quality, meaningful research is no simple matter; some even consider it an art form.

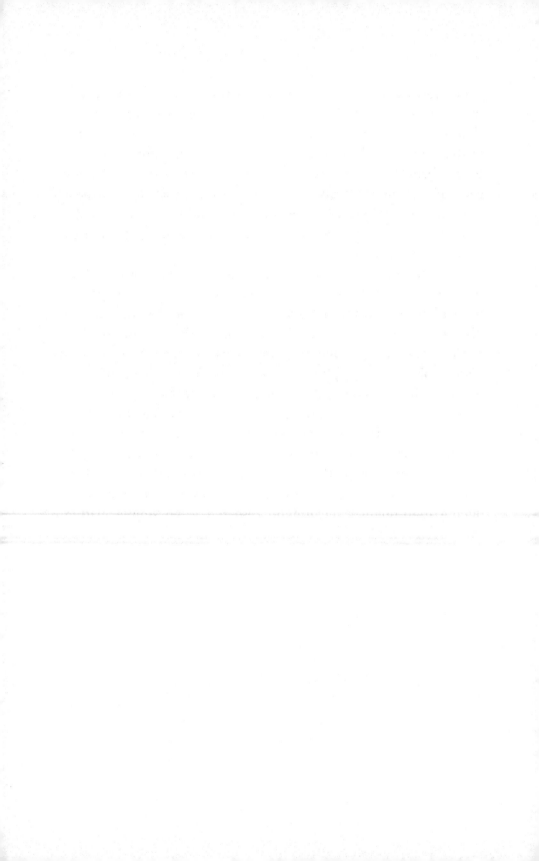

5

PURPOSELY BIASED SCIENCE: EPIDEMIOLOGY AND VACCINE SAFETY

"There are three kinds of lies: lies, damned lies, and statistics."

Mark Twain

In the previous chapter we introduced the medical field of epidemiology, its capabilities and limitations. In this chapter we will look at how medical and scientific bodies make use of biased epidemiological research to present an illusion of vaccine safety to the public. We will document this claim through in-depth analysis of a number of well-known vaccine safety studies from the past fifteen years, highlighting their fundamental flaws and describing the circumstances surrounding their publication.

The previous chapters exposed some of the systematic ways medical authorities and vaccine manufacturers cover up the true extent of vaccine adverse events. Given what we already know, it would be reasonable to suspect that the medical establishment would not, when necessary, shy away from initiating and promoting further biased research to achieve this objective. But in order to convince the vigilant reader that that is indeed what is happening, we must first answer some inevitable questions: Why would the medical establishment encourage biased vaccine safety research? How can the establishment control the outcome of vaccine safety research? Why would researchers and academics cooperate in producing biased science? Why would medical journals publish faulty or biased studies? And how could scientific studies be systematically biased without the public catching on?

Answering these questions is essential if one wants to understand exactly how the medical establishment uses epidemiological studies to preserve vaccines' reputation. Therefore, before delving into the specifics of certain vaccine safety studies, we will devote the next few pages to outlining the context in which these studies are performed and published. Once one learns how science funding works and how vaccine safety research is conducted and published, it will not be possible to dismiss specific researchers' breaches of the scientific code of ethics as the actions of a few "bad apples". By putting our examples of faulty studies in context, taking into account the relevant players and the motives that drive them, a coherent picture emerges of a deliberate and systemic process used to generate a complex of misleading scientific research designed to cover up the truth about vaccine safety.

Back to the 1990s

Toward the end of the 1990s, after a relatively quiet decade and a half, concerns about vaccine safety began to re-emerge in the United States. This period of relative tranquility was preceded by the turbulence of the '70s and early '80s, when the media focused on the purported harms of the DTP, or "triple-vaccine" (a vaccine against diphtheria, tetanus and pertussis). National headlines followed the 1982 airing of the TV documentary *DPT: Vaccine Roulette*, which included footage of children who suffered severe adverse reactions following DTP vaccination.[1] Across the Atlantic, similar stories about the DTP vaccine were published in the UK as early as the mid-1970s. These stories, backed by credible testimony from renowned doctors, sparked a public outcry that led the British government to suspend DTP vaccination for several years.[2] Despite media chatter, however, and the support of a handful of maverick doctors and researchers, re-examination of DTP safety was limited in scope and depth. Public debate at the time was almost entirely confined to mainstream media – television, newspapers, and medical journals. Any information that reached the public was pre-filtered and edited, as was the norm in those days, making it difficult for parents of vaccine-injured children to make their case publicly, find like-minded parents, and win allies to their cause.

Once the DTP storm subsided, medical authorities enjoyed a quiet period that ended abruptly in the late 1990s. Public interest this time around was focused on the MMR – another triple vaccine (for measles, mumps and rubella) – and the mercury-based preservative thimerosal used in many of the routine childhood vaccines. Concerns about the MMR arose in the UK in 1998 with the publication of a paper by Dr. Andrew Wakefield and colleagues in *The Lancet* medical journal. Wakefield and his 12 co-authors suggested that the MMR vaccine might have caused autism and inflammatory bowel disease in some children who regressed developmentally following MMR vaccination.[3] At nearly the same time in the United States, the FDA calculated, for the first time, the amount of mercury infants were receiving in routine vaccinations and discovered that the cumulative amount far exceeded the threshold considered safe by various government health agencies. Following these findings, even before the information reached the public, a number of US health organizations recommended removing thimerosal from childhood vaccines.[4] The establishment's sudden interest in removing mercury from vaccines caught the attention of some parents of autistic children. These parents were already collaborating in efforts to identify the causes behind the huge rise in autism rates and to find effective treatments for their children.[5] The parents' activities led to lively public discourse regarding an apparent link between vaccines and autism that culminated in a series of Congressional hearings from 2000–2002.[6]

The renewed public interest in vaccine safety issues (and particularly in the vaccine–autism link) accelerated during the next decade after the breakout of the internet in the early 2000s. The trickle turned into a creek, then into a mighty river, creating a new and unprecedented challenge to those in charge of the vaccine program. Newly created websites, mailing lists, and online forums enabled parents to discuss their children's adverse vaccine reactions in ever-increasing numbers. The internet also enabled parents to gather vaccine-related information more easily and share it with other parents. Everything related to vaccines and vaccine policy, from the real risks of vaccine-preventable diseases to the dubious tactics of pharmaceutical companies, became the focus of intense online discussion. This information, which had, for the most part, been accumulating dust in the basements of public libraries, virtually inaccessible to the average parent, became available to anyone with an internet-connected computer. In addition, the Web became an amplifier for physicians and researchers who dared to criticize institutional vaccine policy.[7] Thanks to the internet, these "rebel" professionals could now reach parents directly, bypassing the "old" media that had, until then, served as a de facto buffer between them and the general public.

Within a few short years, through vigorous collaborative efforts coordinated through the internet, parents and researchers accumulated a large body of knowledge critical of vaccines and vaccination, based in large part on rational, science-based, and compelling claims. The once tiny group of non-vaccinating parents expanded rapidly, growing louder and ever more critical, until they became a force to be reckoned with.[8] Health authorities like the CDC could no longer ignore the parents. They had to go on the offensive, and they did so by putting science – and more precisely, epidemiology – at the forefront of the battle.

Epidemiology to the Rescue

Health authorities' response to the growing public criticism of vaccines was largely framed as "the (rational) scientists vs. the (emotional) parents". According to this narrative, on one side of the debate stood science, represented by dignified experts who cited published research and echoed official health guidelines, while on the other stood parents (mostly mothers), who lacked formal relevant training and based their views on personal anecdotes and quack doctors' publications.[9] To enhance this narrative, authorities began commissioning studies on numerous vaccine-related topics to "beef up" the surprisingly small body of vaccine safety research and ostensibly provide decisive scientific answers to each and every criticism raised by parent advocacy groups.[10]

The authorities had several courses of action to choose from for their surge of vaccine safety research efforts. One obvious theoretical option would be to devise and conduct specialized medical tests and examinations on the infants and children allegedly harmed by vaccines in an attempt to better understand the biological factors and mechanisms underlying their medical conditions. If common features between the injured children emerged, they could further investigate them to identify exactly what was causing the damage – a vaccine, a particular vaccine ingredient, a combination of a vaccine and specific medical conditions, or even something unrelated to the vaccine itself.

As we saw in chapter 2, however, this line of investigation has never appealed to the medical establishment. Even today, after more than 60 years of scientific research in the modern era, there are very few mainstream physiological studies investigating vaccine adverse events. The establishment's evident dislike for this line of inquiry is hardly surprising. Such studies could potentially draw scientific and public attention to injured children and to the alleged link between their injuries and the vaccines they received. Another tricky aspect of this approach, from health authorities' perspective, is the relative difficulty of ensuring results favorable to vaccines. Physiological studies are largely based on standard biomedical tests, which are performed using instruments that produce precise numerical results. Attempting to "fix" such test results can be risky for researchers, since it is usually quite simple to send samples for retesting to another, independent, laboratory.

A "safer" research approach, then, would be to fund research that would look for, and find, non-vaccine factors responsible for the adverse reactions blamed on vaccines. US health authorities, for example, allocated more than a billion dollars over the past decade or so to study the (non-vaccine) causes of autism, most notably genetics.[11] But despite the vast resources invested in the search for "the autism gene", the results have been quite disappointing. Genes alone, as it turns out, can explain only a tiny fraction, if any, of the huge rise in the autism rate.[12]

While physiological (genetic) research has failed repeatedly to deliver a convincing blow to the growing public criticism of vaccine safety, epidemiology – and, more specifically, retrospective observational studies – have turned out to be health authorities' most effective tool in the public relations battle. Within a few years, dozens of vaccine-related epidemiological studies were conducted, funded by interested public and private entities. These studies approached vaccine safety from various angles and seemingly affirmed and reaffirmed vaccination's clean bill of safety. Many studies addressed the suspected link between vaccines and autism. Others focused on refuting the alleged link between vaccines and chronic illnesses such as diabetes, asthma, and allergies. For every critical claim made by parent advocates, one or more epidemiological study soon appeared, presenting evidence that seems to clear vaccines of all charges. Thus, vaccine proponents could use these studies to emphatically deny the link to vaccination of virtually any alleged vaccine injury. With epidemiological science ostensibly backing their position, officials could credibly claim that "science did not find a link between vaccines and disease or condition X."[13] The torrent of epidemiological studies that began in the late 1990s continues to flow to the present day, ever increasing, as the public controversy over vaccines intensifies.

Opportunistic Retrospective Observational Studies

As described in the previous chapter, epidemiology deals with the study of population-level disease and is therefore ideal for making sweeping assertions about vaccine safety (although those assertions obviously depend on the quality of the studies). You may recall from chapter 4 that epidemiological studies can be distinguished by the intervention factor (interventional or observational), and the time-perspective factor (prospective or retrospective). Generally, interventional studies are more reliable than observational studies, and prospective studies yield higher quality results than retrospective studies.

Retrospective observational studies are relatively inexpensive and easier to perform. In addition, they have one more distinct feature that is crucial to the discussion that follows: Their results can be rather easily "adjusted". This point becomes clear when comparing retrospective observational studies to randomized controlled trials (RCTs), the industry's "gold standard"[14] and the staple of the vaccine licensing process.

Random allocation of subjects into trial and control groups, as well as concealment of the participants' grouping throughout the trial (blinding), considerably limits researchers' ability to skew, intentionally or otherwise, the results of an RCT. Unfortunately, these advantages do not apply to retrospective observational studies.

Unlike in RCTs, where subjects are allocated to groups by "coin flip", in retrospective observational studies researchers allocate the subjects according to their own criteria. Researchers can easily tweak selection criteria as they see fit, adding subjects to one group, removing them from another, or moving subjects from one group to another. Even when researchers formally declare that they have randomly allocated subjects – for example, in selecting members of the control group in a "case-control" study – we have only their word for it. Unlike clinical trials, non-interventional epidemiological studies are not inspected by government officials or any other formal body. Consequently, in most, possibly all, vaccine-related retrospective observational studies, there is no one who monitors researchers' conduct and ensures that they adhere to the formal research plan and ethical standards.

A retrospective observational study is inferior to the RCT in another crucial aspect: blinding. In a retrospective study, where relevant events have already occurred and the data to be analyzed already exists, researchers can "massage" the results to achieve a predefined outcome. One technique already mentioned above is moving subjects between groups to change the resulting comparison between the groups. RCTs, on the other hand, are prospective, which means the data doesn't exist at the time of subject allocation. Hence, it is much more difficult, and frequently impossible, for researchers to affect the outcome by fiddling with the group allocation process. To do so, they would need to accurately predict in advance how certain participants would react to the trial interventions, which isn't usually feasible.

Though many retrospective observational studies are "controlled", meaning they include a control group similar to an RCT, this, by itself, does not necessarily ensure credible results. Unlike in an RCT, researchers select who goes in the control group, which means they control the study's "baseline". Thus, with subjects' data available to them, researchers can assign participants to study groups, run the statistical analysis, examine the outcomes, and reassign the participants if they don't like the results. Since data analysis is fully computerized, they can easily repeat this process until desirable results are obtained.

The guidelines for retrospective observational studies, unlike RCTs, are quite flexible. As demonstrated in chapter 1, in order to come up with favorable safety results in pre-licensure clinical trials, manufacturers have to apply a rather ingenious workaround: testing a vaccine against a control group that receives a

different vaccine (or a similar compound). The strict requirements of the trials – a control group, randomization, and
blinding – gave rise to this devious method for clearing the
required safety bar. Retrospective observational studies, however, are exempt from these restrictions, which means that
researchers who wish to control a study's outcome have a much
easier task.

But why would scientists ever wish to purposely bias research
results? Isn't the discovery of scientific truth, and that alone, the
purpose of their endeavors? Aren't they bound by the lofty ideals
of the scientific code of ethics, which demands that scientists
perform their work with honesty, objectivity, and integrity?

The Pure Science Myth

Even in our day and age, when information flows more freely
than ever before, many people still cling to a naïve view of
science and the way it is practiced. Science is still regarded by
many as trustworthy and objective, largely free of the internal
politics, power struggles, vested interests, fraud, and corruption
that plague other arenas. According to this view, which we call
"The Pure Science Myth", scientists are faithful professionals,
diligently toiling in the lab, exercising cold logic, objectivity, and
a well-developed sense of skepticism, all for the sake of providing a better future for humanity. Unlike most other
professionals, scientists are expected to put objective truth before
personal gain and self-interest, and if they ever fail to do so, they
are to be harshly condemned by their peers.

The Pure Science Myth is deeply embedded in our culture.
Elementary school children are told stories of the early days of
science and its champions – Marie and Pierre Curie, Louis
Pasteur, Alexander Fleming, and many others[15] – not to forget
Edward Jenner, inventor of the first vaccine.[a] These heroes, we
were taught, have laid the foundation for modern science, to

---

[a] The smallpox vaccine, invented in 1798.

which we owe our present-day prosperity. These seeds sown in early childhood are continuously nurtured by the formal bodies that govern and manage science. Thus, official publications of scientific institutions paint an idyllic picture of the scientific process, omitting any mention of internal politics, pursuit of self-interest, ego battles, financial motives, and the like, as if science were magically devoid of these harmful, yet ubiquitous, human realities.[16] The occasional corrupt scientist is depicted as an outlier, a "bad apple" who must be disciplined for science to maintain its hard-earned and well-deserved reputation.[17]

The discourse inside scientific circles, however, is rather different. Scientists themselves are well aware of the considerable gap, or even chasm, between the ideal and the way science actually works (described below).[18] Outwardly, however, to the general public, they maintain the rosy fiction. It can hardly be denied that, like any other institutional discipline, science is money-driven and significantly affected by greed, self-interest, and other human flaws.[b] Thus, it is not at all surprising that research institutions and individual scientists occasionally deviate from the scientific ideals of objectivity, collaboration, and the uncompromising search for truth. But outliers exist in every field of human activity, and as long as any institution's or individual scientist's dishonest behavior can be attributed to personal ambition or an absence of moral fiber, it should not tarnish the reputation of science as a whole. Unfortunately, the ethical challenge presently facing science isn't merely preventing and punishing scientific misconduct on the part of the occasional rogue scientist. The real problem in science goes much deeper and has broader implications. In fact, it is fundamental to the way in which modern science is conducted.

Scientific research costs huge amounts of money that mostly come from government and corporations. Without funding,

---

[b] A sample quote: "Science, I had come to learn, is as political, competitive, and fierce a career as you can find, full of the temptation to find easy paths." Paul Kalanithi, neurosurgeon and writer (see reference 18).

there can be no science. The National Institutes of Health (NIH) alone is responsible for the allocation of a yearly biomedical research budget of $32 billion.[19] This budget is spent on building labs, purchasing research equipment, and paying scientists' salaries. But medical research budgets, however large, are not unlimited. As such, the institutional (or business) entities in charge of allocating research budgets set their own criteria and priorities, which, of course, align with their agendas and interests.[20] Thus, as one might expect, research money is directed toward studies that are consistent with, or at least do not oppose or contradict, the policies of the funding body.

Again, there can be no scientific research without funding. Researchers cannot operate without grants that allow them to purchase appropriate equipment, hire research assistants, perform trials and tests, and so on. Any researcher, even one holding a permanent ("tenured") position in an academic institution, must keep raising money to continue working.[21] Professional reputation and institutional status are largely contingent on the ability to secure funding,[22] which makes researchers fully dependent on the research funding institutions. A scientist, however talented, cannot attain sustained scientific success without mastering the art of winning research grants. The powers that be must view the scientist's work favorably; thus research proposals must be consistent with the funding institution's policies. A research proposal that could threaten the sponsor's interests is very likely to be turned down.[23] A scientist whose current research challenges the interests or policies of the research funder is likely to find that the money source dries up. Thus, scientists soon learn it is in their own best interests to align their research proposals with their sponsors' expectations.[c] Failure to do so would result in the grant being awarded to a colleague who better anticipated the sponsor's intentions and adjusted the research proposal, and its expected results, accordingly.[24]

---

[c] This phenomenon was even given its own term: "funding bias".

Since they possess the power to decide how research budgets are allocated, funding institutions effectively control the path that science takes, each in its respective area of responsibility. Often, they do not even have to express their views and intentions explicitly. Scientists will do their utmost to identify which way the wind is blowing and adjust their research proposals accordingly.

One could argue, perhaps, that institutions funding medical research have no clear preferences or vested interests in many, or even most, research areas, in which case they would allocate their research budgets according to strictly professional and objective considerations. For all we know this might be true, but if there is one enterprise in which the medical establishment has a clear, decisive, and unequivocal agenda – it is to promote vaccination.

Establishment-Serving Vaccine Science

Vaccine research is funded almost entirely by government bodies and the pharmaceutical industry, both of which have very clear vested interests in the success of the vaccine program.[25] [d]

A vaccine manufacturer, like any commercial company, is primarily focused on making profit. Accordingly, it aims to sell as much of its product as it can, and for the highest possible price. News stories or scientific papers depicting vaccine products in a negative light could seriously hurt a company's image and sales. Additionally, a defective or harmful vaccine could mean heavy fines imposed by the government.[26] So it is hardly surprising that a vaccine manufacturer, as a business entity, has no interest in funding or publishing scientific research unfavorable to its products. Hence, the studies they fund will almost always present vaccines in a positive light. Studies with negative

---

[d] Another source of substantial funding is charitable organizations, most notably, Gavi, the Vaccine Alliance (formerly the Global Alliance for Vaccines and Immunizations), which is funded by Bill and Melinda Gates.

results are likely to never see the light of day.[27] Researchers employed by pharmaceutical companies, whether company employees or academics hired to perform a specific study, understand the rules of the game well and follow them obediently. A Washington Post article aptly describes the established norms of the field: "When the company is footing the bill, the opportunities for bias are manifold: Company executives seeking to promote their drugs can design research that makes their products look better. They can select like-minded academics to perform the work. And they can run the statistics in ways that make their own drugs look better than they are. If troubling signs about a drug arise, they can steer clear of further exploration."[28]

Health authorities, for their part, have their own vested interest in the vaccine program. They regard vaccines as one of the greatest achievements of public health, and medicine in general.[29] Unlike pharmaceutical drugs, medical devices and most medical treatments – all of which are marketed mainly by their manufacturers – the childhood vaccine program is promoted directly, and almost exclusively, by health authorities. In the US national vaccine recommendations and policies are issued by the CDC, and state legislatures carry them out. As they direct and promote the vaccine program, these authorities would be the first to be blamed for any harm caused by a childhood vaccine. It is small wonder, then, that health authorities are not eager to fund studies that could link approved and marketed vaccines to adverse events. Why would they? Criticism would undoubtedly be directed at them, as it should be. This self-preservationist tendency to avoid funding research critical of vaccination strengthened from the late 1990s onwards, as public debate on vaccine safety heated up once again.

Their strategy to shore up trust in the vaccine program, then, is to convince the public that "the science on vaccines is settled" and that laypeople should accept the "scientific consensus" of "vaccine experts". A spokesperson for the health establishment will patiently explain that the vaccine topic is extremely complex, and the average parent simply cannot make sense of it at all. Medical decisions should be based on expert advice, which in turn is firmly based in science.[30]

The truth of the matter, however, is that vaccine science isn't even remotely objective. The medical establishment conceals from a credulous public the grim reality that vaccine science is largely funded by interested parties which produce studies that advance the funder's agenda, not the public's.

This strategy capitalizes on the pervasiveness of The Pure Science Myth that the medical and scientific establishments have cultivated for many decades. This false narrative has been used for years to shore up the vaccine program's reputation and to advance vaccine manufacturers' profit margins. Thus, it serves those invested in the vaccine program well, as well as the scientific and medical professions in general, which enjoy generous funding and high public esteem. Most people are unaware that the institutions funding vaccine science are not objective, their motives are not pure, and the science they fund is neither impartial nor objective.

Institutionalized Research Falsification

Before we look at a representative sample of vaccine safety studies, let's do a short recap of the main points presented so far in this chapter.

The present surge of vaccine skepticism, which has been increasing since the late 1990s, requires the medical establishment to work harder to maintain the vaccine program's reputation. In response to claims from parents and advocacy groups, health authorities have commissioned dozens of studies, most of them epidemiological, intended to provide scientific evidence of vaccine safety. Health authorities, along with pharmaceutical companies, control most of the vaccine safety research budget. Thus, authorities and vaccine makers fund research projects which are likely to support their agenda. Most of their studies have been retrospective and observational, the easiest type of epidemiological study to manipulate. Since securing research funds is so fundamental to a scientist's career, there is never a shortage of researchers willing to adjust their results to align with the funding institution's agenda. Thus, even while exploiting science's longstanding reputation for integrity, authorities promote deceptive, manipulated research to a credulous public as decisive proof of vaccine safety.

For the most part, these contrived studies are tailored to address prevailing critical claims, such as "vaccines cause autism", or "the HPV vaccine may lead to autoimmune disease". The publication of these studies is typically accompanied by an orchestrated public relations campaign in the mainstream media to saturate the airwaves with the idea that "vaccines are [still] safe" and the criticism directed at them was found, once again, to be scientifically baseless. The orchestrators of this media campaign rightly assume that most parents will be either unable to access the original paper or will not bother to read it. The few who do read the paper will be unlikely to comprehend its scientific jargon or able to expose its flaws and biases.

Manipulated or falsified scientific research is, unfortunately, not uncommon. A review of studies that examined the issue found that almost 15% of scientists reported that their colleagues had falsified research results at least once. More than 70% reported that their peers had performed other dubious research activities. The review author also noted that, given the sensitivity of the issue, it is quite likely that the real numbers are higher than those reported.[31] Obviously, this data indicates this is not the aberrant behavior of a few "bad apples" and implies a systemic problem that is a direct result of the manner in which scientific research is funded and conducted.

There are two main techniques used to manipulate epidemiological research: manipulation of the raw data and/or manipulation of the statistical analysis of the raw data.

Epidemiologists can tailor their research data set to support their desired outcome in numerous ways. They can select a small group of subjects in advance whose data will yield the desired outcome; select a large group and exclude those subjects that do not fit the desired outcome; use partial or unverified data that fits the desired outcome; specifically select a group of subjects and claim they were randomly selected; fiddle with selection criteria to change group composition, and more.

The statistical analysis phase also allows a great deal of flexibility. Researchers can process and reprocess the set of data using a variety of statistical techniques, choosing the one that produces the desired outcome. In addition, they can deliberately make erroneous or inappropriate calculations and then omit them from the published paper. They can also opt to include only calculations which show favorable results and exclude others that yield less desirable results.

Five "Doctored" Vaccine Studies

Now let's look at five vaccine safety studies. We will analyze, among other things, the authors' conflicts of interest, study flaws, data manipulation techniques used, and how these studies were used to influence public opinion on vaccine safety. This small, yet representative, sample will demonstrate the deceptive way in which parties with vested interests use science to bolster vaccines' public image.

Madsen 2002: MMR Vaccine and Autism

Paper name: "A Population-Based Study of Measles, Mumps, and Rubella Vaccination and Autism"[32]

Journal and publication year: *New England Journal of Medicine*, 2002

Lead author: Kreesten Meldgaard Madsen

Type of study: Cohort retrospective observational study

Short description: a cohort study that examined the records of over half a million Danish children born between 1991 and 1998. The study compared the rate of autism between children vaccinated with the measles, mumps, and rubella vaccine (MMR) and those that were not vaccinated with the vaccine. The researchers found that the autism rate in both groups was almost identical, slightly lower, in fact, in the MMR group. The size of the study population and the fact that it included all Danish children born in the specified period led the authors to declare that "this study provides strong evidence against the hypothesis that MMR vaccination causes autism."[33]

Media and establishment response: The 2002 study by Madsen and colleagues is one of the most cited studies in the field of vaccine safety. The paper was published in a prestigious medical journal (*NEJM*) and received ample media attention.[34] It is referenced by many institutional webpages concerning the "debunked" link between vaccines and autism, including the websites of the CDC, the WHO, and the American Academy of Pediatrics (AAP).[35] The 2011 IOM report, discussed in chapter 2, names Madsen 2002 as one of only five vaccine–autism studies that met the quality threshold set by the committee.[36] Each of the aforementioned organizations maintain, echoing the authors, that the study presents "strong" evidence against the alleged link between vaccines and autism.

Conflicts of interest: At the time of publishing, seven of the eight authors were employees of the Danish Epidemiology Science Center research group, which has been awarded numerous generous CDC research grants since the year 2000. The group was headed by Danish researcher Poul Thorsen, who has been "wanted" since 2011 by the US Office of Inspector General. Thorsen, who is still a fugitive from justice,[e] was also a coauthor of the Madsen 2002 study. He was indicted for pocketing a substantial portion of the research budget allocated to the group by the CDC.[37] The Danish study group headed by Thorsen was highly productive, releasing a succession of epidemiological studies within a few short years whose findings were fully in line with the CDC's official stance that vaccines do not cause autism or other neurological syndromes.[38] The eighth author of the

---

[e] As of July 2020.

paper, Diana Schendel, was a CDC employee.[39]

The Madsen 2002 study was largely funded by a CDC grant.[40] At the time the CDC commissioned and funded the study, it was under intense public pressure due to parents' claims that vaccines caused their children's autism. The CDC categorically denied the link then, as it does today.[41] Despite its supposedly neutral position as a government institution, the CDC has an obvious bias when it comes to vaccines. It is hardly surprising that the federal agency responsible for the childhood vaccination program firmly and consistently denies any link between vaccines and autism, as well as any link to other neurological and chronic disorders. A CDC-funded study proving a link between vaccines and autism, or even merely suggesting one, would likely spell disaster for the organization, not to mention open a Pandora's box that could potentially obliterate the entire vaccine program.

Study flaws: The Madsen 2002 study demonstrates one of the methodological limitations of epidemiological research, namely its inability to provide conclusive results concerning rare phenomena. The IOM 2011 report alludes to this limitation, noting that "…studies [...] can fail to detect risks that affect a small subset of the population."[42] Although Madsen 2002 examined the health records of over half a million Danish children, the relevant group – children diagnosed with autism – was comprised of only 263 kids vaccinated with MMR and 53 that were not.[f] Given such a small group of relevant subjects, the results are extremely sensitive to any errors or biases in data collection. Though the records of 537,303 subjects were inspected, the MMR status had to be incorrect for as few as 15 autistic children, a meager 0.003% of the study population, for the study results to be completely reversed. The fact that the results were so sensi-

---

[f] For the sake of simplicity, the discussion above refers only to those children whom the researchers classified under the definition of "autistic disorder" and omits the group of children classified under "other autistic-spectrum disorders" (77 children not MMR-vaccinated and 345 MMR-vaccinated). The analysis in the text is valid for both groups.

tive to such a small number of errors is a serious limitation that the authors seemed to be aware of and (partially) tried to address.

Of the myriad bits of information collected on the study subjects, there were two critical details that had to be correct in light of the discussion above: (a) whether the child was diagnosed with autism and (b) whether the child had received the MMR vaccine. In order to verify subjects' autism classification, the researchers specifically examined a sample of the relevant registration files and concluded that they were reasonably accurate.[43] However, when it came to the second important detail – whether or not children had received the MMR – the researchers didn't do any additional verification of the data. The subjects' MMR vaccination status was taken from a national database that received notifications from family physicians after vaccinating children at their clinics.[44] Given the study question and context, underreporting of MMR vaccination would not be unreasonable. For example, a family doctor who vaccinated an infant with MMR at his clinic only to witness the child's severe reaction could have chosen not to report the vaccination to the national database out of practical or emotional reasons. If the child were later diagnosed with autism, the missing MMR vaccination record would put the child in the unvaccinated autistic group, rather than the vaccinated autistic group. Rather than verifying their data, Madsen and colleagues noted that they "assume that the data on MMR vaccination are almost complete, since general practitioners in Denmark are reimbursed only after reporting immunization data to the National Board of Health."[45] But in a study with such a small number of relevant subjects, where inaccuracies for only a handful of children would make such a dramatic difference, why didn't the researchers make the extra effort to verify the MMR vaccination status? And how could anyone say the results of the study provide "strong evidence" when they rely entirely on the authors' assumption that the relevant data was correct?

The questions regarding the researchers' objectivity, given

their conflicts of interest and negligent handling of vaccination data, become even more pronounced when considering the statistical methodology they used to obtain their results.

What stands out in the Madsen 2002 study, quite astoundingly, is that the raw data plainly contradict the study's conclusion. The Danish data, presented in Table 2 of the paper, actually show a 45% higher risk of autism in MMR-vaccinated children, compared to the non-MMR-vaccinated. Suspiciously, after the researchers manipulated the data, the trend was reversed to indicate an 8% lower risk of autism in the MMR-vaccinated children.[46] **To repeat, while the raw data imply a higher risk of autism among MMR-vaccinated children, the study's final results indicate the opposite.**

How did the Madsen 2002 authors end up with a slightly reduced autism risk in MMR-vaccinated children, when the raw numbers showed a substantially increased risk? The answer is "adjustments". The researchers statistically "adjusted", i.e. manipulated, the raw data based on children's characteristics such as age, gender, birth weight, and socioeconomic status.[47] What were the exact calculations applied in these statistical adjustments, and why were they needed? The authors provide no answers.

Omitting a detailed account of statistical "adjustments" from a published paper is not unusual in and of itself. Such details are rarely included in a published paper due to lack of space and readership interest. However, Madsen 2002 is different because the adjustments made to the raw data reversed the study outcome. Under such circumstances, it is appropriate, even imperative, for the authors to provide a reasoned and detailed explanation of their "adjustments" and to justify the reversal in their conclusion. But not only was no explanation provided, the authors also failed to mention that their adjustments reversed the conclusion that could be drawn from the raw data.

Summary: World-leading health organizations consider the 2002 Madsen study "strong" evidence of the absence of a link between the MMR and autism. The study was funded by the

CDC, a staunch denier of the vaccine–autism link, which is hardly surprising given its role as the US's primary vaccine marketer and defender. All authors save one, herself a CDC employee, belonged to a Danish research group that was established and heavily funded by the CDC and headed by a man who is now a fugitive wanted for fraud. Although the authors boasted that their study included more than half a million children, they did not bother to verify the single piece of information most crucial to the study's validity – the MMR vaccination status of the autistic kids. This raises serious questions concerning the accuracy of the data as well as the researchers' ethics. Even worse, it turns out that the study's raw data actually indicated an increased risk of autism for children who had received the MMR, but the researchers managed to reverse this undesired association by performing undisclosed statistical manipulations.

DeStefano 2013: Vaccine Antigens and Autism

Paper name: "Increasing Exposure to Antibody-Stimulating Proteins and Polysaccharides in Vaccines Is Not Associated with Risk of Autism"[48]

Journal and publication year: *The Journal of Pediatrics*, 2013
Lead author: Frank DeStefano
Type of study: Retrospective case-control study

Short description: A case-control study that compared the cumulative number of antigens in vaccines given to 256 autistic children with those received by 752 non-autistic children. The study found that the amount of vaccine antigens to which children were exposed in both groups was almost identical and concluded that increasing exposure to vaccine antigens was not associated with higher autism risk.[49]

DeStefano 2013 is a classic example of a vaccine safety "spin study", that is, a deliberately biased institutional study designed to provide a seemingly scientific answer to a popular vaccine criticism. In this instance, the argument, often brought up in vaccine online debates, was that infants receive too many vaccines and that their cumulative effect had never been properly studied. The paper's publication was accompanied by a media campaign. The news media reporting on the study, assisted by the lead author, went out of their way to imply that science had thoroughly examined the above argument and found it to be false.

Conflicts of interest: The study was funded by the CDC.[50] Two of the three authors were CDC employees. The lead author, Frank DeStefano, is a veteran employee and senior CDC manager who had previously published several vaccine safety studies, all of which, unsurprisingly, found that vaccines are indeed safe.[51] While working on this study, DeStefano headed the CDC Immunization Safety Office, and he still holds this position as of this writing.[52] Given that any scientific finding disputing the safety of vaccines would hit the CDC's Immunization Safety Office first, it is hard to think of a government official more likely to be conflicted with respect to vaccine safety than Frank DeStefano. If it ever became scientifically confirmed that vaccines did cause autism, public outrage, directed first and foremost towards the CDC and its Immunization Safety Office, would be enormous. But even though DeStefano and the agency he works for have the most to lose from studies criticizing vaccine safety, and even though both have been assuring the public for decades that "vaccines are safe", DeStefano disingenuously declares in the paper that he has "no conflicts of interest".[53]

Media and establishment response: As soon as it was published, DeStefano 2013 received widespread exposure in the US media. News stories that appeared simultaneously in various media outlets were all beating the same drum: The new CDC study unequivocally refutes the parental concern that too many vaccines may cause autism. For example, the headline of the story that appeared on the NBC website read: "New study finds no link between 'too many *vaccines*' and autism."[54] In the article, DeStefano himself was quoted as saying: "This study looked into the concern that receiving too many *vaccines* at one doctor's visit or too many *vaccines* during the first two years of life may be linked to the development of autism. We found they're not related." The article also noted that DeStefano expressed hope that the new study would convince parents that there are no safety issues with the CDC's vaccine program and they should vaccinate according to the official schedule. "The number of *vaccines* in the current immunization schedule is what's needed to protect children," he concluded. "It's not too many for a child's immune system."[55] (The emphasis on the word *vaccines* above does not appear in the original piece. See explanation below).

Similar stories appeared in other mainstream media websites such as *Forbes*, *TIME Magazine*, *National Public Radio* (*NPR*), *Medical News Today*, and *CBS*.[56] All of the articles repeated the message that the study found no link between the multitude of child vaccines and autism, and that it provided further proof that vaccines are safe. All expressed a similar expectation that the publication of this study would ease parents' concerns and lead them to resume vaccinating their children according to official recommendations. No outlet expressed any criticism of or even shred of doubt about the study, the vaccine program, or the CDC's vaccine policy. The conflicts of interest of the main author and the funding agency were never mentioned.

And, of course, there wasn't a single word about the awkward fact that the study didn't actually investigate the question the media claimed it had definitively answered: Could "too many vaccines" be causing autism?

Study flaws: The emphasis on the word *vaccines* in the above quotations from NBC is meant to highlight the deliberate deception perpetrated by the study authors and their media collaborators. The reality is that DeStefano 2013 did not explore whether "too many *vaccines*" could lead to autism, but rather the supposed effect of "multiple *antigens*" on the development of autism (and its results are meaningless anyway, as shall be explained later). The paper's title, as well as many other references in the text, explicitly states that it is the number of vaccine antigens that was examined,[g] not the number of vaccines.[57] The distinction between the two is important: The antigen, typically composed of fragments of bacteria or virus, is arguably the principal component of a vaccine, as it is the one that triggers an immune response intended to provide future protection from disease. However, the antigen is just one of numerous substances inside a vaccine vial. Vaccines typically contain a host of other ingredients that serve various functions, such as preservatives, stabilizers, adjuvants, and more. Some of these ingredients are known to be highly toxic (aluminum, mercury) or carcinogenic (formaldehyde). The adverse biological effects this conglomeration of biological and chemical ingredients could potentially have on an infant's body have never been studied in depth, not individually and not in combination.

Thus, parents' concerns do not focus specifically on the potential adverse effects of antigens, but rather on the full range of vaccine ingredients, including those known to be toxic or carcinogenic and those whose effect on an infant's body has not been sufficiently studied. They worry that the growing number of vaccines recommended by the CDC exposes infants to a medley of foreign substances that could harm them. The antigen is but one of these substances, and not necessarily the most harmful.[h] Although DeStefano and coauthors seem well aware of this – stating that "a recent survey found that parents' top vaccine-related concerns included administration of too many vaccines during the first 2 years of life"[58] – they nevertheless chose to investigate the association between the total amount of vaccine antigens and autism, rather than try to address the issue

---

[g] The authors alternatively use the terms "antigen" and "antibody-stimulating proteins and polysaccharides." In the specific context of the paper, these terms are interchangeable, as all refer to substances in vaccines that stimulate an immune system response.

[h] The total number of antigens in the vaccine schedule has never been a significant part of the public discourse, and DeStefano 2013 is the first study to address it. Paul Offit and colleagues, it seems, were the first to make cumulative antigen calculations in a 2002 paper.

that is really concerning parents: the potential consequences of too many childhood vaccines. Why didn't the authors address the link between the number of vaccines and autism and thus provide a direct response to the real parental concern? This question was never answered in the paper or in subsequent media interviews.

Putting aside the inappropriateness of the research topic chosen by government officials whose primary role is to oversee the safety of vaccines, an even more troubling aspect of DeStefano 2013 was the sly manner in which the media spun it. Though the link between vaccines and autism was never really explored by the researchers, the media, assisted by an eager DeStefano, was quick to oversell the study results as putting parental concerns to rest. As shown above, media headlines echoed the same counterfeit message, proclaiming that the study found "no link between the number of vaccines and autism." Moreover, DeStefano, who as lead author surely knew better than anyone what the study was really about, shamelessly repeated this false narrative in some of the news stories.

We have established, then, that DeStefano 2013 did not investigate, or even attempt to investigate, the question attributed to it by the media and its lead author. Instead of exploring the link between "too many" vaccines and autism, as publicly stated, it really looked into a potential link between the number of antigens and autism. But what did the study really examine and what did it actually "prove"?

The researchers propose the total number of antigens in vaccines as a measure of the overall level of immune system stimulation, or immune system response, triggered by vaccination.[59] The validity of this proposition requires evidence in its own right, but the paper presents none. Moreover, its lack of validity becomes apparent when we look at how the cumulative loads were calculated: The researchers multiplied the number of antigens in each vaccine dose by the number of doses each child received for each vaccine administered in the first two years of life. This simplistic and crude calculation, which seems to have been invented specifically for the purpose of this study, is based on the unfounded and highly improbable assumption that disease antigens in different vaccines evoke equivalent immune responses. For example, according to the paper, the DTP vaccine with its 3,000 antigens presumably evokes an immune response 3,000 times greater than that of the hepatitis B vaccine, which contains just a single antigen.[60]

In fact, the researchers are well aware that merely adding up the number of antigens in vaccines as a measure of immune response is nonsensical, and they point out some of its weaknesses, stating that "admittedly, this approach assumes that all [antigens] in a vaccine evoke equivalent immune responses," and "moreover, the calculations do not take into account the number of epitopes per antigen or the immunologic strength of each epitope."[61] Despite the improbability of their assumption and its lack of scientific support, the researchers note that they "think" that their method provides a good estimate of the antigenic load of vaccines and proceed to examine its supposed effect on autism development.[62]

Another glaring weakness of this "antigen counting" calculation, which the authors neglect to mention, is the role played by vaccine adjuvants. In some inactivated vaccines, the bacterial or viral materials that serve as antigens cannot, by themselves, elicit a sufficient immune response to prevent disease. In these vaccines, a substance called an "adjuvant" is usually added to the mix. The adjuvant stimulates the immune system so it responds to the antigen more intensely and for a longer period of time. Adjuvants can also be used to reduce the quantity of antigens required in some vaccines. Thus, the intensity of immune response to adjuvant-containing vaccines is largely dependent on the adjuvant used – its mode of action and its quantity – and less on the antigen itself. Therefore, in order to assess the strength of the immune response elicited by vaccines, whatever that actually means, one must include the adjuvant in the calculation in one way or another. Similarly, it is not unreasonable to assume that other vaccine ingredients may also affect the level of antigenic stimulation induced by the vaccine. Yet, despite the key role adjuvants play in the strength of immune response to vaccines, they are not even mentioned in the paper.

One might conclude, then, that the DeStefano 2013 study failed twice: Not only did it fail to investigate the real parental concern, the link between "too many vaccines" and autism, but also the question it did look into – vaccine antigenic load and its association with autism – was so simplistically and poorly studied its results are scientifically worthless.

One last point worth making regarding DeStefano 2013 is this: Even if we ignore the study's glaring flaws, what did it actually find? The difference in the number of vaccine antigens to which the study subjects were exposed is largely due to the fact that the diphtheria-tetanus-pertussis (DTP) whole-cell vaccine was replaced with the newer acellular vaccine (DTaP) during the study period.[63] The older whole-cell vaccine contained over 3,000 antigens per vaccine dose, while the newer acellular vaccine contains only 4-6 antigens per dose. [64] This is the main reason behind the large differences in the cumulative number of antigens to which study subjects were exposed, as all of them, it seems, were vaccinated with one of these two vaccines.[i] That is, if there were an insight to be gained from the study results (ignoring its salient flaws) it would be this: The risk for autism did not significantly change for children vaccinated according to the recommended schedule after the DTaP vaccine replaced its DTP predecessor. Naturally, since the study population was quite small, this conclusion must be taken with a grain of salt.[j]

---

[i] The researchers do not indicate otherwise. They also cite the typhoid vaccine as a factor in differing antigen exposure levels, but the effect of this vaccine is negligible as only four doses were given (in total) to study subjects (see Table 1 in the paper).

[j] In addition, DeStefano 2013 used the case-control study method. This method allows researchers to obtain the results they aim for by carefully selecting the control group. This technique will be discussed in detail in the analysis of the next study (Grimaldi 2014).

Summary: DeStefano 2013 is a classic example of a vaccine safety "spin study". It was never intended to advance scientific knowledge but rather to be a battering ram for vaccine proponents to counter a specific claim often made by parents questioning the safety of vaccines. The study supposedly answered the parental concern that the large number of vaccines their children were receiving might have a negative impact on their health, and, specifically, might lead to autism. Yet the study didn't investigate this hypothesis at all. Instead, the researchers chose to study the supposed effect of the total number of antigens in vaccines on autism development, using a dubious and scientifically baseless calculation. After reaching the desired result, the authors collaborated with the media to promote a false narrative to the public. Media news stories unanimously affirmed that DeStefano 2013 disproved the suggested link between "too many vaccines" and autism, though such a link was never even investigated.

The study was funded by the CDC and two of its three authors were CDC employees, including the lead author who was the head of the center's Immunization Safety Office. This raises serious questions as to the ethical conduct of the governmental agency entrusted with vaccine safety. It is equally concerning that such a glaringly flawed study hasn't drawn so much as a smidgen of criticism in medical and scientific circles.[65]

Grimaldi 2014: Gardasil and Autoimmune Injury

Paper name: "Autoimmune Disorders and Quadrivalent Human Papillomavirus Vaccination of Young Female Subjects"[66]

Journal and publication year: *Journal of Internal Medicine*, 2014

Lead author: Lamiae Grimaldi-Bensouda

Type of study: Retrospective case-control study

Short description: The study examined whether vaccination with the human papillomavirus (HPV) vaccine Gardasil is a risk factor for subsequent development of autoimmune diseases in girls and young women. The researchers compared the vaccination rate in a group of girls and young women with autoimmune diseases to the respective rate in a control group they selected. The rate of vaccination with Gardasil in both groups was similar, which led the researchers to conclude that the vaccine does not increase the risk of autoimmune diseases examined in the study.

Conflict of interest: A cursory glance at Grimaldi 2014 seems to indicate it is a standard academic study in the field of vaccines; most of its authors are either medical doctors or academics. However, the "Conflicts of interest" and "Funding" sections of the paper tell a different story. The study was funded by Sanofi Pasteur MSD,[67] a French company jointly owned by the pharmaceutical giants and vaccine manufacturers Sanofi Pasteur and Merck (known in Europe as MSD). The joint company is responsible for production and marketing of vaccines in Europe, including the Gardasil vaccine.[68] In addition to providing research funding, the company also paid the members of the scientific committee overseeing the study.[69] Furthermore, about half of the study authors had previously received grants and payments from numerous pharmaceutical companies, including the vaccine manufacturers Novartis, GSK, Merck, and Sanofi Pasteur.[70]

Such a long and varied list of conflicts of interest typically raises questions about the researchers' motives and their ability to be objective. However, in the case of Grimaldi 2014, the reality is even grimmer than usual. The paper's "fine print" reveals that the study was actually conducted by a private company called LA-SER, and that its lead researcher (Grimaldi-Bensouda) and two other researchers (Rossignol and Abenhaim) were company employees (Abenhaim is also the company's manager). LA-SER provides services and consulting to the pharmaceutical industry. Its website boasts that five of the world's eighth largest pharmaceutical companies are clients. The company specializes in pharmacoepidemiology, the epidemiology of pharmaceutical products, and one of the services it provides is "cutting edge outcomes research designed to demonstrate the benefit to patients that products and health technologies provide." In other words, the company sells epidemiological studies that make its clients' products look good. As part of the service it provides, the company handles all aspects of epidemiological research, from designing studies to writing them up and submitting them for publication.[71]

It turns out, then, that the seemingly innocent academic study exploring the link between Gardasil and autoimmune diseases was actually commissioned and sponsored by the vaccine's manufacturer and performed by a private company that specializes in delivering favorable epidemiological studies to its clients.

Media and establishment response: Unlike the previous two studies, Grimaldi 2014 did not receive much media attention. However, it did find its way into CDC publications. A weekly CDC report refers to the study as evidence of Gardasil's safety.[72] Another official document, a parent information leaflet recommending the vaccine published by the CDC and the American Academy of Pediatrics (AAP), also refers to Grimaldi 2014, among other studies.[73] Needless to say, these publications do not bother to mention that the study was ordered by the vaccine manufacturer and delivered by a private company that promises to make friendly pharma companies' products look better.

In addition to CDC publications, Grimaldi 2014 has been frequently cited in the medical literature since it was published. The paper is currently referenced by no less than 84 different medical publications.[74]

Study flaws: Grimaldi 2014 is a retrospective observational study of the case-control type. In a case-control study, the researchers select a "case" group that includes subjects with a specific medical condition (e.g., men in their 50s who have lung cancer or girls with autoimmune disease), and a control group made up of subjects without the condition. Every subject in the case group is matched with one or more subjects from the control group, who have similar personal characteristics (age, gender, place of residence, etc.). The researchers then check the exposure of both groups to the factor under investigation (such as cigarette smoke or Gardasil vaccination). If the data indicate that the case group was significantly more exposed to that particular factor than the control group, this adds weight to the assertion that the factor is indeed a cause of the relevant medical condition. Thus, if the case group of men in their 50s with lung cancer had a much higher exposure to cigarette smoke than the healthy control group, this would indicate that cigarette smoke could well be a cause of lung cancer.

The obvious weakness of a retrospective case-control study is that it is fairly easy to skew its results by deliberately selecting control group members. For example, if the researchers wish to conclude that Gardasil does not lead to autoimmune disease, they can simply assign a high proportion of vaccinated women with no such disease to the control group. In this way, the condition investigated (autoimmune disease) would appear to not be affected by the factor considered (vaccination with Gardasil), as both case and control groups are highly vaccinated, though they differ in their autoimmune disease status. Such a research maneuver is not difficult to accomplish since a case-control study's control group typically includes no more than a few hundred subjects usually drawn from a repository of tens or hundreds of thousands of individuals.[k] Because the researchers had full access to the data on the group with autoimmune diseases (the cases), they already knew the group's Gardasil vaccination rate. Hence, they could easily have assembled a control group with a vaccination rate that matched or surpassed this number, while publicly declaring they had made a random selection.

Evidently, a case-control study is particularly prone to selection bias. By carefully selecting case and control groups, one can quite easily control the study's outcome. But did the researchers do that for Grimaldi 2014? Can we find evidence of a deliberate-

---

[k] In the Grimaldi 2014 study, the control group included only 850 subjects. In the DeStefano 2013 study, the control group included 752 subjects.

ly biased selection of subjects in their paper?

Data for both cases and controls in Grimaldi 2014 were obtained from a private medical database owned by the same company that conducted the study (LA-SER).[75] The case group consisted of girls and young women with autoimmune disease, and for each case four female subjects with similar characteristics (age, place of residence, etc.) were allocated to the control group. That is, the control group subjects were also selected from the same medical repository as the cases, one that is not necessarily representative of the entire population. According to the researchers, the controls were selected randomly. However, we have only their word as proof, as research conduct in general, and specifically for this study, is not supervised by any official body. In addition, the Gardasil vaccination status of study subjects – most of them, at least – was available to the researchers.[76]

Because the case group consisted of subjects with autoimmune diseases, the control group should have been made up of healthy subjects, or, at least, those who did not have autoimmune disease. Then, according to the case-control study methodology, the Gardasil vaccination rate of both groups should have been compared in order to determine whether the data supported the hypothesis that Gardasil vaccination was a risk factor for autoimmune disease. However, Grimaldi 2014 did not follow the standard case-control study design. Instead, the controls the researchers selected for each case were acceptable as long as they did not suffer from the same autoimmune disease as their matching case.[77] For example, a (case) girl with lupus could have been matched with four (control) girls with any other autoimmune disease but lupus (such as type 1 diabetes, for instance). This is comparable to doing a case-control study that explores the association between smoking and cancer by comparing a case group consisting of patients with lung, laryngeal, or pancreatic cancer (smoking is a risk factor for all three) with controls who could have any of these three diseases as long as it isn't the same as their matching case. Naturally, such a study would not find a significant difference in the percentage of smokers between the two groups and could thus conclude that smoking isn't a risk factor for cancer.

The $64,000 question, then, is what was the health profile of Grimaldi 2014's control group subjects? Were they a group of generally healthy girls and young women, as appropriate for this particular study, or was this group selected precisely because of its high incidence of autoimmune disease? One cannot find a straightforward answer to this essential question in the paper, since the researchers, oddly enough, do not tell us how many control subjects suffered from autoimmune disease.[1] However, the paper's Table 1 reveals valuable clues for solving the mystery:[78] (a) It is noted that 72.5% of cases took seven or more medications during the two years preceding the diagnosis of their disease. This figure seems reasonable for girls suffering from medical conditions later diagnosed as autoimmune disease. Surprisingly, an almost identical rate of 72.9% of control group subjects were taking seven or more medications in the same time frame. (b) About 15% of controls had "at least one chronic comorbidity." The notes for the table list these comorbidities as diabetes, Crohn's disease, ulcerative colitis, cancer, epilepsy, multiple sclerosis, and more. The comorbidity rate in the control group was even higher than the case group's 12.6%. Moreover, the exact meaning and significance of the phrase "at least one chronic comorbidity" is difficult to decipher. We know that study cases were selected because they had autoimmune disease, so 12% of them having another chronic disease seems plausible. But what does "chronic comorbidity" mean for controls? This vague wording seems to mean that the control group subjects were just as sick with autoimmune disease as their case counterparts, in addition to having slightly more frequent comorbidities.

The glaring omission of essential information about autoimmune conditions in control group subjects, as well as the clues

---

[1] The authors dedicate a full page(!) to listing all the physicians who assisted in data collection for the company's database (Grimaldi 2014, p. 10) but much less space to the study subjects' relevant medical data.

indicating that the controls were quite sick, make it appear as if the researchers purposely biased their control selections. The trick, it seems, was to assign controls who were at least as sick as their matching cases, just with different diseases. If that's the case, considering that the Gardasil vaccination rate was slightly higher in the control group, it seems that the study's raw data indicate that Gardasil probably is a risk factor for autoimmune disease. But the authors, delivering on their employer's promise to make customers' products look good, masterfully buried this result under heaping piles of deceptive statistics.

Summary: Grimaldi 2014 is a vaccine safety study commissioned and sponsored by the vaccine's manufacturer and marketer and conducted by a private company that specializes in delivering studies that underscore the benefits of customer products. In light of the above, it is likely that the study outcome was agreed upon by the parties before work began, as both shared a common business interest to present Gardasil in a positive light. The researchers chose a convenient case-control design, which facilitates manipulation of the outcome by careful selection of controls. In the case of Grimaldi 2014, the researchers seem to have selected a control group as ill as the case group, or even slightly sicker. It's no wonder that the Gardasil vaccination rate was similar in both groups.

To be sure, neither company's conduct deviates from standard business practices and norms: One company pays for a service, and the other provides it. However, this method of operation is not, and should not be, considered ethical in the realm of medical research. A private company manufacturing tainted scientific research promoting its customers' medical products does not advance scientific knowledge, but in fact hinders it. That a "cooked" study such as this one was published by a respected medical journal and is widely cited in the scientific literature, as well as in publications of leading health agencies, is deeply disturbing. This signifies an acute failure in the way medical science, and vaccine science in particular, is managed, conducted, and publicized.

McKeever 2004: Vaccines and Allergic Disease

Paper name: "Vaccination and Allergic Disease: A Birth Cohort Study"[79]

Journal and publication year: *American Journal of Public Health*, 2004

Lead author: Tricia M. McKeever

Type of study: Retrospective observational cohort study

Short description: McKeever 2004 examined the association between the administration of DPPT[m] and MMR vaccines and the development of asthma and eczema in British children. The researchers examined the records of nearly 30,000 children between 1988 and 1999 and found that children vaccinated with DPPT were 14 times more likely to be diagnosed with asthma and 9 times more likely to be diagnosed with eczema than children who had not received that specific vaccine. Children vaccinated with MMR were 3.5 times more likely to be diagnosed with asthma and 4.5 times more likely to be diagnosed with eczema than children who were not MMR-vaccinated. The researchers dismissed these findings, however, on the pretext that "this association was present only among children with the fewest physician visits and can be explained by this factor" and concluded that "our data suggest that currently recommended routine vaccinations are not a risk factor for asthma or eczema."[80]

Conflicts of interest: Cannot be determined since the paper does not contain "Conflicts of Interest" or "Funding" sections.[81]

Media and establishment response: The study did not receive any media coverage and does not seem to be referenced by publications of official health bodies. This is not surprising, given the high correlations between vaccines and allergic disease that the study revealed.

Study flaws: In the paper's first paragraph, the authors describe their motive for conducting this specific study: "An

---

[m] DPPT is a vaccine for diphtheria, pertussis, polio, and tetanus.

unexplained increase in the prevalence of allergic disease has occurred in the developed world in the past few decades. During the same period, there has been an increase in mass immunization, leading to the hypothesis that certain vaccines may increase the risk of allergic disease."[82] And what is the authors' position on this hypothesis? Are they willing to objectively examine the data, or are they prejudiced in favor of some preexisting outcome? One need only read to the end of the paragraph to find the answer. The association between vaccines and allergies must be studied, the authors write, "because a perception that vaccination is harmful may have an adverse impact on the effectiveness of immunization programs."[83] This sentence reveals that an outcome linking vaccines to allergic disease would be unwelcome to the authors, since it would negatively affect public support for vaccination. Is this predisposition the reason behind the authors outright dismissal of the strong correlation found in the study between the two vaccines and asthma and eczema morbidity?

As mentioned above, children who were vaccinated with MMR or DPPT vaccines were diagnosed with asthma and eczema at rates 3.5 to 14 times higher than children who were not vaccinated with these vaccines. This unequivocal finding should have led the researchers to conclude that the data strongly suggest a link between vaccines and allergies. Instead, they explain away this link, claiming it does not really exist but is rather an artifact of bias in the data. The statistical correlation, they say, was particularly strong for children, vaccinated and unvaccinated, who visited their family doctor no more than three times in the first six months of life. That correlation was much lower for children who had visited their doctor more often as infants. Children who rarely see a family physician tend to be less vaccinated, the researchers explain, and are less likely to be diagnosed by their doctor as suffering from eczema or asthma.[84] In other words, the authors suggest that the low rate of allergic disease in children who were not vaccinated is not genuine. These children, they imply, suffer from asthma and eczema as often as vaccinated children, but, because they visit their family doctor less often, most of them are not formally diagnosed.

McKeever and colleagues' offhand dismissal of the robust correlations found in their study is most puzzling. First, if unvaccinated children who visit their family doctor less often have a significantly reduced chance of being diagnosed with allergies, why are vaccinated children who also visit their doctor less often diagnosed at a rate many times higher?

Second, the researchers assume a causal relationship between the number of visits to the doctor and the rate of diagnosis: The less a child visits the doctor, the less likely they are to receive a diagnosis of allergy. However, this arbitrary assumption, for which the paper presents no supporting evidence, seems to reverse the direction of the causal arrow: Common sense would suggest that children need fewer doctor visits... when they are healthy. Indeed, the causal relationship on which the authors base their argument could be turned on its head: Children with fewer allergies tend to see their doctor less often.

Third, is it reasonable to assume, as the researchers do, that children who were struggling to breathe or covered in oozing rashes would not be taken to a doctor? How were these kids treated for their condition without a doctor's diagnosis? Or do the authors suggest that they were left untreated? (Keep in mind that all the children in the study visited their family doctor at least once during the first three months of life).[85]

None of these issues are addressed in McKeever 2004, which further underscores the arbitrariness of the authors' utter dismissal of their own findings. In fact, the authors do not provide any additional information – data, evidence, or scientific reference – to substantiate their claim that the strong statistical correlations between vaccination and allergic disease is artificial and can legitimately be explained away as a data anomaly.

The researchers' bias toward a finding of no association between vaccines and allergy is also reflected in the "Discussion" section of the paper, where they review previous studies on the topic (and manage to upset two researchers whose findings they misrepresented).[86] Although they cite a number of studies that found a correlation between vaccines and allergies (along with some that did not), and although their own raw data provide strong support for this correlation, they bizarrely conclude with an emphatic and unequivocal denial of this link, stating that "current vaccination practices do not have an adverse effect on the incidence of allergic disease."[87]

Summary: The McKeever 2004 study demonstrates how researchers whose work could potentially provide valuable clues to advance understanding of serious and unexplained medical conditions – the soaring allergy rate, in this case – are quick to dismiss obvious conclusions if they are harmful to vaccines' reputation. According to The Pure Science Myth, scientists examine data with absolute objectivity, not allowing their preconceptions to influence their work. In stark contrast to this ideal, McKeever 2004 affirm their commitment to preserving the public image of the vaccine program in advance, and then proceed to arbitrarily dismiss findings which indicate strong correlations between the studied vaccines and allergies.

This study's main contribution to science, then, is that it demonstrates the staggering ease with which findings that are unfavorable to vaccine dogma can be discarded. It seems that scientists who opt to contravene the fundamental principles of science and blatantly distort the conclusions of their own research will not face any adverse professional consequences, provided that their actions, scientifically unethical as they may be, lend support to the vaccination program.

Fombonne 2006: MMR Vaccine and Autism

Paper name: "Pervasive Developmental Disorders in Montreal, Quebec, Canada: Prevalence and Links with Immunizations"[88]
Journal and publication year: *Pediatrics*, 2006
Lead author: Eric Fombonne
Type of study: Ecological retrospective observational study
Short description: Fombonne and colleagues examined medi-

cal data of children, born between 1987 and 1998, who attended English-speaking schools in Montreal, Canada.[n] The researchers compared the children's yearly rate of autism to the MMR vaccine coverage rate and found that while the rate of autism was on the rise during the research period, the rate of MMR vaccination was trending slightly downwards. This led the researchers to conclude that the MMR vaccine is not a risk factor for autism.[o]

Conflicts of interest: Eric Fombonne, the lead researcher, conducted a series of studies on autism and vaccines starting in the late 1990s, all of which provided support for the institutional stance that vaccines do not cause autism.[89] Fombonne provided paid counseling to vaccine manufacturers and also appeared on their behalf as an expert witness in the Vaccine Injury Compensation Program, part of the US Court of Federal Claims ("Vaccine Court").[90]

Like the authors of McKeever 2004, the authors of Fombonne 2006 do not conceal their firm support of the vaccination program. In the discussion section of the paper they dispense with any semblance of objectivity, stating that "children with autism and their younger unaffected siblings should be vaccinated. Unvaccinated children are at much higher risk of contracting measles and suffering from its sometimes severe or lethal complications."[91]

Media and establishment response: The study was published in 2006 and was covered by news and medical websites, as well as the websites of various health organizations.[92] Lead author Fombonne was interviewed for some of the news stories and issued statements that sweepingly denied any link between vaccines and autism, such as "our study once again rules out MMR as a cause for autism,"[93] and "we hope this study will

---

[n] Most of Montreal's population speaks French.

[o] The Fombonne 2006 study also examined the correlation between the rate of autism and thimerosal (mercury) in vaccines. Although there are serious flaws in that part of the paper as well, this chapter does not deal with them for space considerations.

finally put to rest the pervasive belief linking vaccines with developmental diseases like autism."[94]

In addition, the study is frequently cited in the scientific literature – 243 references by medical publications as of the time of writing.[95] Interestingly, one of the references is in a review authored by none other than Frank DeStefano, head of the CDC's Immunization Safety Office.[96] The IOM 2013 report, which we will review in the next chapter, also mentions Fombonne 2006, stating that it is one of only four studies that might help to better understand the link between vaccines and autism. The authors of the report note that, while it is an ecological study, "the data was interpreted carefully".[97] However, the earlier IOM 2011 report, reviewed in chapter 2, actually dismissed Fombonne 2006 on the grounds that it was an ecological study "lacking individual-level data".[98]

Study flaws: Fombonne 2006 contains so many faults, it would take at least a full book chapter to detail them all. Hence, the analysis below will focus on the most prominent and outrageous of them all: Fombonne and his co-authors made a severe methodological error and appear to have deliberately misrepresented the source of their data. In order to fully comprehend the statistical error, we will first examine a hypothetical epidemiological study:

Due to concerns raised by the public, American researchers investigated the association between smoking and lung cancer. They decided to examine the rates of smoking and lung cancer among the employees of a restaurant chain in the city of Philadelphia because relevant information for this chain was available and fitting for an epidemiological inquiry. The researchers found that the rate of lung cancer in the restaurant workers increased consistently and significantly between the years 1987–1998 and wanted to determine whether the rate of smoking also increased in parallel. To this end, they examined data from statewide smoking surveys conducted by the Pennsylvania Department of Health. These surveys indicated that, during the period in question, the smoking rate among Pennsylvania residents actually decreased slightly. In other words, while the rate of lung cancer among the employees of the restaurant chain in Philadelphia rose steadily during the period under review, the percentage of smokers in all of Pennsylvania actually decreased slightly. After analyzing their data, the researchers concluded that smoking does not cause lung cancer.

This conclusion may seem reasonable, but it isn't really.

The percentage of smokers among employees of the Philadelphia restaurant chain has but a loose connection, if any, to the percentage of smokers in the entire state. This rate could have gone up or down or remained constant during the period under review, regardless of the statewide rate. In order for the study to have any scientific validity, the researchers obviously had to compare the percentage of smokers among the employees of that restaurant chain in Philadelphia with the occurrence of lung cancer in the exact same group of people.[p]

Strange as it may seem, the invalid research method described above is exactly the one used in the Fombonne 2006 study. Fombonne and coworkers found that the number of autistic children in the English-speaking school district in Montreal (1987-1998)[q] consistently increased over time. This data was compared to the MMR vaccination rate – not among the autistic children they were actually studying, nor among the children registered in the English school district, and not even among the children of the entire city of Montreal. According to the paper, the autism rate in the English-speaking schools of Montreal was compared to the MMR vaccination rate of children residing in the Canadian province of Quebec (where Montreal is located).[99] But as in the hypothetical Philadelphia, so in real-life Montreal: It makes no sense to assume that the vaccination rate

---

[p] We assume, for the purpose of the hypothetical example discussed, that smoking may cause lung cancer in the short term, so that an increase in the number of smokers will be manifested within a few months in an increase in the rate of lung cancer patients.

[q] The study found 180 autistic children in total, only about 15 children per age cohort.

obtained from a survey of the entire child population of Quebec province[r] is identical to the vaccination rate of children attending English-speaking schools in Montreal. The vaccination rate in these schools could rise or fall during the period under review, remain constant, or change according to some obscure pattern, regardless of the provincial rate. Why, then, would the researchers use an irrelevant vaccination rate, instead of obtaining the true MMR vaccination rate of the study subjects?

If this seems all too strange, well, take a deep breath. This weird story of research misconduct gets even more bizarre.

Despite the researchers' claim that they compared the rate of autism in children of English-speaking schools in Montreal to the rate of MMR vaccination in the province of Quebec, a year after the study was published the real source for the MMR vaccination data was revealed. It was not obtained from surveys of the Quebec province, as stated in the paper, but from Quebec City, its capital.

The data's misattribution was discovered by an independent vaccine researcher named F. Edward Yazbak, a retired American pediatrician and grandfather of an autistic child. Dr. Yazbak contacted health authorities in Quebec and submitted questions pertaining to the vaccination rates quoted in the Fombonne 2006 study. The response delivered by the Quebec Public Health Department was authored by the same official who provided the vaccination data to Fombonne and colleagues.[100] The letter confirmed Yazbak's suspicion that the MMR vaccination data on which the paper was based came from Quebec City, not the province of Quebec.[101] The discovery made by Yazbak, that Fombonne 2006 compared the rate of autism in a school district in one city (Montreal) to the MMR vaccination rate in a different city (Quebec City), emphasizes even further the absurdity of the researchers' statistical calculations. In terms of the hypothet-

---

[r] According to the paper, the MMR vaccination rate in the province of Quebec is based on an annual government survey of five-year-old children (Fombonne 2006, p. 4).

ical study mentioned earlier, this is equivalent to comparing the rate of lung cancer in the employees of the Philadelphia restaurant chain with the rate of smoking among residents of Harrisburg, the capital of Pennsylvania.

Upon receiving the formal response of the Quebec health authorities, Yazbak wrote a letter to *Pediatrics*, the medical journal that published the Fombonne 2006 study. In the letter he detailed the information in his possession which indicated the paper contained a serious error or perhaps even a deliberate misrepresentation. A copy of the letter was forwarded to Fombonne, who declined to address the accusation. Although its lead author did not bother to explain the glaring contradiction between the data source cited in the paper and the actual source, Gerald Lucy, editor of *Pediatrics*, refused to publish Yazbak's letter. In his reply to Yazbak, Lucy said, "I believe the evidence of no link between MMR and Autism is sufficient. It's not worth publishing more on this subject. We will not be publishing this exchange of correspondence."[102] Yazbak's letter was never published in *Pediatrics* or any other medical journal.

Another important insight to be gained from Fombonne 2006 concerns the relative validity of the results of ecological epidemiological studies which analyze populations. Let us suppose that the Fombonne 2006 study was conducted faithfully and correctly, that is, it compared the rate of autism in the Montreal English-speaking school district with the MMR vaccination rate of the same population. Suppose, moreover, that the rate of autism among the children of the study population increased during the study period, while MMR uptake decreased slightly, leading the researchers to emphatically conclude that the MMR vaccine does not cause autism. Would the researchers' conclusion be reasonable? Can a study of this type justify such a decisive conclusion?

The answer to both questions is "no". Epidemiological studies, especially those looking at the population level, cannot confirm or disprove a causal link, and therefore, the strength of their results is relatively low. This becomes clear when we consider the vaccination status of the 180 autistic children who were the focus of Fombonne 2006. The researchers, oddly enough, made no effort to determine whether these children received the MMR or not, even though they had a complete list of their names[103] and they reported extensively on other personal characteristics. They devote just a single sentence of nine words to this crucial statistic: "Individual immunization data were not available for study subjects."[104] Was that really true, or did they look at the vaccination data for these children and choose not to publish it? Did the researchers prefer not to include the MMR vaccination status of those 180 autistic children because it would "mess-up" their predetermined study outcome? If, for example, vaccination data for the study's autistic children revealed that MMR uptake for this particular group of children was actually rising throughout the period, that would obviously have reversed the results of the study.

Similarly, let us suppose that the researchers interviewed the parents of those 180 autistic children and found that, say, 80% of them had a marked developmental regression following MMR vaccination. Conducting such interviews would yield more robust and convincing evidence of a link between MMR and autism than a population-level correlation discovered through an ecological epidemiological study. However, no information regarding autistic developmental regression following MMR was collected by the researchers.[105] Instead, they went all the way to Quebec City, 235 miles from Montreal, to obtain MMR data for that city's children and used it to provide bogus support for the assertion that MMR does not cause autism.

Summary: It requires a considerable stretch of the imagination to consider the work of Fombonne and his coauthors "science". It is even more difficult to accept that the study was peer-reviewed and published in a leading medical journal and that its scientific record, and the reputations of its authors, remain unblemished to this day. It is highly disturbing that the editor who published the study ignored evidence of malfeasance and chose to protect the study and its authors as well as the reputation of his own journal. All of the above stand in stark contrast to the ethos of science, which places scientific truth above personal, commercial, and even government interests.

The Fombonne 2006 study provides a striking example of the informal rule of vaccine safety research: No matter how contorted or fallacious a study may be, it will receive full support from the medical establishment as long as it supports the vaccine safety dogma.

Medical Journals and Peer Review

The first part of this chapter described the marked contrast between the scientific ideal and real-life science. Scientific research is expensive, and budgets are not inexhaustible. Therefore, researchers, whose livelihoods and professional status depend to a large extent on research grants, are forced to align their research proposals with the agenda of their funding bodies, typically government agencies or pharmaceutical companies. The result of this reality is evident in the sample of vaccine safety studies reviewed above – deeply flawed, misleading science that serves the vested interests of funders instead of the truth.

It is important to remember, however, that securing funding and conducting research is not the end of the line for scientists. They still need to publish their work in medical journals, and the more prestigious the journal, the better. According to The Pure Science Myth, medical journals apply a rigorous screening and review process that ensures the quality of the studies they publish. A study that passes this high editorial bar and is published by a legitimate medical journal is thus awarded a stamp of approval that attests to its adherence to science's methodological standards and ethical guidelines.

The obvious question, then, is how did this quintet of purposely flawed studies ever make it through that rigorous screening process? Why and how did prestigious journals such as *NEJM* and *Pediatrics* print studies with such glaring faults? Why would leading medical journals put their hard-earned reputations at risk by publishing flawed research? And yet another question: For the flawed studies that somehow slipped through and got published, where was the critical post-publishing academic discourse that was supposed to expose their shortcomings, correct their mistakes, and demand answers from their authors?

Contrary to The Pure Science Myth and the impression deliberately cultivated by the scientific establishment, medical journals are quite limited in their ability to ensure the quality of scientific papers submitted for publication. The main tool, or process, that journals use for this purpose is called *peer review*. According to this process, which varies slightly from journal to journal, a candidate paper is evaluated by a handful of professionals who specialize in the same research area as the study. These reviewers read the paper, rate its quality, and if the need arises, raise issues requiring correction or clarification. To maximize objectivity, reviewers' identities are kept secret so that study authors cannot contact them or try to otherwise influence their evaluation.[s]

In theory, this gentlemanly arrangement may seem like an effective way to assure the quality of scientific papers. In practice, however, it is an unreliable process and its capacity to deliver on its promise is dubious at best. In fact, according to a review of the relevant published research on the topic, the scientific validity of the peer review process itself has never been established.[106] Richard Smith, a former editor of the *British Medical Journal (BMJ)*, conducted his own small experiment to test the quality of his journal's peer-review process: "At the BMJ," he writes, "we did several studies where we inserted major errors into papers that we then sent to many reviewers. Nobody ever spotted all of the errors. Some reviewers did not spot any, and most reviewers spotted only about a quarter."[107]

---

[s] Some journals go even further in their quest to avoid bias and hide the names of the study authors from the reviewers as well.

The mediocre quality of reviewers' work should not be surprising considering the conditions under which it is done. Peer review places a considerable burden on reviewers, as it is typically performed on top of their regular work. Furthermore, as the vast majority of medical journals do not pay for peer review,[108] reviewers are rarely compensated for their time and effort. In addition, the task must be completed within a relatively short period of time so as not to delay the paper's publication. But the biggest difficulty reviewers face in detecting errors is the fact that submitted papers rarely contain all the relevant data or the full details behind their calculations. Thus, reviewers cannot verify the quality of the data, the accuracy of the calculations, nor the calculations' appropriateness or rectitude.

This problem becomes even more acute when dealing with purposely biased research. In these studies, researchers typically make an effort to conceal the study's faults by presenting partial or vague information (recall the omitted autoimmune disease statistics for the control group in Grimaldi 2014 and the crucial statistical calculations missing from Madsen 2002). Thus, the authors minimize the likelihood that reviewers will uncover the study's intentional errors. "Peer review sometimes picks up fraud by chance," remarks Richard Smith, "but generally it is not a reliable method for detecting fraud because it works on trust."[109]

In fact, given the dynamics of the current peer-review process, even if reviewers had full access to study data their bias detection yield would not significantly improve. In order to identify all, or most, of a study's errors, reviewers must carefully inspect the data and repeat the calculations performed. They essentially need to repeat large chunks of the work originally performed by the study authors. Obviously, given their time constraints and the fact that they are not financially compensated, this is not even remotely feasible for most reviewers. Richard Smith notes that *BMJ* editors have tried once or twice to review the raw data of a study only to find the task "difficult, expensive, and time consuming."[110]

The peer-review process has many other disadvantages, as

Smith aptly notes: "In addition to being poor at detecting gross defects and almost useless for detecting fraud, it is slow, expensive, profligate of academic time, highly subjective, something of a lottery, prone to bias, and easily abused."[111]

Unfortunately, peer review, the prepublication process implemented by medical journals for assuring the quality of published papers, does not live up to its reputation as an effective barrier to bad science. So what happens when flawed or fraudulent studies manage to sneak their way through the cracks? Does science provide a mechanism to retroactively identify and rectify bad published research? Is there any collective body of scientists out there, as The Pure Science Myth tells us, which keeps probing published research, weeding out studies that fail to meet the scientific standard?

Here, too, the answer is "no".

John Ioannidis, a renowned researcher at Stanford University who specializes in analyzing the scientific method, explains that scientists have no motivation to critically examine the work of their peers: "There's no incentive for scientists or other stakeholders to make a very thorough and critical review of a study, to try to reproduce it, or to probe systematically and spend real effort on re-analysis. We need to find ways people would be rewarded for this type of reproducibility or bias checks."[112] One might add, on top of Ioannidis's pointed remarks, researchers typically have even less incentive to perform "a very thorough and critical review" of a vaccine safety study. Publicly challenging institutional vaccination policies could severely impair their chances of receiving future research grants and would likely provoke harsh criticism from supervisors and peers.

Those scientists who, nevertheless, wish to review their peers' work thoroughly usually face another obstacle: obtaining the raw data for the study. There is no law or regulation compelling researchers to provide the original data they used to other researchers. Moreover, the data used to generate medical research in general, and epidemiological research of vaccines in particular, is usually stored in medical or other institutional computer systems owned by public bodies or health sector corporations. These entities lawfully reserve the right to restrict access to their data for reasons of medical confidentiality or private property. Thus, they can limit at will the reevaluation of questionable studies that make use of data they own and whose outcomes support their agenda.

Editors of medical journals, as well, have limited motivation to encourage critical discourse of studies they published. According to The Pure Science Myth, one of their primary roles is to serve as guardians of scientific truth, including, of course, the research published under the auspices of their own journal. Correcting bad published research is good for science, the Myth asserts, and beneficial to the reputation of the journal as well. In practice, however, encouraging criticism of your own published research is a double-edged sword. Too much of it could seriously, and possibly irrevocably, damage a medical journal's reputation.

It is also important to remember that medical journals are an integral part of the medical-academic world. They maintain close working relationships with pharmaceutical companies, researchers and academics, and official health bodies. Because this world is united by its unreserved support for vaccines, journal editors have nothing to gain by swimming against the current, even if that means tolerating the occasional breach of scientific ethics.[t] Just as researchers and doctors who produce purposely biased vaccine safety research are not chastised or even reprimanded, medical journals rarely, if ever, pay any price for the publication of these studies.

Counter Arguments

"Researchers would not risk their careers by intentionally publishing incorrect or biased research." – Indeed, according to The Pure Science Myth, the scientific–academic system punishes

---

[t] A typical example, mentioned earlier in the chapter, is the refusal of the editor of *Pediatrics* to publish the criticism of the Fombonne 2006 study.

scholars who do not follow its ethical standards. In practice, however, one in seven researchers reports having witnessed research results falsified by peers, and over 70% report that their colleagues have performed other questionable research activities.[113] Moreover, as evident from the studies analyzed in this chapter, vaccine safety researchers in particular seem to enjoy unlimited freedom to skew, and even blatantly ignore, standard scientific methodology, as long as they arrive at the "correct" conclusion. This unethical conduct perfectly aligns with the vested interests of the corporations and government institutions that fund vaccine safety research. As long as researchers conform to the agenda of the vaccine establishment, they are protected by the system and their livelihoods and professional reputations remain unscathed. The events that followed the publication of the Fombonne 2006 study illustrate this point well.

"Vaccine safety studies have been published in leading journals and were peer-reviewed. They are unlikely to contain errors, and they are certainly not biased." – As explained in this chapter and acknowledged by the former editor of one of the most prestigious medical journals in the world, the peer-review process is not fulfilling its intended purpose of filtering out erroneous or falsified research. Hence, publication in a medical journal is not a reliable indicator of study quality or veracity. In the words of Richard Smith, former editor of the *British Medical Journal*: "We have little evidence on the effectiveness of peer review, but we have considerable evidence on its defects. In addition to being poor at detecting gross defects and almost useless for detecting fraud, it is slow, expensive, profligate of academic time, highly subjective, something of a lottery, prone to bias, and easily abused."[114]

"The chapter analyzed only a handful of studies. There are many other studies that have ruled out the link between vaccines and various adverse events." – An entire book could be, and should be, dedicated to analysis of biased vaccine safety studies. Due to space considerations, only five were examined in this chapter. Nevertheless, the biased studies reviewed in this chapter are not exceptions to the rule; they are the rule. Some of these studies were conducted by reputable vaccine researchers, including CDC employees and a CDC-funded group. Some of the studies received extensive media coverage and are referenced to this day by websites of leading public health agencies around the world as well as other medical publications. Despite their conspicuous biases and alleged misconduct, they have not been criticized by any medical or scientific officials. Thus, the inevitable conclusion is that these studies demonstrate the accepted ethical norms of vaccine safety research.

"Why don't we see other researchers examine the same data and come up with different results? This is a sign that the original studies are in fact genuine." – As stated in this chapter, vaccine safety research is funded almost exclusively by health authorities and vaccine manufacturers, both of which have clear interests in the success of the vaccine program and will not fund studies that could jeopardize it. In addition, vaccine safety research makes use of medical data that is largely controlled by these health authorities. This prevents "dissident" researchers from accessing this data, thus artificially limiting the publication of vaccine-critical science.

"So, are you saying there's a worldwide conspiracy involving health authorities, vaccine manufacturers, scientists, and medical journals to publish deliberately biased research on vaccine safety?" – When the interests of separate parties clearly overlap and all stand to gain by joining forces, cooperation is to be expected. This chapter described the major parties involved in vaccine safety research, their motives, and vested interests. All parties are acting in furtherance of their own best interests, trying to achieve their goals through any means at their disposal. Nothing is unusual or novel about that. No "conspiracy" is required to explicate these actions.

Summary

Epidemiological studies are the tool of choice for health authorities and pharma companies to maintain a façade of vaccine safety science. They are cheap, relatively simple to conduct, and, above all, their results are easily manipulated.

The five studies reviewed in this chapter illustrate some of the many methods researchers use to manipulate the results of epidemiological studies:

- ✓ Using unsubstantiated data (Madsen 2002).
- ✓ Using irrelevant data (Fombonne 2006).
- ✓ Hiding the real source of the data (Fombonne 2006).
- ✓ Omitting essential data from the paper (Grimaldi 2014).
- ✓ Reversing the trend of raw data by means of undisclosed statistical adjustments (Madsen 2002).
- ✓ Using arbitrary, meaningless, and scientifically baseless calculations (DeStefano 2013).
- ✓ Dismissing inconvenient findings on a speculative or arbitrary pretext (McKeever 2004).
- ✓ Misrepresenting the subject of the study to the public (DeStefano 2013).
- ✓ Using a grossly inadequate research method (Fombonne 2006).
- ✓ Using a research method that facilitates easy manipulation (DeStefano 2013, Grimaldi 2014).
- ✓ Failing to address post-publication misconduct allegations (Fombonne 2006).
- ✓ Overstating the significance of study results (all).

Amazingly enough, this assortment of faults did not prevent any of these studies from being published in leading medical journals or lead to their retraction. No mainstream scientist, academic, or journalist has directed a single critical word toward the studies or their authors. The studies' scientific reputations remain unblemished to this day, and they are frequently cited in the medical literature and publications of health authorities as evidence of vaccine safety. None of those citing the studies ever mention their obvious flaws or the researchers' conflicts of interest.

The blanket institutional immunity afforded to these purposely biased studies and their authors clearly shows that these studies conformed to the appalling ethical norms of vaccine safety research accepted by the scientific world. This fundamentally flawed research is the direct consequence of the way science is currently funded, which ensures researchers' dependency on their funding source, be it government or a pharmaceutical company. The vaccine establishment relies on the fact that the public is unaware of this mechanism and its inherent flaws, which guarantees that vaccine safety science is almost never carried out objectively.

Therefore, in the spirit of the Mark Twain adage that appears at the beginning of this chapter, one should exercise extreme caution when reviewing the conclusions of vaccine safety epidemiological studies – those that have already been published and those that will be published in the future.

Ask your doctor:

• Do you know who funds most vaccine safety research? Are you familiar with the process used to allocate medical research grants?

• Would you expect pharmaceutical companies and government agencies to fund vaccine safety studies that could potentially find serious faults in the vaccines they manufacture, license, and recommend to the public?

• Are you aware that studies published in leading medical journals which ostensibly confirm the safety of vaccines suffer from serious methodological flaws and are fraught with authors' conflicts of interest?

6

THE STUDIES THAT
WILL NEVER BE DONE

Imagine you are watching a TV documentary on the history of cigarette smoking. The show focuses on the public debate regarding the potential health hazards of smoking in the 1950s. According to this fictional account, the US health authorities of the time endorsed cigarette smoking and reassured the public it was completely safe. Scientific consensus, the authorities repeatedly proclaimed, asserted that smoking had no significant health hazards. No association had been found between smoking and a variety of chronic diseases and syndromes erroneously attributed to it by newly formed anti-smoking advocacy groups. To substantiate their claim, authorities presented a long list of epidemiological studies that confirmed the safety of cigarette smoking: A study comparing the health implications of smoking three packs a day versus two packs a day; a study comparing the health of Camel smokers to that of Marlboro smokers; studies comparing the health of smokers of commercial brands with those who rolled their own; and a host of additional studies exploring potential health risks of smoking. All of these studies, from the first to the last, concluded that no association was found between smoking and adverse health issues, and specifically between smoking and the rising lung cancer morbidity.

"The science is unequivocal on the safety of smoking," pronounced health officials and leading scientists of the 1950s over and over again. "No scientific evidence exists linking cigarette smoking and lung cancer or other harmful effects. This case is closed."

Nonetheless, some advocacy groups didn't consider the case closed. Challenging the scientific consensus, these groups carefully examined the science that upheld the safety of cigarette smoking and discovered an amazing and disturbing fact: None of the dozens of epidemiological studies that looked into the issue compared the health status of smokers to that of nonsmokers. There were studies exploring the health consequences of smoking different amounts, different brands, different ingredients, in different geographical areas, and so on. But in every study, each and every one of the subjects was a smoker. None of the studies compared the health of smokers to that of nonsmokers. How could cigarette smoking be deemed safe, the critics wondered, if essential studies comparing the health of smokers to nonsmokers hadn't even been done?

In response to this criticism, establishment representatives acknowledged that smoker vs. nonsmoker studies hadn't been done. But these studies were neither necessary nor feasible, they explained, so they weren't likely to be conducted anytime in the future either. The bottom line, they concluded, is that we investigated this issue thoroughly, and the science is crystal clear and settled that smoking is completely safe. Everyone can go on with their lives. The matter is closed.

What do you, the reader, think about this narrative? Does it seem conceivable that health authorities could determine that cigarette smoking was safe without ever conducting studies comparing the health of smokers to that of nonsmokers?

Well, it shouldn't. This history is indeed fictional, as stated in the opening paragraph. These events never took place because as early as the 1950s, American and British researchers conducted extensive epidemiological studies that compared various health outcomes in smokers and non-smokers. These studies paved the way for official recognition of the harms of smoking in the late 1950s.

As far as smoking is concerned, the requisite studies were performed long ago and the results made public, thus preventing countless cases of smoking-induced cancer. In the field of vaccine safety, however, the scenario described in the TV documentary is not at all fictional but rather a grim reality.

In the previous chapter we saw how epidemiological studies can be used to create an illusion of vaccine safety. Epidemiology's methods and tools give researchers the flexibility to tailor study results to their sponsor's needs. As it happens, government bodies and private corporations fund dozens, if not hundreds, of new vaccine studies every year. These studies reconfirm, time and time again, the institutional claim that vaccines are safe and effective. Surprisingly, though, a specific kind of vaccine safety study, a study that would be considered absolutely essential in any other medical field, has never been done – and probably never will be.

This chapter, therefore, describes the vaccine safety studies that have never been done and the medical establishment's ostensible reasons for not doing them. As we scrutinize the official explanation, you should be asking yourself some questions: Does the reluctance make sense? Is the establishment being candid about the reasons for not doing these studies? Or is there a better explanation for this peculiar scientific neglect? And what is the impact of not doing these studies on the validity of the vaccine program?

Vaccinated vs. Unvaccinated (VU) Studies

The term *vaccinated vs. unvaccinated study* (henceforth, *VU study*) refers to an epidemiological study that compares different health metrics between a group of subjects who were fully and timely vaccinated (according to official recommendations at the time) and a control group of subjects who were not vaccinated at all. A VU study could potentially look at the effect of the childhood vaccination program on the overall health of vaccinees, or, alternatively, on the incidence rates of specific diseases or syndromes, such as asthma or autism.

VU studies are essential to monitoring the safety (and efficacy) of the vaccine program as a whole. As described in chapter 1, the effect new vaccines may have on the safety and efficacy of the overall vaccination schedule is not studied prior to licensing.[1] Pre-licensure clinical trials test health outcomes of the candidate vaccine when given separately, or, at most, in combination with other vaccines that are typically administered at the same doctor visit. None of the trials use a control group of children who are completely unvaccinated. Therefore, they cannot assess the cumulative effect of adding yet another new vaccine to the childhood vaccination schedule.

Many studies of different types are conducted to test the efficacy and safety of a specific vaccine. But even if a particular vaccine were found to be safe on its own, it could still contribute to a cumulative adverse effect on children who receive all the recommended vaccines. No one piece of straw can break a camel's back, but pile on enough of them and a single piece will eventually be the difference between a tired back and a broken one. For example, many vaccines contain adjuvants made of aluminum salts.[a] Aluminum salts are known to be toxic and in certain doses and conditions may accumulate in the body and subsequently lead to neurological or other injuries. A clinical trial of a new aluminum-containing vaccine cannot identify long-term health effects caused by the gradual accumulation of aluminum in an infant's body. The long-term health effects of aluminum adjuvant accumulation in the human body are not yet well known.[b] Aluminum, needless to say, is just one of dozens of

---

[a] An adjuvant, as you may recall, is used in some inactivated vaccines to stimulate the immune system to respond more vigorously to the vaccine antigen (the immunogenic substance of the vaccine).

[b] Keep in mind that these substances are contained in various vaccine products and given to children of diverse genetic makeup, whose overall health can vary significantly at the time of vaccination.

substances found in routine vaccinations.

Clinical trials of vaccines typically do not report chronic syndromes and diseases, such as autism, attention deficit hyperactivity disorder (ADHD), diabetes, or cancer. These conditions develop over a period of months or years, and consequently researchers tend not to associate them with the tested vaccine even if they are diagnosed during the time frame of the clinical trial.[2] Adverse event reporting systems, which monitor the safety of licensed vaccines, also suffer from a similar limitation. Case reports submitted to these systems mostly describe adverse health events recorded several days or weeks following vaccination.[3] A health condition diagnosed many months after vaccine administration is not likely to be attributed to the vaccine and, therefore, will not be reported.

The lack of safety testing of the cumulative effect of vaccines during their approval process, as well as the inherent limitations of adverse event reporting systems, has not attracted the attention of the FDA or CDC. Over the past few decades, many new vaccines have been approved and subsequently added to the routine vaccination program. However, these agencies have not investigated or even considered the potential adverse effects of the growing number of vaccines on the overall health of vaccinated children.

Thus, in order to evaluate the safety of the entire vaccination program, as well as the impact of vaccines on adverse health conditions that develop in the medium and long terms, clinical trials and studies of the safety of individual vaccines do not suffice. To achieve this end, one must conduct studies comparing the health of subjects who were fully vaccinated with the health of those who were not.[c] These essential studies are the "vaccinated vs. unvaccinated" or VU studies.

As we shall see later in the chapter, although numerous vaccine studies are published annually, no VU safety study has ever

---

[c] It is also possible, of course, to include groups of subjects who have been partially vaccinated or vaccinated on a nonstandard schedule.

been officially conducted to determine the impact of the entire vaccine program on the overall health of children. In addition, no such study ever examined the effect the program might be having on the rising incidence of any chronic health conditions.[4] Thus, no government-funded study has ever compared the rate of autism in vaccinated and unvaccinated children.[5] Similarly, no VU studies have been conducted for cancer, asthma, diabetes, learning disorders, ADHD, epilepsy, Crohn's disease and many other life-altering conditions, although all of them have become increasingly common in recent decades. The fact that these fundamental studies have never been done raises serious doubts about the safety and overall benefits of the routine vaccination program, as will be discussed below.

Overall Health Study: Vaccinated vs. Unvaccinated

The US vaccination program has been constructed layer by layer over the past 70 years. Until the middle of the last century only a single vaccine was widely distributed in the United States – the smallpox vaccine. In the late 1940s, the diphtheria-pertussis-tetanus vaccine (DPT) was becoming popular, and in the mid-1950s the polio vaccine was introduced – the first vaccine to be introduced in a nationwide campaign. An ad hoc precursor to the Advisory Committee on Immunization Practices (ACIP) recommended that all American children receive the measles vaccine in 1963. The ACIP was officially formed the following year and has been "calling the shots" ever since, adding more and more vaccine recommendations throughout the subsequent decades, especially following the 1986 National Childhood Vaccine Injury Act. Presently, by the time they are two years old, American children receive up to 28 vaccine doses for 14 different diseases.

Each new vaccine that was added to the schedule in recent decades was previously tested in a series of clinical trials. However, the overall health impact of routinely administering an ever-increasing number of vaccines to American infants has never been studied. In other words, the fundamental question that bothers every vaccine-informed parent – "Will my child be better off fully vaccinated, partially vaccinated, or unvaccinated?" – has never been adequately answered by science. No study that compares the overall health of vaccinated children to that of unvaccinated children has ever been done by the medical establishment.

In the absence of a VU study examining vaccines' impact on overall health, science cannot determine the real net benefit – positive or negative – of the childhood vaccination program. Accordingly, health authorities' repeated mantra of "vaccines have been extensively and thoroughly investigated and shown to be safe and effective" has not been demonstrated. It is entirely possible that the potential benefits of the vaccine program (lower rates of vaccine-preventable diseases) are outweighed by its costs (higher incidence of chronic and other infectious diseases). Until VU studies are done, we won't ever know for sure.

Given the firm and longstanding global support for vaccines, one might expect that VU studies of overall health had been conducted many times over in numerous countries around the world. Different countries have different childhood vaccination schedules, each of which ought to be scientifically studied and its benefits validated. These vitally important studies, however, have never been sanctioned by medical authorities in the US or anywhere else in the world.

The Establishment Avoids Conducting VU Studies

It seems inexplicable that VU studies have not been initiated by the vaccine establishment for so many years. Could thousands of officials, researchers, and medical professionals around the globe have just "not noticed" the complete absence of this crucial piece of vaccine safety research from the medical literature? Well, even if they did, there were plenty of people pointing it out to them. Parents have been demanding VU studies for nearly 30 years.[d] [6] Many believe vaccines to be the prime suspect in the recent huge increase in chronic disease in children, and there can be no vindication until proper VU studies are performed.[7] The reluctance of health authorities to perform VU studies is even more intriguing in light of the continuing decline in public confidence in vaccines. Authorities constantly predict dire consequences from declining vaccination rates, yet they refuse to conduct the one study that could indisputably prove the benefits of the vaccination program and relieve parents' concerns, even as they continually commission the sort of vaccine safety studies discussed in the last chapter that pretend to address parental anxiety.

As a substitute for VU research, every year the establishment funds dozens of studies that look at vaccine safety and effectiveness from (almost) every angle. Some of these studies flirt with the concept of a VU study and, with a sprinkle of public relations magic, are even presented as such. For example, a prominent national autism organization announced in 2015 that "No MMR-autism link [was found] in a large study of Vaccinated vs. Unvaccinated kids."[8] The term "unvaccinated" that appears in the title and is repeated several times in the article, implies that the study included a group of children who were completely unvaccinated. In fact, the study only examined the subjects' vaccination status of a single vaccine, the MMR, and not of the entire childhood

---

[d] In fact, the demand for a VU study is at least 165 years old. In a pamphlet published in England in 1856, John Gibbs wrote about the smallpox vaccine: "The main question for the consideration of science is not whether vaccination be a protection against one form of disease, but what is its general influence upon the constitution? [...] What is the percentage of deaths before a given age, from all epidemics, amongst the vaccinated, as compared with the unvaccinated? What is the percentage respectively of cases of disease of the respiratory organs, of skin diseases, of scrofula, and of convulsions? What is the average duration of life amongst the vaccinated and amongst the unvaccinated? Of a thousand children vaccinated within a given time after birth, and of a thousand unvaccinated, the whole two thousand being placed as nearly as possible in like circumstances, what percentage in each thousand attain the age of puberty? These are statistics with which the advocates of vaccination have never grappled."

schedule. It is entirely possible, then, that the vast majority of the "unvaccinated" children in the study received every dose of every vaccine on the schedule other than MMR.

Another study that some websites claim looked at the overall health of vaccinated children compared to unvaccinated children was conducted in Germany in 2011.[9] However, the study only examined the morbidity rates of several infectious diseases and two types of allergies. Data on almost all the chronic diseases associated with vaccines and other important health-related parameters (e.g., pharmaceutical prescriptions, hospitalization days, deaths, etc.) were not presented in the paper. Although the study examined a very narrow slice of "overall health", and despite its serious methodological limitations,[e] some present it as a study that answers all parents' questions about the risks and benefits of vaccination.[10]

The most notable example of the demonstrable reluctance of health authorities to conduct VU studies is in the field of autism research. Over the past 15 years, dozens of epidemiological studies have been conducted examining the association between vaccines and autism, but not a single one compared the rate of autism in fully vaccinated and fully unvaccinated children.[11] Despite the fact that autism has become a huge social and financial burden on American society, the US medical establishment has stubbornly rejected every opportunity to dive deeper into its root causes by investigating the rates of autism in unvaccinated populations.[12]

In 2005, journalist Dan Olmsted paid a number of visits to Amish country in Lancaster County, Pennsylvania, in an attempt to ascertain whether the rate of autism in Amish communities had risen in sync with the rate in the general population. The Amish, whose lifestyle has not changed much over the past 200 to 300 years, vaccinate their children at a fraction of the national

---

[e] For example, the unvaccinated group had only 94 subjects, a mere 0.7% of the study population of 13,453 children. This raises serious doubts as to the validity of the findings.

rate, as confirmed by surveys conducted by the CDC and others in 2006 and 2011.[13] Contrary to conventional wisdom, Amish parents are not vaccinating less due to religious beliefs but because of safety concerns.[14] Extrapolating from the national autism statistics of the time, Olmsted expected to find several dozen autistic Amish children in the county he visited. However, his search yielded fewer than five kids with autism, and some were quite atypical for Amish children.[f] In a series of articles that have since traveled far and wide,[15] Olmsted published his findings and hypothesized that the low incidence of autism among the Amish was due to their significantly lower rate of child vaccination.

Given that autism is arguably the greatest public health mystery of our time, Olmsted's findings, while anecdotal and unscientific, should have elicited a response from the CDC. In addition to determining vaccine policy, the CDC is also tasked with investigating the root causes of autism.[16] As the CDC wears both hats, it should have enthusiastically hopped on the Olmsted bandwagon and sent a team of researchers to thoroughly investigate this hypothetical correlation between the low vaccination and low autism rates among the Amish. The high proportion of unvaccinated children in the Amish population provided a golden opportunity for scientists to conduct a VU study of autism and other chronic diseases. However, nothing was done. Furthermore, the CDC never officially responded to Olmsted's Amish findings. The CDC's apparent idleness is even more striking in light of the speed and vigor of its actions when outbreaks of infectious diseases erupt in Amish counties. In the period 1991–2005, the agency sent at least four separate investigative teams to carry out epidemiological inquiries in the wake of outbreaks of measles, mumps, pertussis, and haemophilus

---

[f] For example, one girl was born in China and adopted by an Amish family. This girl was vaccinated in her country of origin.

influenzae type B (Hib) among the Amish. [g] [17] It appears, therefore, that the CDC springs into action when dealing with infectious disease in Amish country but takes a pass when it comes to chronic conditions like autism. This difference in priorities becomes even more baffling when you consider the huge economic and social burden of autism, which far exceeds that of the four aforementioned infectious diseases combined.[18]

After completing his tour of Amish communities, Olmsted continued his quest for unvaccinated populations to examine their autism rates. This led him to Chicago, to the Homefirst clinic of Dr. Mayer Eisenstein and colleagues. Homefirst doctors took a rather unconventional approach to medical care that involved home birth and minimal use of prescription medications and vaccines. They didn't know of a single case of autism, they said, among the thousands of unvaccinated children they'd had under their care over more than 30 years of practice.[19] Once more, one would have expected the CDC to jump into action upon hearing the news and send a research team in an attempt to crack the autism riddle. A group of several thousand children without a single case of autism among them might provide an important clue to the mystery that medical science had failed to solve over the past half century. As with the Amish, however, the CDC did nothing, and the opportunity to do a VU autism study died on the vine, again.[h]

Another fortuitous opportunity for a VU autism study came up in 2004 at the Ruppin Academic Center in Israel. Ruppin researchers compared the rate of autism among Israeli children of Ethiopian descent born in Ethiopia with that of those born in Israel.[20] The rate of autism in Ethiopian-descent children born in Israel, who had presumably been vaccinated with all the vac-

---

[g] Interestingly, all of the teams reported a low vaccination rate in Amish communities, less than 25%, which reinforces Olmsted's hypothesis.

[h] The establishment's response to Dr. Eisenstein probably came several years later in the form of an investigation by a Chicago Tribune journalist casting doubt on his professional conduct and credibility.

cines in the Israeli program,[i] was quite similar to the national rate. In stark contrast, in the Ethiopian children who immigrated to Israel at a young age (who were likely not vaccinated in infancy), the autism rate was... zero. Not even a single case of autism was recorded among them. The difference between the groups was not likely to be due to misdiagnosis, as all the children ended up in Israel and would have been diagnosed by the same government-provided screening services. The results of the Ruppin study suggest that environment and lifestyle, much more than genetic disposition, are the main factors affecting the development of autism. Both Ethiopian-descent groups shared similar genes, but autism was evident only in Israeli-born children. The Ruppin researchers, who were studying the assimilation of immigrant populations in Israel, were unaware of the broader significance of their research and its indirect support for the vaccine–autism link. The CDC, unsurprisingly, ignored yet another opportunity to conduct a VU autism study. Unfortunately, the Ruppin study has not been publicly discussed or referenced by any US health agency, and, as might be expected, no funding was allocated for further research on the intriguing Israeli data.

Another immigrant community from Africa, this time closer to home, presented the CDC with one more opportunity to investigate the link between vaccines and autism by means of a VU study. In 2008, news stories began to appear reporting a particularly high rate of autism among children of Somali descent who were born in Minnesota.[21] The autism rate in this group of children was reported to be three to four times higher than the national rate. Furthermore, similar to the children of Ethiopian-descent in the Ruppin study, all the autistic children in the Somali community in Minnesota were born in the United States. None of them were born in Somalia.[22] Some of the children's mothers noted that autism is unknown in Somalia and

---

[i] The Israeli vaccination program is almost identical to the American program.

that the Somali language does not even have a word describing this condition. At the same time, particularly high rates of autism were also found among children in the Somali immigrant community in Sweden.[23] Swedish researchers who reported these findings hypothesized that these high rates may have been caused by a vitamin D deficiency due to the low sun exposure in northern countries.[j] The CDC, yet again, did not seek out causes for the high autism rate among Somali immigrant children in Minnesota or Sweden despite solemn promises made to the Somali community that the issue would be investigated. Indeed, five full years later, the CDC summed up the "project" by publishing a study[24] whose sole contribution was to formally confirm what was already known: The autism rate in the Somali community is significantly higher than average.[k] No study, VU or otherwise, has even attempted to discover what is causing the high rate of autism in the Somali community.

The establishment's reluctance to conduct a VU study to clarify the association between vaccines and autism, which by this time had reached Washington, led two members of Congress to introduce a bill that would compel the US Department of Health and Human Services (DHHS) to conduct such research. But the bills by Congressional Representatives Caroline Maloney and Dave Weldon (in 2007)[25] and Bill Posey (in 2013, and again in 2017)[26] puzzlingly failed to gain any traction even in the first phase of the legislative process. The CDC, it seemed, could once more heave a sigh of relief.

Similar to the way the medical establishment avoids actually researching the vaccine–autism connection, it avoids doing VU studies for other chronic conditions and for overall child health as well. So, instead of giving parents the studies they had been

---

[j] This hypothesis cannot explain the "normal" rate of autism among "veteran" African American children in Minnesota.

[k] The study found an autism rate of 1 in 32 among Somali children. Quite bizarrely, a similar rate of 1 in 36 was found among white children in Minnesota. This finding, whether true or not, provided the formal justification for closing the Somali autism case.

demanding for years, vaccine officials commissioned a shiny new IOM report to officially exonerate them for not doing their jobs properly in the past, and excuse them from ever having to in the future.

The IOM 2013 Report

The public's growing discontent with the continuing lack of scientific research that examines the effects of the entire vaccine schedule placed US health authorities in an awkward position. The loud and repeated demands of parents and advocacy groups to carry out VU studies were amplified by the internet and shined a spotlight on the weakest part of the fortress surrounding the vaccine program.

Human bodies are incredibly intricate, and the range of effects triggered by vaccinating them is broad and complex. To engage in an educated discussion on the topic, you need a considerable amount of knowledge, some of it quite technical. As such, representatives of the vaccine establishment had the upper hand in most online discussions, easily refuting the average parent's criticism of the vaccine program. Nevertheless, the "vaccinated vs. unvaccinated studies" argument posed an exceptional challenge to vaccine proponents. Here was an argument that was fairly simple to grasp, one that could be understood by laypeople with limited scientific knowledge as well as medical professionals. Why hadn't such a study ever been conducted, as they had for cigarette smoking and numerous other health issues? Is there an "inconvenient truth" the medical establishment is keeping under wraps? Questions like these, when left unanswered for too long, raise doubts in parents and erode public confidence in the folks running the vaccine program.

US health authorities had to respond. And what do bureaucrats do when they intend to bury an inconvenient truth? They form a special committee to "investigate" the issue, of course.

And so, in 2009, the Institute of Medicine (IOM) was called in once again to save the day. As described earlier in chapter 2, the IOM is a council of experts advising the federal government on various health issues, including vaccines. This time around the National Vaccine Program Office in the US Department of Health and Human Services requested the formation of a committee to investigate the current science on the safety of the vaccine schedule and the concerns raised by parents. This request followed a recommendation of the National Vaccine Advisory Committee (NVAC) for an external expert committee to look into this issue.[27] In addition, the IOM committee was asked to identify potential research approaches and methodologies that could provide information about the above issue and evaluate them in financial, ethical, and practical terms.[28] In other words: the committee was asked to provide an official and persuasive institutional response to the complaints about the absence of VU studies.

After three years of preparations, finally, the committee convened in 2012 and began its proceedings. In addition to work meetings behind closed doors, the committee held a series of open hearings in which public representatives were given the opportunity to voice their concerns. One year later, the committee published its 237-page report.

It was business as usual. The same unequivocal support for vaccines and the vaccine program expressed in previous vaccine-related IOM reports was evident in the IOM 2013 report as well. The committee proclaimed its allegiance to the institutional dogma on vaccines in the first paragraph of the first chapter of the report: "Vaccines have significantly contributed to worldwide reductions in morbidity and mortality by reducing the incidence of serious infectious diseases. [...] However, as the incidence of vaccine-preventable disease has declined, many do not appreciate the potential of these diseases to reemerge, and the potential adverse effects of the vaccines themselves take on greater saliency among certain stakeholders."[29] The opening paragraph clearly marks the path the rest of the report will take. And, indeed, the report's conclusions, reviewed below, provide firm and unreserved support for institutional lethargy when it comes to investigating the vaccine program as a whole.

Although the IOM 2013 report does not contain any new or particularly interesting information about the benefits of the vaccine program, there are a few good reasons for delving into it. Regarding "the studies that will be never done", the report formally refines and summarizes the vaccine establishment's reasons, or excuses, for not doing VU studies. Moreover, the manner in which the committee defends the establishment position actually exposes its weakness for all to see, while at the same time stamping it with an official seal of approval. An in-depth reading of the report reveals numerous contradictions, unreasonable claims, circular arguments, and – above all – an almost desperate effort to legitimize the inaction of the vaccine establishment. To the critical reader, the report appears to be a masterpiece of bureaucratic doublespeak whose sole purpose is to justify and perpetuate the decades-long institutional refusal to study the safety of the vaccine program.

Let's take a look at some of the more interesting points covered in the report.

Formal Admission

For decades, and more frequently in recent years, the medical establishment has been repeating an unvarying message that goes something like this: The childhood routine vaccine program is the best there is. Its safety and effectiveness have been corroborated in countless scientific studies and by thousands of researchers. Therefore, dear parents, go ahead and vaccinate your children according to the recommended schedule, as this is the best action you can take to protect their health.

All of us, from cradle to grave, are steeped in this message, which is disseminated through many different channels: teachers at school, posters at the doctor's office, articles in lifestyle magazines and news media, TV programs, movies, and the like. All of these informally echo the institutional message, taking its veracity for granted and asking no questions.

And what about the establishment itself? By now, you know that the medical establishment does not provide sufficient scientific evidence to support these safety claims, but you might be surprised to learn that government health agencies don't actually make those guarantees. If you search the websites of the DHHS or the CDC for a statement claiming that the vaccination program of the United States has been tested for its effectiveness and safety, you will not find any. You may come across a webpage asserting that specific vaccines have been tested, individually or with other vaccines given at the same day according to the recommended schedule, or that vaccine adverse events are well monitored.[30] But you will not find a clear and explicit statement arguing that the vaccine program as a whole has been properly tested and found to be safe and effective.

In case you were wondering, this is not a coincidence or indicative of negligence on the part of the CDC or DHHS. Of course, it is easy to believe that a government body might be slightly negligent in making important information accessible to the public through its website. But this is not the current case. A formal statement attesting to the scientific validity of the vaccine program as a whole does not appear on health authorities' websites because these institutions are well aware that it has never been tested. This fact was formally documented in the IOM 2013 report, which details many aspects of the vaccine program that have never been scientifically investigated.

Firstly, the report acknowledges that no studies have ever compared the overall health of fully vaccinated children to that of children who have never been vaccinated. In addition, no VU studies have been conducted on specific health outcomes such as autism or autoimmune diseases.[31] As a rule, the report elaborates, the recommended schedule in its entirety has not been studied. Instead, most vaccine-related research focuses on individual vaccines or combinations of vaccines administered on the same day as recommended by the CDC.[32]

What does the committee mean exactly when saying that the recommended schedule as a whole has not been studied? The report clarifies: "[...] key elements of the entire schedule – the number, frequency, timing, order, and age at administration of vaccines – have not been systematically examined in research studies."[33] Furthermore, when a new vaccine is added to the vaccine schedule, no studies are done to examine its effect on the other vaccines on the schedule. Research to evaluate different variations of the schedule, to ensure it is still "optimal" is also never done (and bear in mind that each country implements its own vaccination schedule, with different vaccine products, doses, and timings, etc.).[34]

But that does not conclude the uncertainty embedded in the vaccination program, the report asserts. Due to a severe lack of relevant scientific research the committee is unable to determine whether vaccine safety concerns have been thoroughly "addressed". Also, it could not make up its mind whether the introduction of better surveillance systems would lead to the identification of "new" vaccine-related safety issues. Furthermore, the report adds, the underlying causes of some of the adverse health conditions for which concerns have been raised – including immunologic, neurological and developmental problems – are not sufficiently understood by medical science.[35]

Another area that is not sufficiently understood, the committee notes, concerns the identification of subpopulations that may be particularly susceptible to vaccine side effects, their characteristics, and specific potential health risks. There is also a shortage of data and diagnostic tools for the early identification of these children, including those born prematurely or those with a family history of autoimmune disease.[36]

"In summary," the report states, "to consider whether and how to study the safety and health outcomes of the entire childhood immunization schedule, the field needs valid and accepted metrics of the entire schedule [...] and clearer definitions of health outcomes linked to stakeholder concerns [...]."[37]

Evidently, the IOM 2013 report officially confirms the claim made by many parents that the safety of the vaccination program as a whole has never been tested. The committee completely rebuts the omnipresent, yet unofficial, institutional claim that the vaccine program has been thoroughly tested and found to be safe and effective. It unequivocally attests that the program's overall safety, as well as key aspects such as the impact of a new vaccine, the number of vaccines, administration timing, recognition of side effects, and identification of vulnerable populations have never been systematically and scientifically studied.

The wide gap between the paucity of science verifying the safety of the vaccine program and the medical establishment's groundless claims of safety is even more puzzling given the huge number of vaccine studies commissioned by the same players in the past few decades. A good example of this is provided courtesy of the committee itself: Since the late 1970s, the IOM has conducted 60 different studies on vaccination. None of them, as the report attests, dealt with the fundamental safety issues discussed above.[38]

Is It Really Impossible to Conduct VU Studies?

Given the massive uncertainty regarding the risks and benefits of the vaccine program and the growing public criticism of vaccine policy, there seem to be plenty of good reasons for the medical establishment to conduct not one but many VU studies. This type of study would be the best validation for the safety and effectiveness of the vaccine program and provide a credible and persuasive scientific answer to parental doubts.

Surprisingly, this seemingly self-evident point of view is not shared by the IOM 2013 committee. While it acknowledges the acute lack of research on key aspects of the program and recognizes the importance of these studies in alleviating parental concerns,[39] the committee devotes most of its efforts to justifying this lack of science with contorted arguments that these studies should not or cannot be performed:

Clinical trials of vaccinated vs. unvaccinated subjects cannot be performed as parents should not be forced to either vaccinate or not vaccinate their children.[40] Indeed, a clinical trial (RCT) of vaccinated vs. unvaccinated children would not be appropriate as it would require random allocation of participants into trial and control groups. Thus, a child whose parents did not wish to vaccinate could end up in the vaccinated group, and vice versa. The ethicality of such a trial is rather dubious, and in any case, researchers would find it difficult to recruit participants.

However, there are no methodological or ethical barriers to conducting non-randomized prospective VU studies or retrospective VU studies.[1] One such study is a non-randomized clinical trial (i.e., a prospective study) comparing the health outcomes of vaccinated vs. unvaccinated children over a prolonged period of time. Since it is not randomized – participants would be assigned to the group of their parents' choice – a trial such as this one would be somewhat inferior to an RCT. Even so, it could provide valuable medical information. Alternatively, retrospective studies of various kinds could be performed. Retrospective research, due to its relatively low cost, is very common in the medical field. A retrospective VU study could examine the medical records of a very large set of children, allocate them to groups according to their vaccination status, and compare various health outcomes between the groups. In fact, most vaccine safety studies, including studies investigating the link between vaccines and autism, are retrospective epidemiological studies of a similar design.

Not vaccinating children in a prospective medical study would be unethical as it would put them at an elevated risk of contracting vaccine-preventable diseases.[41] This argument is logically untenable as it assumes what is yet to be proven. Claiming that not

---

[1] As mentioned in chapter 4, a prospective study (or trial) selects participants and follows them over a period of time, while a retrospective study examines data that already exists.

vaccinating children consigns them to "an elevated risk" presupposes that the overall benefit of the vaccine program has already been properly studied and proved to be positive. But that is precisely what a VU study is supposed to test. Put differently, the IOM 2013 report authors claim it is unethical to do a VU study examining the benefits of the vaccine program because we already know that vaccines are beneficial and therefore they cannot ethically be withheld from trial participants. Seeing this logical fallacy in a report authored by senior medical experts is quite astounding, and even more so when you consider that the report explicitly states that proper research into the safety and effectiveness of the vaccination program has never been done.

This argument is not only nonsensical, it becomes irrelevant as well if the study's unvaccinated group consists solely of children whose parents were not intending to vaccinate them in the first place. In the United States, for example, it is estimated that 0.8% of children are completely unvaccinated, which translates to about 30,000 children in every birth cohort.[42] And in Australia the rate is about 1.5%.[43]

The term "overall health" is undefined. Therefore, one cannot conduct a VU study of overall health.[44] Studies examining the association between smoking and various adverse health conditions were conducted as early as the 1950s. Nowadays, the computer systems used by healthcare providers store a great deal of information about patients. Information reflecting the patient's level of health is easily extracted from these systems. Key metrics could include the number of doctor visits, hospitalization days, emergency room visits, life-threatening conditions, chronic and disability conditions, medications consumed, and more. Most of these parameters are routinely monitored in vaccine clinical trials, and similar information is gathered in retrospective studies. For example, a US study conducted by Jason Glanz and colleagues that was mentioned in the IOM 2013 report[45] looked for a correlation between delaying child vaccination and healthcare utilization rates – hospitalization days, emergency room visits, outpatient visits, and frequency of febrile illnesses.

It is also important to note that the supposed lack of definition for overall health does not apply to VU studies of specific diseases and conditions, such as asthma, diabetes, or autism. These health conditions are well defined with standardized diagnostic codes stored in healthcare providers' databases.

VU studies cannot be performed because there are too few unvaccinated children.[46] As noted above, there are at least 30,000 unvaccinated children in every birth cohort in the United States, a small portion of which would be sufficient for an initial VU study. In fact, the IOM 2013 report mentions at least one information system (VSD) that "has a large enough proportion of unvaccinated children to investigate differences in health outcomes of unvaccinated and vaccinated children." [m][47]

VU studies are too expensive to conduct.[48] The committee claims that VU prospective studies must be conducted over a long period and therefore would be too costly to be feasible; however, the report does not provide financial analysis or any other evidence to support this claim. In addition, the committee seems uninterested in assessing the potential economic benefits of VU studies. The costs of caring for children with chronic diseases are astronomical, and a VU study that could provide important clues toward prevention of these diseases could potentially result in huge economic savings. Moreover, a convincing VU study could also provide scientific proof of the alleged benefit of the vaccine program and (finally) restore skeptical parents' confidence in vaccines. By doing so, health authorities would presumably save the money that they currently spend trying to persuade these parents to vaccinate their children. Counted among these "per-

---

[m] As mentioned in chapter 3, the Vaccine Safety Datalink (VSD) is an information system that draws data from a small number of major health care providers that have agreed to make their customer records available for CDC researchers to analyze and monitor vaccine adverse events.

suasion expenses" are the frequent studies performed to better understand parents' opposition to the current vaccine schedule (more on this below). The IOM 2013 report itself, which presumably cost several million dollars, is another expense directly related to persuasion of reluctant parents. Conducting VU studies would have eliminated the need for the report and would have saved the considerable sums invested in producing it.

In any case, financial costs are not an obstacle to conducting retrospective studies. As you know by now, these studies analyze existing computerized records and are much cheaper to perform than prospective studies. And many dozens of retrospective vaccine studies are conducted annually; the Glanz 2013 study mentioned earlier is but one example. Obviously, allocating funds for retrospective VU studies is economically feasible. It seems the committee agrees with this assertion as the report does not mention retrospective studies in this regard.

Unvaccinated children benefit from the disappearance of vaccine-preventable diseases and therefore a VU study would show biased results.[49] According to this claim, unvaccinated children are not currently exposed to the potential harms of vaccine-preventable diseases, while vaccinated children are subject to the side effects of vaccines. Therefore, a health-outcomes comparison would be biased in favor of the unvaccinated. There is a grain of truth in this assertion, as incidence of a few infectious diseases was reduced considerably thanks to vaccines (see chapter 8 for a detailed discussion of the topic).

The above claim is not an argument against doing VU studies, however; it's just a caveat regarding interpretation of their results. VU studies are essential for true assessment of the overall benefit of the vaccine program at a given point in time. They are especially important now because many parents want to know whether the current vaccine program contributes to children's health or harms it. These parents argue that the large number of vaccines administered to children may reduce episodes of infectious disease, which are typically short-lived, but greatly increases the incidence of chronic diseases. (For instance, as the McKeever 2004 study in chapter 5 suggests, children may be exchanging a bout of pertussis, which is usually limited to a few weeks of coughing and difficulty breathing, for asthma, which can mean a lifetime of gasping for breath.) According to this argument, reducing the number of child vaccines would serve to improve their overall health. VU studies are essential for providing the public with scientific data on this crucial subject. Once these studies were done and their results analyzed, if it turned out that the unvaccinated were indeed healthier, health authorities would have to reconsider their vaccination policy. They would need to find ways to reduce the damage caused by the vaccine program while doing their best to maintain its disease protection benefits. They would have to look for the optimal tradeoff point between infectious and chronic disease burden, rather than continue to assume that reducing incidence of infectious disease to zero is worth whatever it costs. VU studies are the starting point for this process; if they had been done years ago, as they should have, we would already possess extensive knowledge on the subject.

Having said that, the above argument is irrelevant with respect to the chronic illnesses which are concerning parents. Vaccine-preventable diseases are not considered a significant cause of chronic disease. Measles, whooping cough, diphtheria, chickenpox, and other diseases that children are vaccinated against are not significant factors in the onset of chronic conditions such as diabetes, cancer, autism, and ADHD. That is, unvaccinated children do not benefit from any "protection" from chronic illness supposedly provided to them by their vaccinated friends.

The results of VU studies would be of no practical significance due to differences in the lifestyles of vaccinated and unvaccinated children.[50] According to this argument, there is a high probability that the lifestyle, and perhaps even the genetic makeup, of unvaccinated children is fundamentally different from that of vaccinated children. Therefore, even if a large difference in health outcomes between the groups were found, this would not be of much scientific value as the real (confounding) factors at play could not be determined. Unvaccinated children, it is claimed, tend to live in families that adhere to a "natural" lifestyle that typically includes prolonged breastfeeding, organic nutrition, reduced exposure to toxins, and herbal medication usage. Hence, if a study showed that unvaccinated children suffered significantly less from, say, autism and ADHD than the vaccinated, vaccines would be blamed when the disparity may actually be due to other aspects of their "natural" lifestyle.

This argument, despite its seemingly scientific aroma, is not based on evidence but rather on mere speculation as to the characteristics of households of unvaccinated children. To disqualify the potential value of VU studies on that premise, one must firstly establish that the lifestyle of non-vaccinating families is indeed quite homogeneous. However, studies looking into the characteristics of non-vaccinating or partially vaccinating families have failed to identify common salient features.[51] As already mentioned, the number of unvaccinated children in the US population is relatively high – around 30,000 per birth cohort, or 300,000 children up to the age of 10. In the absence of solid evidence to the contrary, it is reasonable to assume that such a large number of children could be stratified in a VU study according to various lifestyle choices. Thus, researchers could make use of conventional epidemiological methods to examine the effects of different lifestyle choices on the measured health outcomes. For example, if a VU study found that the rate of autism in unvaccinated children was significantly lower than in vaccinated children, researchers could perform additional analysis to identify possible confounders. They could, perhaps, divide the unvaccinated group into organic and non-organic food consumers and test the rate of autism in the two groups. If both groups shared a similar autism rate, the researchers could conclude that there was no correlation between the home consumption of organic or non-organic foods and autism. Thus,

they could rule out this feature as a cause of autism. Other
lifestyle characteristics could be analyzed in a similar fashion.
Similar analysis has been carried out for years in numerous
epidemiological studies of vaccination, as well as for other
health-related topics.[n] Thus, in order to reject in advance the
potential benefit of VU studies, it is necessary to demonstrate
that the non-vaccinating population is so homogeneous that
there is no possibility of meaningful secondary analysis. As there
is no well-founded evidence for high uniformity in the unvaccinated, this argument rests on speculation rather than solid
science.

Although the above is quite sufficient to refute the claim in
question, it is important to consider it from another angle.

As we've mentioned before, recent decades have seen a huge
increase in the incidence of numerous chronic conditions in
children, conditions for which medical science has few answers:
no means of prevention, few effective treatments, and no cures.
The total societal cost of these conditions – from research on
effective treatments, to special education costs and loss of parental work days – is astronomical. Autism is a typical example:
Despite the huge sums (over a billion dollars) spent on autism
research,[52] the medical establishment has yet to identify its root
causes, effective treatments, or ways to prevent it.

Yet, astonishingly, the IOM committee advises against doing
VU studies, arguing that if such a study indicated that autism
was much less common in unvaccinated children there would be
no practical use for that information. In other words, the committee opposes studies that could potentially identify a subgroup

---

[n] As explained in chapter 4, researchers in the 20th century found that drinking alcohol was not linked to lung cancer, although a statistical correlation was
found between the two phenomena. Further analysis of the results revealed that
the rate of lung cancer among *non-smoking* alcohol consumers is low while its
rate among *smoking* alcohol consumers is *high* (similar to that of non-drinking
smokers). From this, the researchers proceeded to conclude that the source of the
link between drinking alcohol and lung cancer is that alcohol consumers also
tend to be heavy smokers.

with a significantly lower autism rate, thereby deliberately cutting off an avenue of research that could provide important clues for solving the autism mystery! Identifying a specific group of children, in this case unvaccinated kids, with a significantly lower-than-average autism rate would constitute a scientific breakthrough and provide a springboard for further research into what exactly makes this group different.° Even if it turned out that the causative factor had nothing to do with vaccines but was due to some other common characteristic – particular genes, organic food consumption, or prolonged breastfeeding, for example – that would still constitute an important breakthrough. To date, medical science has failed to identify any such group, and autism research continues to wander in the dark. Autism, of course, is just one example of many. Identification of a less-affected subgroup could advance the scientific research for many other chronic conditions that, like autism, medical science cannot currently prevent or cure.

* * *

Thus, the contribution of VU research to the scientific under-standing of chronic disease would certainly be positive – whether health-related differences were found between the groups or not, and regardless of the homogeneity of the unvac-cinated group. Either way, VU studies would tell us more about the causes of the conditions investigated.

In light of this discussion, it is difficult to fathom the offhand manner in which the committee dismisses the potential benefits of VU studies. It's almost as if the committee is looking for any excuse to avoid recommending that these studies be done. The

---

° For example, Amish children are different from the general population in their lifestyle and, perhaps, even in their genetic profile. Somali descent children in Minnesota who were born in Somalia and their younger siblings who were born in the United States differ only in life circumstances during maternal pregnancy and infancy (and the same is true of children of Ethiopian descent in Israel).

committee's arguments are speculative, not grounded in science, and, ultimately, unconvincing. Thus, contrary to the report protestations, there seems to be no real barrier to conducting VU studies. Support for this comes from a surprising source – the committee itself: "Secondary analyses with data from other existing databases [...] would be feasible, ethical, and a lower-cost approach to investigating the research questions that the committee identified, including research on alternative immunization schedules."[53] Thus, the committee contradicts its own arguments and inadvertently exposes the truth: There are no real obstacles to conducting VU studies – other than the demonstrable reluctance of the medical establishment to perform them.

What to Investigate, Then? The Parents...

Parents' criticisms of vaccine science and policy, referred to as "parental concerns" in the report, receive a great deal of attention from the IOM committee. That's not surprising: After all, it was growing parental criticism of the vaccine program that led to the IOM 2013 committee in the first place, as well as all the other IOM committees that grappled with vaccine safety issues over the past 15 years.

These concerns are not shared by the medical establishment and its representatives, it seems. As the committee notes, the parental concerns "were not expressed by clinicians, public health personnel, or policy makers in the committee's review. Among the last three groups, the childhood immunization schedule is considered one of the most effective and safest public health interventions available to prevent serious disease and death."[54] Contrary to the confidence the medical establishment shows in the vaccine program, the report continues, many parents express distrust "in the quality and thoroughness of vaccine safety research."[55] The problem, then, in the committee's eyes, is not the vaccine safety science per se, as the professionals evidently stand behind it, but rather the parents' distrust of that science. The motivation for setting up the committee was, then, the institutional desire to dispel those supposedly unfounded parental concerns.[56]

As we know, this institutional desire to allay parents' concerns about the safety of vaccines is long-standing. The report notes that between 2002 and 2012, at least 26 studies examined parental concerns with vaccine safety, and 31 additional studies looked into various aspects of vaccine-related communications between health providers and parents.[57] Studies of this sort are still frequently funded by health authorities.[58]

Although the committee is well aware of the copious amounts of money spent studying parental concerns and "vaccine-related communication", it argues that those do not constitute sufficient justification for conducting "expensive" VU studies.[59] In other words, it's appropriate to fund dozens of "parental concern" and "vaccine communication" studies – as well as a multitude of vaccine safety-related IOM committees that cost millions each – but no funding should go to "costly" research that actually addresses parents' concerns. Even worse, at the same time the committee discourages doing the "expensive" VU studies parents want, it recommends further study aimed at improving communication between parents and health providers and building parental trust in the safety of the vaccine program.[60]

Evermore Studying What to Study

From start to finish, the circumstances surrounding the IOM 2013 committee – the motivation for its formation, its mandated activity, the report it produced, and its conclusions – indicate a bureaucratic effort to bury an inconvenient truth.

Firstly, as already mentioned, forming a committee is a well-known bureaucratic tactic to appear to be "doing something" while not actually doing anything. Rather than fund a useful series of VU studies – of Amish communities, of the Minnesota Somali community, of Mayer Eisenstein's patients, and of the VSD system (all of which were possible) – US health authorities established a committee whose job was to convince the public that such research cannot be done.

Secondly, the committee's conclusions were most likely predetermined since the body that commissioned their work – the National Vaccine Advisory Committee (NVAC) – had already produced its own report concluding that VU studies were either unethical or inappropriate. In a 2009 report, the NVAC stated that a VU randomized clinical trial (RCT) would be unethical and that VU observational studies would draw biased results.[61] Evidently, and not unexpectedly, the IOM 2013 committee did not venture outside the boundaries drawn by its commissioning body.

And thirdly, although the committee acknowledges that adequate research into the safety of the vaccine program was never done, it maintains that the program is safe as "there is no evidence that the schedule is not safe."[62] The intrinsic contradiction of this conclusion is obvious: How could the committee determine that the recommended schedule is safe when it knows the studies that could demonstrate that safety have never been done?!

The acute lack of proper research validating the safety of the vaccine program apparently doesn't bother the committee. This paucity in vaccine safety science should have prompted the committee to sound the alarm and call for immediate action to bridge the great knowledge gap. But the studies it recommends are not VU studies – or even any other vaccine safety studies. Rather, the committee calls for various preliminary studies to be carried out before even deciding whether or not to study the safety of the vaccine schedule.[63] And lest anyone reading the report infer any hint of urgency from the above recommendation, the committee is quick to correct that impression: Even before approaching these "preliminary studies", they must be prioritized. And the prioritization process, the committee notes, may prove to be "a challenge" (so be patient, everyone).[64]

In summary of its work, the committee submits five recommendations. Three of them suggest activities that have been ongoing for years anyway: Gather information about "public confidence in and concerns about the childhood vaccination program" with the goal to improve communication between parents and health care professionals;[65] continue funding the VSD system;[66] and refrain from conducting VU randomized controlled trials of the safety of the vaccination program, including studies investigating the safety of alternative vaccination schedules.[67] The remaining two recommendations, which represent a modest degree of innovation, relate to implementation of the aforementioned "preliminary steps" to be completed before any study of the safety of the vaccine program begins. These steps include better defining and characterizing the key components of the vaccine program, vaccine adverse events, and susceptible population subgroups,[68] and "incorporating" the study of the overall safety of the childhood vaccine schedule into the Department of Health and Human Service's "processes for setting priorities for research."[69] Saliently missing are recommendations for studies actually assessing the safety of the vaccine program and the setting of a binding time schedule.

Thus, with a stroke of bureaucratic genius the committee fulfills its mission by burying VU studies under layer upon layer of red tape. The vaccine establishment got exactly what it paid for when commissioning the IOM committee: an official and "scientific" excuse to keep dragging its feet, to stand firm in the steadfast refusal to perform elementary studies that could potentially demonstrate the safety of the vaccine program.

Will Never Be Done: The Real Reason

How can we explain the bewildering attitude of both the medical establishment and the IOM 2013 committee toward VU studies? What possible reason could they have to prevent research that would advance the understanding of pressing medical issues, that is ethically, methodologically, and economically feasible, and that is demanded by an ever-growing number of parents? Why, in the face of increasing parental criticism and reluctance to vaccinate their children, are they not conducting the very studies that could alleviate parents' concerns? And why on earth aren't they performing the studies that could provide concrete scientific proof of the vaunted safety of the vaccine program?

As we have seen, there is no real obstacle to conducting VU studies. There are no valid ethical or economic objections, there is no shortage of unvaccinated children, there are no technical or scientific limitations, and there is no doubt that the results – whatever they may be – would advance the scientific understanding of vaccine safety and chronic disease which is so obviously lacking.

So why, then, have VU studies never been conducted?

Well, the most plausible explanation is that these studies have been done, unofficially, numerous times, but their results have not been made public.

It is inconceivable that informal VU studies have never been conducted. Computerized medical records have been around for years. In fact, many vaccine studies have made use of the information stored in such databases while exploring research questions closely related to the ones that are not being asked. One such example is the Glanz 2013 study mentioned earlier in the chapter, which used the VSD system to explore potential correlations between delaying vaccination and various health parameters.[70] A study by Zerbo and colleagues also used VSD data to analyze the vaccination patterns of children diagnosed with autism and their younger siblings.[71] A pair of 2001 studies, led by our old friend Frank DeStefano of the CDC, examined the rates of asthma and type 1 diabetes in children who were partially vaccinated. Like Glanz and Zerbo, DeStefano and his team examined records from the VSD system. As the IOM committee noted, over 1% of the children in the VSD system are completely unvaccinated.[72]

Since this information has been accessible for many years and since parental vaccine-safety concerns have been keeping establishment officials busy for at least the past two decades, it is inconceivable that health agency epidemiologists have not informally compared the health outcomes of vaccinated and unvaccinated children. The medical establishment can be blamed for many things but irrational behavior is not one of them. Assigning a CDC researcher, for example, the task of quietly checking what the data showed on such a hot topic, would be a "no-brainer" for vaccine policy makers.

If these internal VU studies were indeed quietly performed, as seems very likely, why weren't they published? After all, the end goal for any researcher is to make their work known to the public. There can be only one explanation: **The results were markedly in favor of the unvaccinated**. Dozens of epidemiological studies supporting the efficacy and safety of vaccines are published every year, but none are VU studies, despite the fact that a VU study that demonstrated superior overall health in the vaccinated would provide the ultimate vindication for the vaccine program. If those informal VU studies showed a positive result for vaccines, they would have been published faster than you can say "vaccines are safe and effective!" – no doubt about it. Moreover, the fact that such a study has never been published probably means that these studies found that the health of the unvaccinated was considerably better than that of their vaccinated peers. The gap, it would seem, is too wide to be closed even with "cooked" epidemiological research such as the purposely biased epidemiological studies described in the previous chapter.

This conclusion may seem too far-fetched or harsh to some. But in light of the health establishment's consistent and long-standing refusal to conduct VU studies when the data is right in front of them, it seems the only reasonable explanation.

Counter Arguments

"Vaccinated vs. unvaccinated studies have already been done!" – There have been several disingenuous attempts, mainly by so-called science bloggers on the internet, to convince the public that VU studies of overall health, autism, or other chronic conditions have been already done. Yet the IOM 2013 report "debunks" these claims by explicitly stating that such studies have never been conducted. Read more about this in the chapter's *Formal Admission* section.

"The health authorities are not aware of the need for VU studies." – Parents' request for a VU study goes back at least 25 years. In the 2000s, this demand was publicly raised time and time again. In 2007, a Congressional bill (that failed to pass and has been introduced several times since) was proposed requiring the US DHHS to conduct a VU study. In addition, this request has been repeatedly documented in mainstream studies of parental concerns about vaccines. More on the subject in *The Vaccine Establishment Avoids Conducting VU Studies* section.

"There is no real need to investigate the safety of the entire vaccine program. It is sufficient to establish the safety of individual vaccines." – Safety studies of individual vaccines rarely report chronic conditions that develop over an extended period of time. In addition, because these studies do not include a completely unvaccinated group, they do not and cannot discover the cumulative health effects of the administration of numerous vaccines over time, nor the potential cross-reactions of multiple vaccines. See more information in the *Vaccinated vs. Unvaccinated (VU) Studies* section. In addition, see chapter 1 for details on vaccine pre-licensure safety testing.

"Vaccinated vs. unvaccinated studies are unethical and therefore cannot be performed. Children cannot be deprived of vaccines and parents cannot be coerced into vaccinating their kids." – An RCT consisting of children randomly assigned to vaccinated and unvaccinated groups would indeed violate the medical code of ethics. However, conducting other types of studies would not violate ethical guidelines, and health authorities know it. These include prospective and retrospective observational studies, as well as RCTs examining different vaccination schedules. More about this in the *Is It Really Impossible to Conduct VU Studies?* section.

"Vaccinated vs. unvaccinated studies cannot be performed because there is no applicable definition for the term 'overall health'." – Defining a numerical measure or index of overall health for use in a VU study is quite feasible. This index may be calculated by combining relevant health-related statistics, such as number of doctor visits, hospitalization days, emergency room visits, life-threatening conditions, and chronic and disability conditions. This information has been available for many years in medical data banks and several vaccine-related studies have already made use of it. See also in the *Is It Really Impossible to Conduct VU Studies?* section.

"Vaccinated vs. unvaccinated studies cannot be performed because there are not enough unvaccinated children out there." – According to the CDC, there are at least 30,000 unvaccinated children in every US birth cohort. Moreover, according to the IOM more than 1% of the children tracked in the VSD system, which is run by the CDC, are completely unvaccinated. More about this in the *Is It Really Impossible to Conduct VU Studies?* section.

"Vaccinated vs. unvaccinated study results would not be of scientific value because unvaccinated children also tend to have a more 'natural' lifestyle." – Because the number of unvaccinated children is relatively large (see above), a VU study could select an unvaccinated group diverse enough for research purposes. By using standard epidemiological analytical methods, the preliminary results of a VU study could be further stratified in order to neutralize the effect of any confounding factors. Regardless, a VU study would be very likely to enhance scientific understanding of the health conditions investigated. See more in the *Is It Really Impossible to Conduct VU Studies?* section.

"The Amish population is very different in its genetic and environmental characteristics; therefore, a VU study comparing Amish children to the rest of the population would not yield meaningful results." – On the contrary, studying a genetically different subpopulation that practices a unique lifestyle could be very helpful in unravelling the autism mystery. Interestingly enough, a 2017 study published in the journal *Pediatrics* examined the incidence of vaccine-preventable diseases among Amish and non-Amish children living in the same geographical area. The study examined and compared, among other things, the subjects' vaccination status.[73] It seems, then, that a comparative study examining health aspects and vaccination status of Amish children is fine as long as it deals with "allowed" areas of research (infectious diseases) rather than "forbidden" ones (autism and chronic illness).

"Unvaccinated children benefit from the disappearance of vaccine-preventable diseases, thanks to vaccines and the vaccinated. Therefore, a vaccinated vs. unvaccinated study would show biased results." – This claim carries the implicit assumption that a VU study would indicate that unvaccinated kids are healthier. Without a VU study one cannot evaluate the benefit of the vaccination program. The current mantra of the vaccine establishment is that children should get vaccinated to protect their health. If a VU study found that the unvaccinated were healthier than their vaccinated counterparts, that would compel reevaluation of vaccine policy in order to maximize the health of children.

Additionally, even if the results were biased with respect to some infectious diseases, that would be irrelevant when it comes to chronic conditions such as autism. Vaccination cannot provide any protection from those to the unvaccinated. More about this in the *Is It Really Impossible to Conduct VU Studies?* section.

Summary

"The studies that have never been done" is one of the weakest points in the fortress that the medical establishment has built around vaccine dogma. It highlights the wide gap between the establishment's overwrought safety claims and the reality: the (meager) scientific evidence which support these claims and the straightforward and crucial research that has not been done to prove them.

In stark contrast to the (apparently unofficial) message of the medical establishment that the current vaccine schedule has been thoroughly investigated and reviewed and was found to be the best available, the schedule as a whole has never been properly studied for safety or efficacy. The major features of the program were also never investigated, as the IOM 2013 committee attests. Although numerous vaccines have been added to the childhood schedule over the past 30 years, no studies have ever explored the ramifications of the growing number of vaccinations an infant receives, the age at which they are administered, the frequency and order in which they are given, their effect on susceptible subpopulations, or other key aspects of the schedule.

The pre-licensure vaccine approval process does not evaluate the impact a new vaccine may have on the long-term health of the vaccinee. Clinical trials and post-marketing studies target either an individual vaccine, a specific component of a vaccine, or, at most, one or two additional vaccines administered on the same day. Studies examining the long-term and cumulative effect of routine vaccinations on the health of the vaccinated have never been done by the medical establishment.

Given this lack of supporting science, affirmed by the IOM 2013, anyone claiming that the current vaccine program was tested and found to be the best there is being blatantly deceptive.

Without science-based evidence regarding the health impact of the vaccine program as a whole, health authorities have no real answer to the concerns raised by parents. They can present no solid evidence to refute the hypothesis linking the increase in the number of routine vaccinations to the recent huge rise in the incidence of numerous chronic conditions in industrialized countries. Inexplicably, the vaccine establishment, which vehemently denies this link, has chosen not to conduct those studies that could either confirm or refute it. Despite increasing public pressure from parents, advocacy groups, doctors, and politicians, the establishment stands firm and continues to ignore repeated requests to perform VU studies. This lack of action becomes even more indefensible considering that a credible VU study showing that children vaccinated according to the recommended schedule are healthier than unvaccinated children – as it should, if the program is indeed safe – would likely be instrumental in alleviating parents' concerns.

After many years of inaction, US medical authorities belatedly launched an IOM investigation to examine the issue of the studies that have never been done. The committee's report enumerates the ostensible reasons why studies evaluating the purported health benefits of the vaccine program cannot be conducted. Contradictions, circular claims, unsubstantiated claims, and other baffling assertions abound in the IOM report. Its main theme is that VU studies are not feasible for ethical, economic, and technical reasons, ignoring the fact that similar studies utilizing computerized medical data have been repeatedly conducted for at least two decades. Browsing through the report's 237 pages, it becomes evident the committee's agenda was political, rather than scientific. The committee was tasked with providing the medical establishment with a formal scientific stamp of approval to continue its policy of passivity and inaction with respect to studying the safety of the vaccination program as a whole – and so it did.

There can be no legitimate reason for the establishment's steadfast inaction when so many other vaccine studies are continuously published, including many exploring "parental concerns" and "vaccine-related communication between parents and health providers." In light of the establishment's seemingly inexplicable position on the subject, and considering what we already know about the reality of vaccine safety science from previous chapters, there is only one logical conclusion: VU studies are not being done because the outcome is already known. The vaccine establishment is well aware that these studies would demonstrate to the public that the overall health of unvaccinated children is superior to that of the vaccinated (especially with respect to chronic medical conditions). Findings such as these would imply that vaccines are the main culprit behind the astronomical rise in chronic health conditions in children of the developed world and would likely cause a social and political upheaval of unprecedented proportions, both in the United States and around the globe.

The IOM 2013 report was intended to justify the establishment's policy of not investigating the vaccine program as a whole. Instead, the report exposed the absence of a reasonable rationale for not carrying out the missing research. But more importantly, the report provided formal, institutionally approved evidence for the claim that the effectiveness and safety of the entire vaccination program have never been studied.

At the end of the day, the medical establishment may continue to successfully avoid conducting VU studies till the end of time. But as long as these studies are not done the claim that the "vaccine program is safe and effective" will have zero scientific validity. Additionally, medical science will not have – even after decades of vaccine research – an answer to the most basic question every parent should be asking: "Will vaccination make my child healthier or sicker?"

Ask your doctor:

• Are you familiar with any medical study that compared the overall health of vaccinated children to that of unvaccinated children?

• In the absence of studies comparing the overall health of vaccinated vs. unvaccinated children, what is the scientific evidence for the safety and benefit of the vaccine program?

• In the absence of a study comparing the overall health of children who vaccinated according to the official schedule to that of children who received no vaccines, would you still tell parents their children are better off getting all routine vaccinations? If so, on what grounds?

7

UNSUBSTANTIATED VACCINATION GUIDELINES

"Doctor, aren't seven shots in one visit too many for my baby? I'm not sure he can handle all of these vaccines together."

"Well, you shouldn't worry too much about it, Ms. Davies. These vaccines have been tested in dozens of studies, I can assure you. All were found to be completely safe."

"I don't know … It just seems so much for such a tiny body. How many diseases are you vaccinating him for? Is it ten?"

"Ten is really nothing, trust me. Your baby's immune system handles thousands of viruses and such every time he's out in your backyard. It's scientifically proven that a baby's body can easily handle 10,000 vaccines in a day."

"How about we spread out his vaccines anyway, doctor? He'll get one per visit. What do you think?"

"Well, I don't know, Ms. Davies. Do you really want to come here six or seven times? We can do all of them right now, and he'll be protected from all of these deadly diseases. You know, studies have shown that spreading vaccines out does not decrease the side effects. And those are negligible, anyway. If you delay some of the vaccines, your child will be unprotected for quite some time, and for no good reason. I really can't recommend it."

As the previous chapters demonstrate, there is a wide chasm between what the public is told about vaccine safety and the reality of the matter. Every day it seems, some establishment spokesperson or another beats the "vaccines have been tested in thousands of studies and their safety has proven beyond a shadow of doubt" drum. But these oft-repeated claims are not based on scientific evidence: The science demonstrating the safety of individual childhood vaccines is completely inadequate, health authorities are deliberately avoiding doing crucial vaccine safety studies, vaccine adverse event monitoring systems are flawed by design, and no vaccine program has ever been tested for safety as a whole.

This chapter illuminates yet another aspect of the disturbing gap between the institutional assertion that vaccines are safe, and the scientific basis on which it is ostensibly founded.

Health authorities around the world proclaim that children should be vaccinated according to the routine childhood schedule in their respective countries. Official guidelines dictate the specific vaccines that the child should receive at each doctor's appointment and at what age these appointments should take place. Parents are urged to adhere to the official timeline and make sure their children receive all the recommended vaccines. Despite institutional pressure to stick to these official recommendations – or perhaps because of it – many parents feel the guidelines are not always compatible with the well-being of their child. For example, some parents tend to break up the multiple vaccines scheduled for a single appointment and spread them out over time so as not to overburden their child's immune system. Others may wish to postpone vaccines if their child is not feeling well. These tendencies, which are usually based on intuition and common sense, run counter to official guidelines and often lead to head-to-head confrontations with pediatricians. Medical professionals, as depicted in the imaginary, yet realistic, dialogue at the beginning of the chapter, tend to endorse vaccines and are likely to vehemently discourage any deviation from the official guidelines. With all due respect for parental intuition and "gut feelings", they may say, important medical decisions should be based on sound science and official recommendations. At this point, given the unequivocal recommendation of the doctor, purportedly backed by science and the medical profession in general, many parents will likely proceed to vaccinate their children on schedule despite their apprehensions and concerns.

But should they? Are parents doing the right thing when they cast their doubts aside and comply with their doctors' advice? Do official vaccination guidelines always rely on solid scientific evidence, as physicians frequently tell anxious parents? To answer these questions this chapter will explore the scientific evidence for some common practices advocated by health authorities: Administering multiple vaccines in a single appointment, spacing out vaccines, and vaccinating a baby with a mild illness.

Multiple Vaccines in a Single Visit

Over the past several decades, the number of vaccines on the recommended childhood vaccination schedule has greatly increased.[a] Thus, while vaccine-related well-baby visits have become more frequent, the number of vaccines given at each appointment has also increased. According to the US vaccine schedule an infant can receive up to 9 vaccines against 13 different diseases in a single doctor appointment.[1]

As we saw in chapter 1, every new vaccine must undergo a series of clinical trials to test its safety and efficacy before it is approved for use.[b] It is important to remember, though, that testing the new vaccine by itself is not sufficient, as in most cases it will be administered with several other vaccines at the same

---

[a] As of June 2021, the typical American infant receives 26 vaccine doses against 14 diseases by age two.

[b] Recall that pre-licensure trials are specifically designed to obscure the true adverse event rate of the new vaccine.

doctor visit. Therefore, a vaccine pre-licensure safety trial should also examine the effects of administering the new vaccine along with the other vaccines recommended for the same visit according to the national schedule. The rationale for this is straightforward: Every vaccine contains potent substances whose combined effects on an infant's body cannot be fully anticipated and must therefore be thoroughly tested before it is approved for use. Co-administration of multiple vaccines only magnifies this uncertainty as the number and variety of foreign substances, as well as the ways those substances can interact, are increased. Combining several vaccines could potentially cause serious side effects and even impair the effectiveness of one or more of the individual vaccines. This is not fundamentally different from the need to test the cross-reactivity of multiple therapeutic drugs administered at the same time; such cross-reactivity is responsible, according to various studies, for a significant share of drug adverse events.[2] The requirement for preliminary testing of vaccine combinations is acknowledged, at least theoretically, by health authorities. The CDC website, for one, explicitly states that "[…] when every new vaccine is licensed, it has been tested along with the vaccines already recommended for a particular aged child."[3]

How could a pre-licensure clinical trial test the safety of a new vaccine along with other vaccines scheduled to be given on the same day? One such trial design could involve four different groups: The first group would receive all of the vaccines on the same day, the second just one vaccine per appointment, with a month or so between appointments. The third and fourth groups would receive placebos, mirroring the first and second group, respectively.[c] Adverse events would be monitored up to several

---

[c] Slightly delaying vaccination for the last three groups is ethically acceptable. One example of such a design is this trial:

http://www.ncbi.nlm.nih.gov/pubmed/16567978.

Additionally, children are vaccinated on "delayed" schedules anyway in some countries. For example, in the United Kingdom only 3 doses of the DTaP-equivalent vaccine are given in the first 18 months of life (at 2, 3, and 4 months

months following the last vaccination appointment. After the conclusion of the follow-up period, adverse event rates between the different groups could be compared in order to determine the safety profiles of administering the vaccines at the same time vs. spacing them out.

Untested Vaccine Combinations

The CDC, as we have seen, acknowledges that a new vaccine should be tested along with the vaccines with which it is to be given according to the schedule. But does the CDC consistently enforce its own policy?

As of this writing, the CDC website maintains that "a number of studies" have been conducted to test vaccine combinations, but it does not list which of the vaccine combinations on the US childhood vaccine schedule have been so tested. A World Health Organization document states that vaccine combinations have been studied for "many years" before and after licensing, including "concomitant use studies". However, it too does not specify exactly how and when these combinations were actually tested.[4] Instead, it refers the reader to a 2002 article by Offit and colleagues which aims to provide answers to common parental vaccination concerns. This article argues that administering multiple vaccines in one day does not "overwhelm or weaken the immune system", since studies have shown that concurrent administration of vaccines does not produce a "lesser immune response".[5] That, however, is an efficacy argument, and the safety of concurrent vaccinations is not directly addressed by the authors. Similar to the WHO document that referenced their paper, Offit et al. refer the inquisitive reader to yet another paper, this time a 1994 review by King and Hadler of the CDC's National Immunization Program.[6] King and Hadler performed a comprehensive review of studies testing the combinations of

---

of age), compared with 4 doses in the US. The fourth dose in the UK is given at age three.

vaccines used in the United States in the early 1990s. Alas, since the review's publication, several vaccines have been added to the schedule[d] and others have been replaced with newer versions.[e] Thus, it is now largely outdated, as most of the vaccine products and combinations it covers were discontinued years ago.

It seems, therefore, that neither the WHO nor the CDC is aware of any timely and comprehensive safety assessment for the vaccine combinations currently recommended on the US childhood vaccine schedule. The most comprehensive review they cite, possibly the only one in existence, was published more than 25 years ago and does not cover most of the vaccine combinations given today. More up-to-date information doesn't appear to be available. With no official record of the safety testing of current vaccine combinations, to determine what testing has actually been done, one must scan the medical literature for each of the individual combinations in use and find the studies performed for each of the individual products.

Let's consider, for example, the vaccines an American 15-month old might receive according to the schedule. According to the CDC,[7] at 15 months a child could receive as many as 9 shots for 13 diseases.[f] (Different combinations of vaccine products exist for the applicable diseases, so the number of shots may vary between 5 and 9). A search of the medical literature failed to find any published report of a clinical trial, or even a retrospective study, which looked at the safety of concurrently administering this combination of vaccines.

Thus, in stark contrast to its own assertion that new vaccines are tested with the vaccines that are administered at the same time, the CDC's recommended schedule includes vaccine combinations whose safety has never been tested. Vaccinating with

---

[d] Vaccines added to the routine program in the United States since 1994 include hepatitis A, Prevnar and Prevnar 13, rotavirus, and varicella (chickenpox).

[e] The whole-cell DTP vaccine has been replaced by the acellular vaccine (DTaP).

[f] The 13 diseases are hepatitis B, diphtheria, tetanus, pertussis, Hib, pneumococcal, polio, influenza, measles, mumps, rubella, varicella, and hepatitis A.

this approved combination of shots effectively enrolls American infants in a large-scale vaccine trial without their parents' consent or awareness. Actually, using the term trial here is generous, as the results of this "experiment" are not tabulated and will never be published. Does the concurrent administration of 9 shots against 13 diseases increase, perhaps, the risk of neurological disorders or autoimmune diseases? Neither the CDC nor any other health agency can provide a reliable answer to this question. The CDC's ineptitude, or perhaps negligence, on this matter is aggravated by its inability to monitor the adverse events of these vaccine combinations effectively (see discussion in chapter 3).

Despite the evident lack of research on the potential side effects of recommended vaccine combinations, representatives of the health establishment continue to repeat the institutional mantra that these combinations have been thoroughly tested and found to be safe and effective.

Spacing Out Vaccinations

The lack of science supporting the safety of recommended vaccine combinations has implications for another crucial vaccination decision that many parents struggle with: to space out or not to space out?

A reasonable argument could be made against splitting the administration of a combined vaccine into several different injections. For example, one might argue that splitting the DTaP-polio-hepB vaccine into three separate shots[g] would challenge the vaccinated infant with roughly triple the amount of foreign substances. However, spacing out multiple injections over the span of several doctor appointments, rather than giving all of them at once, would not present this dilemma, as the exact same

---

[g] The DTaP-polio-hepB vaccine can be divided into three separate injections: diphtheria-tetanus-pertussis vaccine (DTaP), inactivated polio vaccine (IPV) and hepatitis B vaccine.

shots would be given, just at different times.

Many parents intuitively feel it is healthier for their baby to receive one vaccine per visit rather than multiple shots. When they express these concerns, however, they typically encounter the definitive declaration that spacing out shots has absolutely no benefit.[8] Separating vaccines in time, a medical practitioner will say, has been thoroughly tested and does not reduce the number or severity of adverse events. On the contrary, they might add, administering multiple vaccines during the same visit may even be better for your child, as common side effects caused by vaccine injection – fever, for example – would occur just once.

Spacing out shots increases the likelihood that infants will not (eventually) get all the recommended doses of all the recommended vaccines, so it make sense for health authorities to discourage this practice. But what about its safety implications? Is there solid science backing the institutional assertion that spacing out vaccines doesn't reduce side effects when compared with concurrent administration?

The concern shared by many parents that receiving multiple vaccines in a single visit can cause serious health damage, comes from life experience and cannot be dismissed out of hand. It is not unreasonable to assume that overburdening the body, and especially that of an infant, can lead to severe damage. We are all familiar with real-life examples. Carrying a 60-pound box up the stairs is arguably more likely to injure one's back than making the trip four times, each with a 15-pound box. Similarly, a single marathon strains a runner's body much more than running 5k races on 10 consecutive Sundays. A baby who is down with the flu and diarrhea is likely to be considerably sicker than a child with just one of those conditions. Similarly, the body of an infant receiving three concurrent vaccine injections absorbs a threefold dose of foreign substances. The probability of an acute reaction in this scenario is likely to be higher than getting three shots separated in time, which would give an infant's body at least a month to recover between injections.

As already shown, some of the combinations of vaccines given in the United States and many other industrialized countries have never been tested for safety. Hence, reliable information regarding the benefits (or lack thereof) of spacing out recommended vaccines over multiple doctor visits is virtually nonexistent. Therefore, the prevalent claim that spacing out vaccinations does not reduce side effects is not based on sound evidence but, perhaps, on the "gut feeling" of the medical establishment. If the establishment wishes to pacify parental concerns that are rooted in common sense and life experience, it had better provide proper scientific evidence to back up its claims.

The Shneyer 2009 Study

It is difficult to reconcile the medical establishment's claim that the vaccine schedule has been thoroughly tested and found to be safe with the apparent lack of scientific evidence to support it. The case of the Shneyer 2009 study further exemplifies the gulf between the health establishment's solemn public declarations that they are doing everything possible to ensure vaccines are safe, and what is really being done.

Elena Shneyer and colleagues[9] at the School of Public Health at the University of Haifa, Israel, compared the safety of administering the MMR and pentavalent[h] vaccines at the same time to administering them on separate occasions.[i] The researchers initiated the study following unsolicited reports from one of Israel's health districts. Nurses from well-baby clinics in that district reported that the rate of adverse events following the combined administration of the two vaccines was substantially higher than when babies were given one per visit.[10] The researchers took advantage of the fact that some children received

---

[h] The pentavalent vaccine is a 5-in-1 shot against diphtheria, tetanus, pertussis, polio and haemophilus Influenzae type b.

[i] The study was conducted in 2004–2005 before the Prevnar vaccine was added to the vaccine program in Israel. At the time, Israeli infants received the MMR and the pentavalent vaccines at 12 months.

both vaccines on schedule (age 12 months), while others received the MMR on time but had to get the fourth dose of the pentavalent vaccine at a later date.[j] At the time of its publication in 2009, this study was the only one investigating the safety of concurrent administration of the MMR and pentavalent vaccines, which are given together to children in Israel as well as in other countries.[k]

Shneyer and colleagues decided on a prospective study design. They followed 102 children who were simultaneously vaccinated with both vaccines and 74 children who were vaccinated at different times.[11] The rate of adverse events in the first group turned out to be 50% higher than in the second group.[12] This significant finding led the researchers to suggest that the Israeli vaccination schedule be modified in order to reduce side effects: "In this study it was demonstrated that the rate of adverse effects in the separately vaccinated group was significantly lower than in the simultaneously vaccinated group. The results of this study do not support the national recommendation of simultaneous vaccinations of MMR and DTaP-Hib-IPV [the pentavalent vaccine]. Rather, our data call for reconsideration of the current policy of simultaneous injections of MMR and DTaP-Hib-IPV – at least until a larger study is conducted."[13]

Shneyer 2009 is a small observational study[l] and on its own cannot be regarded as an unequivocal proof of the benefit of splitting up vaccine combinations into separate visits, or even dividing this particular vaccine pair. However, its results should

---

[j] The fourth dose of the pentavalent vaccine must be given at least six months after the third dose. If a child is late getting the third dose (scheduled at 6 months), the fourth dose also has to be delayed.

[k] The package insert of GSK's pentavalent vaccine states that this combination has never been tested. Since the Shneyer 2009 paper was not widely publicized outside of Israel, it is likely that the authors of the insert were not familiar with it.

[l] Although, as a prospective study, in which researchers select study participants before collecting the data on adverse events, Shneyer 2009's design is superior to the retrospective study design that is more common in vaccine safety research.

not be ignored, either, as was the case. It's been over a decade since the publication of Shneyer 2009, and even though it created a notable media stir at the time,[14] the Israeli Ministry of Health seems to have ignored it completely: It did not initiate follow-up studies, nor did it mention the study's results or conclusions in any of its formal publications. Needless to say, neither did the CDC nor any other international health agency. Epidemiological studies such as Shneyer 2009 are relatively inexpensive and straightforward to perform. It is difficult to explain why the Israeli Ministry of Health, and other health agencies around the world, which regularly proclaim their commitment to maintaining the safety of the vaccination schedule, would neglect to conduct subsequent studies looking into the safety of combining these two injections.[m] It seems that the authorities prefer having (almost) no safety science to having appropriate science reporting the "wrong" results.

10,000 Vaccines in One Day

The practice of administering multiple shots on the same day raises another important question: Is there an upper limit to the number of vaccines an infant should receive in one day? How many vaccines, against how many diseases, can be safely administered to a child during a single visit to the pediatrician?

As surprising as it may seem, according to the website of the Immunization Action Coalition (IAC), a nonprofit organization that collaborates with the CDC to promote vaccination, there is no such limit. The coalition's site bluntly declares that "there is no upper limit for the number of vaccines that can be administered during one visit."[15] No opposing statement can be found on the CDC website or those of other national or international health agencies. The lack of such a guideline implies that an

---

[m] Since the late 2000s, children in Israel and many other countries routinely receive yet another vaccine (Prevnar) at their 12-month visit, making this issue even more crucial.

infant could theoretically receive any number of shots against any number of diseases – be it 5, 10, or 20 – at any one time.[n]

The medical establishment's supposition that there is no upper limit to the number of vaccines that can be simultaneously administered is as nonsensical as it is unscientific. It has never been clinically tested or otherwise proven, since injecting infants with an increasing number of vaccines simply for the sake of identifying their maximal tolerance level would be both scientifically unethical and immoral.

While there is no science backing the idea that there is no limit to the number of vaccines a child can safely receive, some vaccine proponents have repeatedly referred to it as a proven fact. According to this view, "a baby's immune system could handle as many as 10,000 vaccines" (and some even raise the bar to 100,000 vaccines at the same time).[16] The most vocal proponent of this claim is Dr. Paul Offit, a vaccine expert at the Children's Hospital of Philadelphia and the co-inventor of a rotavirus vaccine. In a 2002 article meant to provide an institutional response to parents' vaccination concerns, Offit and colleagues wrote: "Each infant would have the theoretical capacity to respond to about 10,000 vaccines at any one time."[17] Although this statement by Offit and colleagues runs contrary to common sense and seems to be using the term "vaccines" misleadingly (as will be shown below), it is often repeated and presented as a scientifically proven fact by health organizations around the world.[18]

As it turns out, the presumed safety of giving an infant "up to 10,000 vaccines at one time" is not founded on vaccine science at all. Rather, it is based on a theoretical assumption as to the number of organisms (bacteria, viruses, etc.) to which the infant's immune system can respond at any given time.[19] And this assumption, in turn, is based merely on theoretical computations involving various immune system parameters and has no physio-

---

[n] The practical limit is the number of vaccines currently approved for use, with very few restrictions on specific vaccine combinations.

logical evidence to back it up.

Furthermore, the leap from "10,000 organisms to which the immune system could respond to" to "10,000 vaccines an infant can tolerate" is fundamentally flawed, as it rests on the erroneous assumption that a bacterium or virus is somehow equivalent to a vaccine. It may have made sense, in the context of this discussion, to equate a live organism to a weakened or inactivated vaccine antigen, but not to a vaccine in its entirety. As you may recall from the chapter 5 discussion of the DeStefano 2013 paper (which also advantageously blurred the distinction between vaccine and antigen), the antigen is the specific vaccine component, typically a weakened bacterium or virus, whose job is to trigger an immune response that will confer protection against the real disease. However, in addition to the antigen every vaccine contains many other potent substances whose effects on the body are not fully understood and are, thus, potentially harmful. Thus, for example, the DTaP-Ipv-Hib vaccine includes the following list of ingredients (besides the antigens for the five diseases against which the vaccine protects):

> lactose, sodium chloride, aluminum adjuvant (as aluminum salts), Medium 199 (as stabilizer including amino acids, mineral salts and vitamins) and water for injection, residual formaldehyde, polysorbate 80, potassium chloride, disodium phosphate, monopotassium phosphate, glycine, and trace amounts of neomycin sulphate and polymyxin B sulphate.[20]

It follows, then, that the terms vaccine and antigen are not interchangeable when discussing vaccine safety. Thus, transforming the theoretical assertion that "the immune system can simultaneously respond to 10,000 organisms" to the practical rule-of-thumb that "an infant can tolerate 10,000 vaccines" is both scientifically unfounded and misleading. There's no logical reason to assume that an infant, or even an adult, could handle the concurrent administration of ten vaccines without significant harm, let alone a hundred or a thousand of them.

Is the immune system capable of responding to 10,000 antigens simultaneously? Neither Dr. Offit nor any other scientist has managed to conclusively prove this claim, even if it does have some theoretical computational merit. But publicly proclaiming that giving infants 10,000 vaccines at the same time would pose no health risk, while knowing full well this claim has no evidential or even theoretical basis, is outrageously deceptive and dangerous.

Vaccinating a Baby with a Mild Illness

Vaccinating an infant with a "mild" illness – such as a cold, low fever, stomachache, or ear infection° – is yet another vaccination guideline that seems to defy common sense for some parents. Many believe it is best to wait until full recovery before stressing the child further with their scheduled vaccines. A round of vaccines, they fear, could exacerbate the child's illness or cause worse side effects compared to vaccinating a fully healthy child.

Yet this parental concern, too, is generally met with a decisive negation by the vaccine establishment, which asserts that a mild illness should not prevent routine vaccination. An official guideline document from the CDC and the American Academy of Pediatrics states that "vaccines are safe and effective when given to children with mild illness" and that "vaccines do not make a mild illness worse,"[21] and most medical professionals take the truth of these statements for granted.

Why does the medical establishment insist on vaccinating infants who are physically unwell? The likely explanation seems to be apprehension that delaying vaccinations to a time when a child is fully healthy may disrupt their vaccination timeline and leave them vulnerable to diseases from which they could have been protected.[22] The underlying assumption is that infants are

---

° Vaccination during an acute illness is not recommended by health authorities.

frequently ill during their first year of life, so fitting vaccination rounds into "full-health" windows may prove to be impractical.

Thus, the health establishment emphasizes the importance of timely vaccination and resolutely dismisses parents' fear of increased risk when vaccinating a sick child. Once again, however, it is reasonable to ask for the scientific evidence underlying this counterintuitive guideline. Is it founded on robust scientific evidence, or could it too stem from an institutional "gut feeling" or administrative whim?

The official guidelines from the CDC and AAP (mentioned above) do not provide any medical references supporting the recommendation to vaccinate mildly ill children on time. Browsing the CDC website, as well as those of other leading health agencies, also failed to locate backing evidence. Finally, a thorough search of the medical literature did return a single-page paper in the form of a Q&A that reviewed the scientific knowledge on the subject at the time it was published in 2011 in *Paediatrics & Child Health*.[23] The paper was written by experts from the Vaccine Evaluation Centre at the BC Children's Hospital in Vancouver, Canada. The authors scanned the scientific literature for "evidence that minor illnesses are not a contraindication to most vaccinations"[24] and found that the research base on this topic was extremely poor. Discussing inactivated vaccines, the authors note that "no publication in recent decades has assessed administering inactivated vaccines to mildly sick children."[25] As for attenuated (live) vaccines, the authors mention a handful of studies of only one (MMR) of the three live vaccines on the American vaccine schedule.[p] Further examination of the cited papers on the MMR reveals that all but one looked exclusively into efficacy aspects of vaccination during mild illness, and not into safety.[q] The sole study examining the safety of the MMR

---

[p] Three live attenuated vaccines are currently included in the US vaccination program: rotavirus, MMR, and varicella. There are currently two different products available for each of them.

[q] One reference leads to a CDC document that includes additional references to studies conducted on the measles vaccine, rather than the MMR vaccine.

in children with mild illness was comprised of only 157 children[26] and, according to one critic, was of somewhat low quality.[27]

Surprisingly, although their comprehensive review of the medical literature yielded only one small study of just a single vaccine that investigated the safety of vaccinating infants with a mild illness, the authors conclude the review by stating, "In summary, the health care provider should be reassured that mild illness is not a reason to delay routine vaccination. Many good-quality studies have provided strong support for the recommendation."[28]

Offit and colleagues, authors of the aforementioned 2002 article on parental concerns, also devote a paragraph to vaccination during mild illness, asserting that it is safe and effective.[29] To back up their claim they cite four studies: Two only examined the MMR vaccine (also mentioned in the Canadian 2011 Q&A article discussed above), and the remaining two investigated the single measles vaccine which has not been available in the US since 2009.

Thus, a search of the medical literature reveals that the institutional recommendation of vaccinating infants with a mild illness, whether with a specific vaccine or a combination of vaccines, is not evidence-based. With the exception of one weak study of the MMR vaccine, no studies have investigated whether vaccinating mildly ill infants increases the risk of serious side effects, exacerbates the severity of the illness, or prolongs its duration.

Counter Arguments

"There is no reason to believe that administering multiple vaccines in one day can exacerbate vaccination side effects." – When dealing with a medical intervention that is recommended for all infants there is no room for speculation or assumptions. The safety of a universally applied medical procedure must be robustly proven prior to its approval, and even more so if the intended recipients are healthy infants. The CDC itself understands this and (misleadingly) declares that each new vaccine has been tested along with the other vaccines that may be concomitantly administered according to their recommended vaccine schedule.[30]

"It isn't feasible to test all possible vaccine combinations. The number of vaccines in the routine program is too great to test each vaccine along with any other vaccine." – This claim is theoretically correct if one refers to the maximal number of possible combinations of available childhood vaccines. In practice, however, the number of combinations to be tested in each country is limited by the (small) number of competing vaccine products (i.e., same vaccine from different vendors) and the specific vaccines recommended for a given age. In any case, administering vaccines in combinations that have never been tested is gambling with infants' lives. At a minimum, health authorities are ethically bound to share this information with parents and cease falsely declaring that these combinations have been tested and found safe.

"Combinations of vaccines do not need to be tested before approval. If any safety issues arise following routine use, they will be identified by the computerized systems monitoring vaccine adverse events and handled appropriately." – This claim implies that it's okay to approve new medical interventions for infants, or anyone else for that matter, without adequate testing as long as post-licensure injuries will be monitored by health authorities. That is as nonsensical as it is immoral and also contradicts the CDC's assurance that pre-licensure tests of vaccine combinations are performed. In addition, as described in chapter 3, current vaccine adverse event reporting systems in the United States and elsewhere cannot provide adequate real-time information regarding the true risks of combining vaccines.

"It is good enough to test just a partial vaccine combination. For

example, if three vaccines A, B, and C are given simultaneously, and the two combinations A+B and B+C have been tested, that is sufficient." – This is merely a speculative claim that has no scientific merit. It defies common sense, the precautionary principle, and the vast experience gleaned from the history of pharmaceutical drug use. The effect of a new ingredient added to a vaccine, or a new vaccine added to a vaccine combination given to infants, cannot be determined in advance and, therefore, must be thoroughly tested before approval. Deviating from this fundamental principle will likely result in colossal health disasters. Regardless, the CDC itself emphasizes the importance of such testing when it declares that every new vaccine has been tested along with the vaccines with which it is routinely administered.

"The practice of spacing out vaccines was studied, and it turns out it doesn't reduce the extent of side effects." – The research dedicated to the practice of spacing out vaccines is insufficient, at best. There are also studies, such as the Shneyer 2009 study discussed in this chapter, which found that spacing out vaccines did lower the rate of adverse events. As we already know, the safety of some combinations of vaccines routinely given in the United States and other countries has never been tested. Hence, there is no data on whether splitting up these combinations would or would not affect the rate of adverse events. It is worth adding that one cannot generalize about vaccine combinations. Each and every combination has to be studied on its own.

"The Shneyer 2009 study is not of high quality because it is only a 'survey' in which data was collected by means of telephone calls." – Data collection by telephone interviews is an established and common practice in prospective studies, and even in vaccine clinical trials.[31] If the Shneyer 2009 study were dismissed on the grounds of utilizing telephone interviews, many vaccine safety studies which are widely cited would have to be discarded as well. In any case, due to the importance of the study question, even if the research method Shneyer and her colleagues used were not optimal, that would not justify the complete disregard of the Israeli and international health agencies.

"Guidelines are not modified due to the results of one small study. Guidelines are set based on an extensive body of research." – That is theoretically correct. However, in the absence of an extensive body of research regarding childhood vaccine combinations, the findings of the only study (Shneyer 2009) that examined a common combination given at age 12 months should be taken very seriously, especially if it indicates a higher rate of side effects for the combination. There is, perhaps, no immediate reason to modify guidelines when such a study appears. However, its alarming results necessitates follow-up studies to further investigate and clarify the issue, something that has not been done to date.

"There are no studies showing that vaccinating a mildly ill baby can exacerbate vaccines' side effects, and there is also no known biological mechanism that might explain why this should happen." – When it comes to medical interventions given to all infants there is no room for speculation. General guidelines for medical interventions applied to healthy children must be strictly evidence-based. The safety of the practice of vaccinating infants during mild illness is virtually unstudied: Apparently, only one small, low-quality study for just a single vaccine has been conducted. Thus, the absence of scientific evidence of any harmful impact of this practice on vaccine side effects is hardly surprising. Given the distinct lack of research on this subject, the medical establishment should, at the very least, make it absolutely clear to parents that the recommendation to vaccinate mildly ill children is not based on scientific evidence.

"One vaccine that was studied and found to be safe for administration to infants that are mildly ill proves that vaccines in general are safe in similar circumstances. It is not necessary to test

all vaccines." – Each and every vaccine is uniquely constituted out of specific ingredients in particular amounts and is intended to have different effects on the body. Just as every new vaccine must be specifically tested in a clinical trial before it is approved for use, so the vaccine's effect on mildly ill children must be separately tested.

Summary

With the addition of numerous vaccines to the routine child-hood program in recent decades, simultaneous administration of multiple vaccines has become increasingly common. Nowadays, two or more vaccines are administered at most well-baby visits, and each vaccine contains a number of potent chemical and biological substances, some of which are known to be toxic or carcinogenic.

Although the CDC declares that vaccine combinations have been tested as part of the process of approving a new vaccine, in practice, most of them have not. Scientific research on the safety of simultaneous administration of multiple vaccines combinations is quite limited. An Israeli study found that the administration of two vaccines at the same time, as recommended by the Israeli Ministry of Health, increased the amount of side effects by 50%, yet this study was ignored by health agencies in Israel, the United States, and elsewhere. Nevertheless, the authorities continue to maintain, without adequate scientific proof, that administering multiple vaccines simultaneously poses no additional risk because "an infant's immune system can handle up to 10,000 vaccines at one time." In addition, they recommend vaccination of infants with mild illness, though the scientific evidence as to the safety of this practice is also virtually nonexistent.

Ask your doctor:

• Do you know of any studies that have examined the safety of the simultaneous administration of 9 vaccine injections against 13 different diseases to a 15-month year-old infant?

• Are you familiar with any studies that have shown that spacing out vaccines does not reduce the number and severity of side effects?

• Do you believe that administering 10,000 vaccines in one day to an infant is safe? If you do, can you provide studies that have demonstrated the safety of this procedure?

• Do you know of any studies that examined the safety of the recommendation to vaccinate infants with mild illness? If not, what is the scientific evidence on which the CDC relies in determining that this would not increase the risk for vaccine injury?

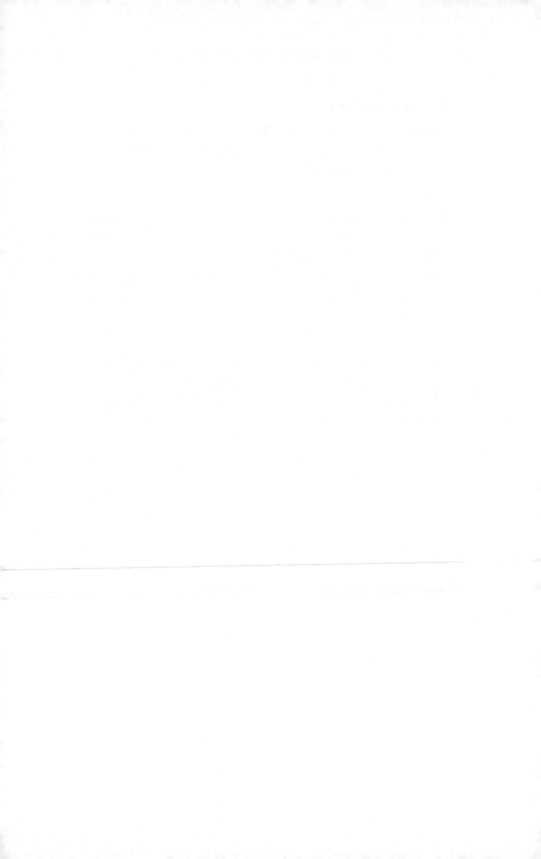

PART II

FOUNDING MYTHS

A myth is a semi-true story whose main purpose is to instill common beliefs and values in a group of people. Humans have utilized myths for their social ends for thousands of years, and even now they still play a central role in public life.

Like other present-day governmental bodies, the medical establishment does not shy away from cultivating and disseminating myths that serve its interests. One such myth has already been discussed in the first part of the book. "The Pure Science Myth" is exploited by health authorities to persuade the general public, particularly "rebellious" parents, to accept its manufactured vaccine-safety science as gospel. The intent behind this myth is to establish and instill the perception that science operates in an objective and disinterested way, and, since it is by far the best decision tool at our collective disposal, one should accept its decrees regarding vaccination efficacy and safety.

The Pure Science Myth, put to good use as it is by the medical establishment, is but one of several employed in the vaccine wars. Several other myths, specific to vaccination, are promoted by the establishment. These myths contribute to the formation of a positive public mindset about vaccines and constitute a protective barrier, a "vaccine" if you will, against viewpoints that challenge the institutional dogma. By cultivating these myths, the medical establishment seeks to sanctify vaccines, thereby delegitimizing any criticisms, ultimately excluding them entirely from public scrutiny.

The second part of this book tackles some of the more prominent myths of vaccination, the stories we are first told in kindergarten, when we are too young to question their veracity, and that we hear over and over again once we become parents and continue hearing throughout our lives.

8

THE DISAPPEARANCE
OF
DISEASE

Most people would probably admit that their knowledge about vaccines (and their effects) is sketchy at best. Vaccination is such a complex topic that the average person is content to leave vaccination decisions to qualified medical professionals. Despite their lack of detailed knowledge on the subject, if asked, most people would probably also vehemently proclaim that "vaccines have saved millions of lives by eradicating the dreadful diseases of the past!"

The idea that vaccines have freed humanity from the deadly diseases of yore is deeply ingrained in our collective consciousness. Growing up, we all heard stories of horrible infectious diseases that killed millions throughout history in Europe and the United States but have almost entirely disappeared in modern times "thanks to vaccines". This is as common as common knowledge gets. Everyone knows we have the medical profession and vaccines to thank for our (relatively) disease-less lives, right?

Unfortunately, "everyone" is wrong.

Historical evidence uncovered in the second half of the 20th century shows, clearly and unequivocally, that the narrative of "life-saving vaccines" is largely fictitious. As it turns out, vaccines played only a limited role in reducing the burden of infectious disease in modern times. Although the historical facts are already well established in the scientific community, health authorities continue to – knowingly – use this false narrative to enhance the image of vaccines, as well as to glorify the medical profession's role in eradicating disease.

Another popular myth often coupled with the "life-saving vaccines" narrative is that our present collective health, and our children's health in particular, has never been better. For this good fortune we should be ever grateful to modern medicine and public health administrators. But is our health really as good as public health officials and pharmaceutical companies would have us believe? It's highly doubtful. In fact, history shows that during the second half of the 20th century – after most of the major infectious diseases of the 19th century had all but disappeared – Western children experienced a consistent and sustained rise in chronic illness that paralleled the increasing use of vaccines. Despite the fact that this rise has been well documented for several decades and seems to be picking up momentum with time, public health authorities display a surprising lack of concern and a disconcerting helplessness in the face of it.

This chapter explores the historical circumstances that led to the disappearance of infectious diseases which terrorized humanity up until the mid-20th century.[a] In addition, it provides a brief description of the ascent of chronic illnesses that have severely impacted millions of children in the past 60 years and are hurting more and more kids in industrialized countries each and every passing year.

---

[a] The analysis in this chapter will not include smallpox and polio. The story of these two diseases is particularly complex. A separate chapter is dedicated to polio.

The Decline in Infectious Disease Mortality

Between 1955 and 1975, Dr. Thomas McKeown, a physician by training and head of the social medicine department at the University of Birmingham,[1] published a series of articles that challenged the orthodox view of the factors responsible for the dramatic modern decline in infectious disease mortality in industrialized countries. Prior to McKeown's groundbreaking publications, the scientific consensus held that most of this decline was due to advances in medicine from the late 19th century onwards and, more specifically, to the widespread use of medical drugs and vaccines.[2] McKeown and his colleagues, however, examined official mortality data from England and Wales from the early 18th century to 1971 and came up with very different conclusions.

The first article in the series, published in 1962, examined mortality records for the 19th century, dating back to 1838.[3] The researchers discovered that during the period in question mortality from some of the most prominent infectious diseases of the time declined significantly despite the utter lack of medical measures for preventing or treating them.[b] "The nature of infectious diseases was not understood before 1850," McKeown writes. "Infectious organisms affecting man were not identified until the last quarter of the nineteenth century, and specific prevention or treatment is unlikely to have had much influence on the national death rate before the introduction of chemotherapy in the 1930s."[4] (Chemotherapy in this context refers to therapeutic drugs in general.)

The most noteworthy decrease in mortality was in tuberculosis, which was the deadliest disease of the era. Tuberculosis mortality decreased by almost 50% in the second half of the 19th century.[5] Other infectious diseases whose mortality declined steeply in this era include typhoid, whose death rate dropped by

---

[b] Smallpox is unique in this context. In his later writings McKeown even cast doubt on the role the Jenner vaccine had in reducing mortality from this disease.

close to 80%; scarlet fever, which also decreased by about 80%; and the bowel diseases dysentery and cholera, whose mortality had cumulatively dropped by approximately 30%.[c] As noted above, medical science had not yet developed a vaccine or effective cure for any of these diseases, so the steep drop in mortality, as McKeown aptly points out, had to be due to other factors.[6]

In 1975 McKeown published another article, this time examining 20th century mortality in England and Wales (1901 to 1971). According to the English government's official data, the overall mortality rate steadily decreased during that period,[7] with deaths from infectious diseases accounting for about three-quarters of the total decline.[8] Although effective infectious disease treatments first appeared in the mid-1930s with the introduction of sulfonamides[d] in 1935 and antibiotics in 1941, more than half the decrease in infectious disease mortality (56%) was recorded before 1931.[9] For example, mortality from scarlet fever (caused by streptococcus bacteria), decreased by about 90% from the turn of the century to 1935, the very same year Prontosil, the first of the sulfonamides, was available for general use.[10] Mortality from intestinal diseases (such as dysentery) also decreased by a similar rate in the first three decades of the 20th century.[11]

We know from McKeown's analysis of 19th century data that mortality from tuberculosis was cut in half by the end of the 19th century. An effective treatment (streptomycin) didn't become available until 1947, by which time the mortality rate had already dropped by another two-thirds since the start of the

---

[c] Mortality from tuberculosis decreased from an average of 277 per 100,000 cases per year in the decade 1851–60 to an average of 141 per 100,000 in 1891–1900. Typhoid mortality dropped from 89 to 18 cases per 100,000 over the same period, and mortality from scarlet fever dropped from 77 to 15 per 100,000, while bowel disease mortality dropped from 99 to 71 per 100,000.

[d] Sulfonamides are a family of medicines used for treating infectious diseases that preceded the development of antibiotics.

20th century.[e] Tuberculosis vaccination in the UK began in 1954, and by 1961 mortality had dropped to zero. Drug treatment, McKeown notes, made a significant contribution to reducing tuberculosis mortality only after 1947, and it is highly likely that the downward trend would have continued even without it.[12]

Now let's look at trends in mortality rates for diseases for which we have vaccines. McKeown notes that the decline in mortality of pertussis (whooping cough) began in the late 19th century. In the 20th century, a drop of about 86% occurred before 1938, when sulfonamides first appeared (and in any case, he adds, the efficacy of sulfonamides and antibiotics against pertussis is still unclear). The pertussis vaccine only became widely used in Britain in 1952. McKeown does not specify a concrete figure, but we can infer that by that time the mortality rate had already dropped by more than 90% compared to early-20th century rates.[13]

Measles mortality in Britain did not decrease significantly until the second decade of the 20th century; 1915, however, marked the beginning of a rapid decline in measles mortality, a half-century before the vaccine was introduced in 1969. Measles deaths, for the most part, are caused by secondary bacterial infections that would now be treated with antibacterial drugs, yet approximately 82% of the reduction in measles mortality occurred before 1935, when sulfonamides were first used.[14]

As was the case with measles, diphtheria mortality did not decline in the second half of the 19th century, but rather increased. At the turn of the 20th century, antitoxin, a drug for the treatment of diphtheria was introduced, and a corresponding gradual decline in mortality followed. Another decrease in mortality occurred following the introduction of the diphtheria vaccine in 1941.[15] Diphtheria is the only major disease for which the decline in UK mortality occurred in parallel with the widespread use of either an effective drug treatment or a vaccine.

---

[e] That is, about 5/6 of the drop in tuberculosis mortality since 1850 was achieved even before the introduction of drug treatment for the disease.

Even in the case of diphtheria, however, McKeown is still hesitant to ascribe the decline in mortality to these medical measures: "It is tempting to attribute much of the decline of diphtheria mortality between 1901 and 1931 to treatment by antitoxin, and the rapid fall [in death rates] since 1941 to immunization. Nothing in British evidence is seriously inconsistent with this interpretation," he writes. "However," he continues, "experience in some other countries is not so consistent. Moreover, as already noted, other infections declined in the same period in the absence of effective prophylaxis [i.e., preventive measure] or treatment."[16]

Whether or not the sharp decrease in diphtheria mortality in the 1940s is attributable to the vaccine, vaccines' overall contribution to reducing mortality from infectious diseases in 20th-century Britain was no more than marginal. The cumulative decrease in mortality from these three vaccine-preventable diseases, pertussis, diphtheria, and measles, accounted for only about 10% of the overall decline in infectious disease mortality during the period under study, and, as we've seen, only a small part of that cumulative decrease can be attributed to vaccines.[17] Apart from the vaccines for these three diseases, other vaccines in wide use during the 20th century had only a negligible impact on the overall mortality decline, as McKeown notes. Mortality from polio and tetanus had always been relatively small, owing to their low prevalence, whereas common diseases such as rubella, mumps, and chickenpox, rarely caused death.[18]

Yet another paper published by McKeown and colleagues – this, a 1972 study looking into the causes of modern-age mortality in four other European countries (Sweden, Ireland, France, and Hungary) – reached similar conclusions: "Although data for the nineteenth century are seriously deficient," McKeown writes, "analysis by cause of death for the four countries and England and Wales leaves little doubt that the decline of mortality was due to a reduction of deaths from infectious disease, almost wholly until 1900 and predominantly after that time... [Yet] it was not until 1935 [...] that therapy became available which reduced mortality from infection to an extent that could be expected to lower the national death rate."[19]

As might be expected, McKeown and his colleagues' unorthodox conclusions stirred up quite a controversy in academic circles, and various aspects of their work were heavily criticized. Notably, however, the criticism focused on aspects that were largely inconsequential to this chapter's subject matter.[f] Even the most adamant critics of McKeown's work did not question the credibility of his data[20] and essentially accepted his assertion that medical interventions (i.e., medicines and vaccines) played only a marginal role in reducing mortality from infectious disease in England and Wales during the 19th and 20th centuries.[21]

McKeown's conclusions gained greater support in the late 1970s when Americans John McKinlay and Sonja McKinlay (a married couple, he a Boston University sociologist and she a Harvard mathematician) applied similar research methods to US mortality data. The two published a 1977 paper presenting their analysis of official US mortality figures for the period 1900–1973.[g] Similar to the results from England and Wales, the US data also exhibited a significant drop in the overall mortality rate in the 20th century, the main cause of which was the steep decline in mortality from infectious disease.[22]

The McKinlays' analysis of US mortality data indicated that most of this decline was achieved prior to the widespread use of vaccines. The diphtheria mortality rate, for example, plummeted 87% from the start of the 20th century to 1930, the year the McKinlays estimated that its first treatment, antitoxin, became widely available in the US.[23] General use of the diphtheria vaccine did not begin until the late 1940s (as a component of the diphtheria-tetanus-pertussis vaccine – "DTP").[24] Thus, it is

---

[f] For example, there were those who disputed McKeown's assertion that the overall population increase was due to a decrease in mortality, rather than an increase in births. Others claimed that McKeown had partially misinterpreted the data and, thus, overestimated the role the rise in living standards played in the decline in mortality from infectious diseases.

[g] Official mortality data has been recorded in the United States since 1900.

reasonable to assume that over 90% of diphtheria mortality reduction took place prior to extensive use of the vaccine. The authors note that mortality for pertussis, another component of the DTP vaccine, dropped by 50% before 1930, the year the McKinlays used for the introduction of the vaccine.[25] [h] Since the pertussis vaccine was also not widely distributed until the DTP was developed in the late 1940s, this strongly suggests that the bulk of the decline in pertussis mortality was not due to its vaccine either. Most impressively, measles mortality dropped almost 99% by 1963, the year measles vaccination commenced in the United States.

Like McKeown before them, McKinlay and McKinlay also note that the major reduction in US infectious disease mortality in the 20th century occurred prior to the introduction of effective medical interventions. "In general," they conclude, "medical measures (both chemotherapeutic and prophylactic) appear to have contributed little to the overall decline in mortality in the United States since about 1900 – having in many instances been introduced several decades after a marked decline had already set in and having no detectable influence in most instances."[26]

Two decades later, the McKinlay findings were twice confirmed by CDC researchers. In 1999, Dr. Gregory Armstrong and colleagues at the CDC's Infectious Disease Center, published a paper in the *Journal of the American Medical Association* (*JAMA*), in which they presented official US infectious disease mortality data for the 20th century (1900–1996).[27] US mortality figures are maintained by the CDC's National Center for Health Statistics and are considered to be the best and most complete of their kind.[28] The charts in the paper demonstrate that infectious disease mortality in the US had already dropped by about 90% from the turn of the century to the late 1940s[29] when the first vaccine came into general use (the aforementioned diphtheria-

---

[h] The McKinlays were generous with their estimate of 1930. The first truly effective pertussis vaccine was developed in 1932 by Kendrick and Eldering, who did not begin their field trial until 1934.

tetanus-pertussis vaccine).[30]

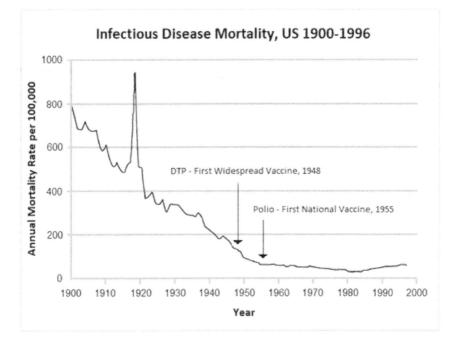

Figure 8-1: Mortality from infectious disease in the United States (1900–1996)

Infectious disease mortality in early childhood (0-4 years) also decreased similarly, as shown in Figure 8-2 (see next page).[31] Mortality from the nine leading infectious diseases dropped dramatically by the end of the 1940s, again, with no significant contribution made by vaccines. The chart also shows that by the mid-1970s, the collective child mortality rate of these diseases dropped to almost zero, even though at the time the US offered vaccines for only three of the nine major diseases.[i]

---

[i] The nine diseases included in the chart are pneumonia/influenza, tuberculosis, typhoid, dysentery, syphilis, AIDS, pertussis, diphtheria, and measles. Only the last three had childhood vaccines that were in use prior to the 1970s.

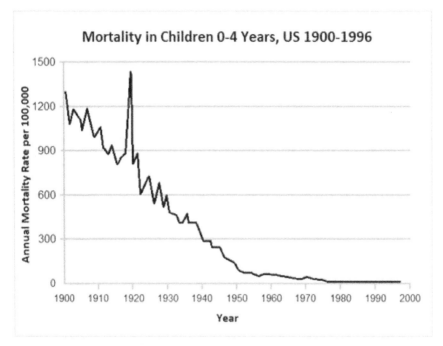

Figure 8-2: Mortality rate from infectious diseases in children aged 0-4 in the United States (1900-1996)

A separate chart (figure 8-3, next page) presents the decline in 20th century mortality for the three childhood diseases with vaccines that were available in the United States.[32] Again, it is obvious that the majority of the decline occurred before the respective vaccines were introduced. In addition, mortality rates have fallen similarly for diseases such as dysentery and typhoid (see figure 8-4), even though vaccines for those were never introduced in the United States.[33]

A year after the publication of the Armstrong study, a team of researchers at Johns Hopkins University and the CDC's National Center for Health Statistics reaffirmed its conclusions. Dr. Bernard Guyer and colleagues write that "nearly 90% of the decline in infectious disease mortality among US children occurred before 1940, when few antibiotics or vaccines were available. [...] Vaccination," they conclude, "does not account for the impressive declines in mortality seen in the first half of the century."[34]

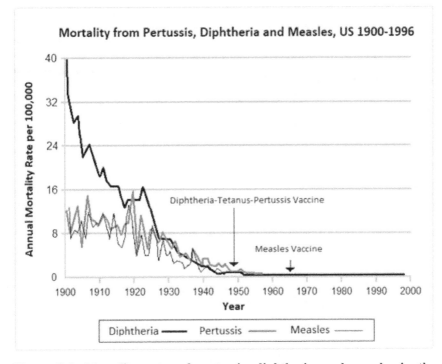

Figure 8-3: Mortality rates of pertussis, diphtheria, and measles in the United States (1900–1996)

Thus, official mortality figures from Britain and the United States (as well as data from a handful of other European countries) indicate that the vast majority of the reduction in infectious disease mortality had already transpired by the mid-20th century, before vaccines were widely used.

The data is patently clear: Vaccines, as well as medical drugs, had only a marginal impact on the decline in infectious disease mortality. Furthermore, it is quite probable that the downward trend in mortality would have continued even in the absence of vaccines, albeit, perhaps, at a slower rate. In Britain, for example, the death rates for pertussis and measles continued to drop until the years their vaccines were introduced – 1952 and 1969, respectively.[j] [35]

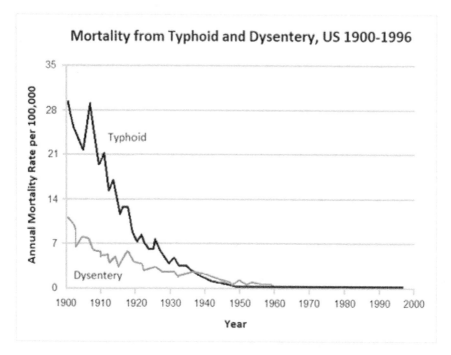

Figure 8-4: Death rates from dysentery and typhoid in the United States (1900–1996)

The Decline in Infectious Disease Morbidity

Compared to the mortality data reviewed in the previous section,

---

[j] Between 1941 (the year in which the diphtheria vaccine was introduced in Britain) and 1952 (the year in which the pertussis vaccine was introduced), pertussis mortality decreased from a three-year average of 1,286 cases per year (1940–42) to 458 (1949–51). This is a drop of approximately 2/3 that likely would have been credited to the pertussis vaccine had it been introduced in 1941. Similarly, between 1941 and 1969 (the year the measles vaccine was introduced), a sharp drop-off was recorded – from a three-year average of 820 measles deaths (1940–42) to 77 (1966–68), a decline of about 90%. [In fact, the resulting drop in mortality rate would have been even greater, especially for measles, if the calculation allowed for population growth in Britain during the period in question.]

morbidity statistics (the number of reported cases) for the US and UK are more recent and less accurate.[36] In Britain, historical morbidity data is available from the late 19th century. In the United States, reports of infectious disease morbidity from all states began to be consistently gathered in 1925, whereas national mortality data has been available since 1900.[37] According to the CDC, historical morbidity data should be taken with a grain of salt, as reporting integrity and accuracy vary from disease to disease and depend on various factors.[k] However, as we shall see shortly, handled with due care, the data can be helpful in analyzing historical morbidity trends.[38]

Unlike the historical decline in infectious disease mortality, on which they had only a marginal impact, vaccines did play a significant part, though not an exclusive one, in the decline in infectious disease morbidity. Most of the major infectious diseases of the 19th century are no longer considered significant public health threats, and vaccines played a prominent role in reducing morbidity for some of them. For example, though the declines in deaths due to diphtheria and pertussis in the US began as early as the first quarter of the 20th century, the reported incidence remained high – tens of thousands of cases per year for diphtheria and hundreds of thousands for pertussis – until the introduction of the triple vaccine (diphtheria-tetanus-pertussis) in 1948.[l] [39] In Britain, a similar trend was observed: A consistent drop in diphtheria morbidity began in the early 1940s with the introduction of the vaccine,[40] whereas a marked decline in pertussis cases began after 1952, the year in which the DTP vaccine was introduced.[41]

Measles also exhibited a similar pattern: Although the mor-

---

[k] For example, for minor illnesses such as mumps, the number of reported cases is significantly lower than the actual number of cases. For other diseases, many infections may be subclinical (meaning there are no apparent symptoms) and would therefore not be reported.

[l] The decline in diphtheria morbidity began as early as the mid-1930s, with the introduction of a (single) diphtheria vaccine for use in several areas of the US.

tality rate dropped sharply in the first half of the 20th century, the morbidity level remained fairly stable (hundreds of thousands of reported cases a year). The introduction of the measles vaccine in the mid and late 1960s in the US and UK, respectively, resulted in a sharp decline in morbidity and a further steep drop to a level of only several thousand cases a year following the introduction of the MMR (measles-mumps-rubella) vaccine (figure 8-5).[m]

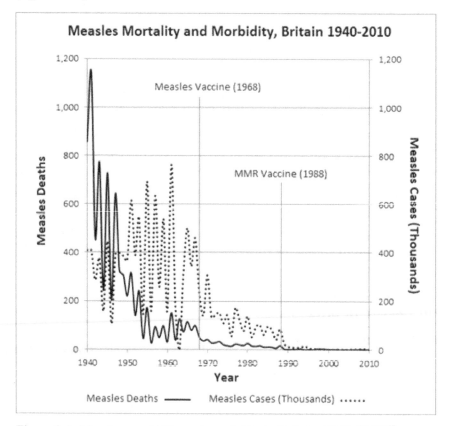

Figure 8-5: Measles morbidity and mortality in Britain (1940–2010)[47]

These large reductions in disease incidence for diphtheria, pertussis, and measles make the vaccines look impressive. How-

---

[m] The MMR vaccine was introduced in the United States in the 1970s and in the United Kingdom in the late 1980s.

ever, these were not the only diseases exhibiting dramatic declines in morbidity in modern times. Other diseases, for which no effective medical preventive or intervention was developed, have also been largely eradicated. Cholera killed thousands in Britain in the second half of the 19th century but virtually disappeared in the 20th century in both the US and UK. Annual case-counts for typhus fell to the single-digit level in Britain as early as the second decade of the 20th century, and in the United States to a mere few dozen cases per year in the early 1960s.

Incidence of typhoid fever, one of the most dreadful diseases of the 19th century, also decreased in the UK to fewer than a thousand reported cases a year as early as the 1940s and reached a similar level in the US in the late 1950s.[42]

Tuberculosis incidence also dropped significantly in the 20th century despite the lack of an effective vaccine.[43] In the UK, tuberculosis morbidity decreased from 100,000 a year in 1912, to less than 70,000 cases per annum in the late 1920s.[n][44] The tuberculosis vaccine (BCG) only became available in the UK in the early 1950s.[45] In the US, the annual incidence dropped from approximately 100,000 cases a year in the 1930s to below 30,000 in the 1970s, even though the tuberculosis vaccine was never routinely given to American children.[46]

For dysentery and scarlet fever, two other prominent diseases of the 19th century for which no effective vaccine has ever been used, the UK morbidity level declined during the 20th century as well. More than 100,000 scarlet fever cases were recorded annually between 1912 and 1915, and only a few thousand a year by the beginning of the 21st century. Dysentery morbidity dropped from tens of thousands of cases a year in the 1950s and 1960s, to 267 cases in 2010, the year mandatory reporting of the disease

---

[n] From 1931 to 1962, no data was collected in the UK for tuberculosis. In 1963, fewer than 20,000 cases were recorded. The data is not sufficient to determine how much of the decline from 70,000 to 20,000 cases per year occurred prior to the vaccine's introduction in the early 1950s.

ceased.[o]

Other notorious diseases also recorded dramatic declines in morbidity in the 20th century without the help of mass vaccination. In the United States, malaria and syphilis morbidity decreased significantly from the late 1940s onwards.[48] Spraying of DDT, which began in the US shortly after World War II, killed the mosquitoes that carried malaria, resulting in a sharp decline in morbidity – from 100,000 cases a year in the 1930s to a few dozen in the 1960s.[49] The drop in syphilis morbidity began when antibiotics began to be used for treatment and contagion prevention.[50] Scurvy and pellagra, lesser-known historical diseases caused by nutritional deficiencies, were almost completely eliminated in the first half of the 20th century.[51]

In addition to successfully reducing morbidity levels of diphtheria, pertussis, and measles, vaccines had other notable achievements in the second half of the 20th century, though mostly for diseases that are relatively mild or rare. A vaccine for tetanus, a deadly but rare disease, was introduced in the United States in 1948. The previous year only 560 cases of the disease were reported (about 0.4 cases per 100,000) in the whole country.[p] The gradual decline in tetanus morbidity (to about 30 cases a year) since 1948 may be attributable to the vaccine.[52] In Britain, too, tetanus wasn't considered a major public health threat as can be deduced from the fact that official morbidity reporting didn't even begin until 1969 (the vaccine was introduced 15 years earlier).[53]

Vaccination's impact on morbidity reduction is more apparent for mumps and rubella (see figure 8-6 on next page). Official morbidity reporting for these relatively mild diseases didn't begin until shortly before their vaccines were added to the national vaccine programs (the mid-1960s in the US and the late 1980s in the UK). Widespread use of the MMR vaccine signifi-

---

[o] In the United States there was still a relatively high level of dysentery and scarlet-fever morbidity during the 20th century.

[p] Official reporting of tetanus morbidity began in the US only in 1947.

cantly reduced morbidity levels of these two diseases. In the US, the MMR vaccine introduction in 1971 resulted in a large drop in mumps morbidity – from more than 100,000 cases a year at the beginning of the decade to about 15,000 cases a year toward its end. Similarly, rubella morbidity decreased approximately 75% during the 1970s.

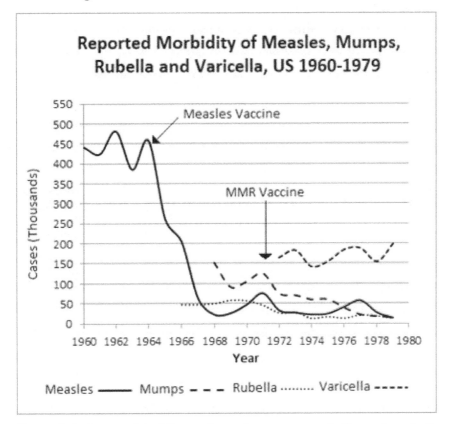

Figure 8-6: Reported incidence of measles, mumps, rubella, and varicella (chickenpox) in the United States (1960-1979)

By comparison, incidence of varicella (chickenpox), a disease whose epidemiological characteristics are quite similar to those of mumps and rubella and for which there was no vaccine in the 1970s, remained high in the US throughout the decade.

This discrepancy reinforces the notion that vaccines played a primary role in reducing the morbidity of mumps and rubella.

Britain experienced similar success with the MMR vaccine in the 1990s. Mumps cases plummeted from about 20,000 annually in 1989 to about 2,000 in the year 2000. Rubella morbidity decreased by a similar rate.

In summary, it seems that vaccines played a significant role, though not a principal one, in reducing infectious disease morbidity in the United States and Britain during the 20th century. Of the nine major infectious diseases of the 19th century, only three (diphtheria, pertussis, and measles) experienced declines in morbidity that could be ascribed to vaccination. The other six, as well as additional diseases such as malaria, disappeared or came close to it for other reasons. To their credit, vaccines were also responsible for a considerable decline in morbidity of some of the milder diseases (mumps, rubella).

Real Reasons for the Decline in Infectious Disease

The official record shows that vaccines made only a marginal contribution to reduced mortality from infectious disease and played a significant, but not primary, role in reducing morbidity. If not vaccines, then what was primarily responsible for the drastic reductions in infectious disease mortality and morbidity observed in the United States and Britain in late 19th and early 20th centuries?

Following the publication of McKeown's research, the academic consensus holds that the major contributors to the decline were improvements in sanitation and hygiene, a rise in the standard of living, better nutrition, and the gradual introduction of medical interventions during the 20th century.[54] In the following pages we will look at what "better sanitation and hygiene" means and how lifestyle changes in the modern age have led to such dramatic improvements in public health.

Improved sanitation. The term sanitation, in the context of this discussion, refers to actions taken to maintain cleanliness in the public domain, especially sewage treatment and delivery of clean drinking water.

In the major cities of Europe and the United States centralized sewer treatment systems were practically nonexistent until the mid-19th century. In most homes, wastewater and excrement were discharged into privy vaults or cesspools.[q] [55] Accelerated urbanization in the 19th century led to a huge influx of city dwellers and an increase in population density, which in turn led to a considerable surge in the amount of sewage requiring treatment. Over time, it became clear to the municipal authorities that traditional sewage management, which relied on private facilities with no central planning or control, was not equipped to handle the increased load, nor could it prevent contamination of local reservoirs. Wastewater from privies and cesspools occasionally overflowed and flooded nearby areas, penetrating groundwater basins and polluting the drinking water, thereby posing an environmental hazard which was a frequent cause of disease outbreaks.[56]

The load on the outdated sewer systems of large cities further increased with the gradual introduction of water pipes and toilet facilities in houses. Now, in the absence of modern sewage systems, the growing quantity of wastewater was handled by diverting it to nearby streams or rivers, where many city residents got their drinking water.[57]

A typical example is the city of London, where a number of cholera epidemics broke out in the mid-19th century following the contamination of drinking-water reservoirs. Dr. John Snow, a British physician who studied the London cholera epidemic of 1854, discovered that most cholera patients had consumed drinking water from sewage-contaminated sections of the River Thames, while residents of neighborhoods that received their drinking water from unpolluted sections of the river did not fall ill.[58] Twelve years later, when yet another cholera epidemic struck London, William Farr utilized a technique similar to the one employed by Snow and was able to pinpoint the specific

---

[q] Privy vaults and cesspools were, essentially, pits dug into the ground near houses to contain the occupants' excrement.

cause of the plague. Farr overlaid the map of London with the distribution areas of the companies that supplied the drinking water. Thus, he was able to identify the source of the epidemic as a sewage-contaminated reservoir, unlawfully soiled by one of the municipal water suppliers.[59]

The work of Snow, Farr, and others provided convincing evidence of the close link between sewage-polluted drinking water and the emergence of epidemics. This link spurred municipal authorities to construct central sewage systems. Such a system was completed in London in the 1860s following the enactment of a law in Parliament.[60] Consequently, the aforementioned 1866 cholera epidemic was the last to strike London. Similarly, in the United States, a succession of cholera and typhus epidemics in the mid-19th century convinced city leaders of the need for central sewage systems. By the end of the century, such systems had been established in most of the major cities of the United States.[61] In addition, centralized water purification systems, which filtered and chlorinated water to make it safe for drinking, were also introduced in large American cities at the turn of the 20th century.[62]

The establishment of major sewer systems in large cities led to a drastic reduction in epidemics of food- and water-borne diseases in the last third of the 19th century. Harvard University researchers Cutler and Miller point out that advancements in water quality are credited with the disappearance of typhoid from the United States in the first third of the 20th century.[63] McKeown notes that improvements in sanitation accounted for about one-third of the reduction of all deaths from infectious diseases in the second half of the 19th century, and one-sixth of all deaths in the 20th century. He attributes this trend to a sharp decline in deaths from intestinal diseases (typhoid, cholera, dysentery, and others).[64] Simon Szreter, otherwise McKeown's most prominent critic, actually agrees with him on this point, writing: "There can be little doubt that the first two-thirds of the 19th century witnessed an increasing incidence of such diseases, which was directly attributable to the unplanned proliferation of overcrowded cities and towns lacking even the most basic sanitary facilities such as proper water supply and waste disposal systems. Conversely, the ensuing disappearance of water-borne diseases in the last third of the century was due to the eventual provision of adequate sanitary facilities, long delayed but finally implemented."[65]

Another factor contributing to improved cleanliness of urban areas was the gradual disappearance of horses from cities. In the 19th century, horses were the main means of transportation, and the excrement that clogged city streets as a result was a serious health problem. An average urban horse produced approximately 25 pounds of feces a day, much of it scattered on the streets.[66] Horse feces provide a fertile substrate for the growth of tetanus bacteria.[67] This, coupled with the occasional fallen horseshoe nail, meant conditions were favorable for contracting deadly tetanus. Making matters worse, horse dung in the streets attracted swarms of flies, which played a key role in the transmission of intestinal diseases such as typhoid.[68] City horses posed health hazards even after the termination of their earthly chores. Life was harsh for urban horses, and average life expectancy was as low as four years. Thus, it was common in 19th-century cities for horses to collapse and die on the street. New York City, for example, cleared some 15,000 horse carcasses from the city's streets in the year 1880 alone.[69]

Horses gradually disappeared from the urban scene. As early as the middle of the 19th century, horses began being replaced as "motors" in mechanized production, and by the end of the century their role in public transport, which was now powered by electricity, had also ended. In the early decades of the 20th century, first in the United States and later in Europe, cars took over horses' final urban role — private transportation — which finally emptied city streets of horses.[70]

Improved hygiene. Researchers studying the history of infectious disease (such as McKeown) sometimes use the terms *sanitation* and *hygiene* interchangeably. In this chapter, *hygiene* will be used to denote the actions that individuals take in order to reduce their own exposure, or that of family members, to disease-causing organisms (pathogens).

Science discovered pathogenic organisms in the last third of the 19th century with the work of Koch, Pasteur, and others, the founding fathers of the field of microbiology. During that period the concept of hygiene – that is, that cleanliness was of paramount importance in the prevention of infectious disease – began to take hold. Basic hygiene practices such as washing hands, bathing frequently, wearing clean clothes, and keeping food clean are taken for granted today but were virtually unheard of in the late 19th century.

The history of typhus exemplifies the role personal hygiene played in reducing morbidity. Typhus, a highly contagious and deadly disease, has been historically linked to poverty and unsanitary conditions. It often broke out in conditions where good hygiene was scarce: in prisons, in armies during war, during periods of famine and drought, and the like.[71] Since both the cause of the disease and its mode of transmission were unknown, there were no effective means for preventing its spread. These mysteries were eventually solved in 1909 by a French physician and microbiologist named Charles Nicolle, who served as the director of the Pasteur Institute in Tunis. While observing at a local hospital, Nicolle noticed that typhus patients were no longer contagious after arriving at the facility, where they were stripped of their street clothes, scrubbed, and dressed in hospital garb. His conclusion was that typhus was spread by lice on the patients' bodies and clothing, and experiments he conducted on monkeys proved that this was indeed the case.[72] Nicolle's discovery – that typhus is transmitted by body lice[r] – marked the beginning of the end for a disease that had taken a heavy toll on humanity throughout history.

In order to prevent infectious disease outbreaks, we must

---

[r] The cause of the disease is a bacterium called *Rickettsia prowazeki*, which is transmitted through the secretions of the lice in contact with the skin and eyes (Schultz 2009, p. 2).

know how a disease is transmitted, but awareness alone is often not enough. Poverty, filth, and overcrowding, conditions which affected most urban populations during the 19th century, provided an ideal setting for the spread of infectious diseases that were transmitted through human secretions.[73] With the improvement in living conditions in early 20th century – such as running water in homes, more spacious housing, and improved means of storing food – personal hygiene also improved, resulting in a further decline in the incidence of infectious diseases.[74]

Fresh and healthy food. Until the second half of the 19th century, food supplied to cities in the United States and Europe was mostly local and seasonal. Local farmers, shepherds, hunters, and fishermen took their produce to the city market in boats and horse-drawn carts.[75] The absence of reliable means of transportation or refrigeration technology meant most urban dwellers ate very little in the way of fresh food. In the cold months, even the affluent were accustomed to eating spoiled or stale food. In summer, the produce was more varied, but the food rotted rapidly.[76]

Naturally, a poor and unbalanced diet renders the body more susceptible to disease. Severe vitamin C deficiency is the direct cause of scurvy, which plagued many seafarers in previous centuries. Lack of vitamin B3 and vitamin B1 plays a key role in pellagra and beriberi, respectively. These diseases are caused by an acute deficiency of a specific vitamin, but less pronounced deficiencies can weaken the body's resistance to some diseases – measles, for example. McKeown mentions the consensus among researchers that risk of death from measles (but not the risk of catching it in the first place) is highly influenced by the quality of the patient's diet. In the UK, he adds, the measles mortality rate is much higher in poorer populations than in affluent ones. Similarly, measles mortality rates in developing countries are significantly higher than in developed countries.[77]

City dwellers' poor nutritional status began to change in the second half of the 19th century, when a succession of inventions and technological developments changed the face of transportation in general and the field of food transportation in particular. In the United States new canals and railroads enabled food to reach cities from afar while maintaining its freshness and quality. The introduction of refrigerated railroad cars meant fresh food products, including dairy and meat, could be dispatched year-round throughout the country. Steamboats made international trade cheaper and more reliable, thus leading to a significant increase in the variety of food products that flowed into major cities.[78] In addition, improvements in ice-making technology and home refrigeration made it possible to preserve food for longer periods of time once it reached the consumer.[79]

These technological advancements led to continuous improvement in the variety and quality of food available to city residents. However, these developments also had a downside. The rapid development of food transportation and marketing was not accompanied by pertinent regulations preventing the distribution of spoiled or toxic food to markets. Safety issues in food production arose from time to time, in the production and supply of milk, for example.[80] Congress took on these issues, and in the last third of the 19th century several laws were enacted to regulate the activities of the food and pharmaceutical industries. Finally, the Food and Drugs Act was passed in 1906, and the Bureau of Chemistry in the Department of Agriculture (later the Food and Drug Administration – "FDA") assumed responsibility for its enforcement. Among other things, the law prohibited the inclusion of contaminated, rotten, hazardous, or foreign substances in foods.[81] The United Kingdom also enacted similar laws during that period.[82]

The development of modern medicine. As we have seen, it was not until the second half of the 19th century — thanks to the innovations of Joseph Lister, Ignaz Semmelweis, Florence Nightingale, Louis Pasteur, Robert Koch, and others — that hygiene's importance in preventing infectious disease became apparent.[83] As such, most invasive medical procedures performed in the 19th century (surgery, for example) were extremely dangerous for patients. The rooms in which operations were performed were not sterile, and doctors did not bother sterilizing their hands, clothes, or tools between treating one patient and the next. A hospital stay always involved a high risk of contracting an infectious disease, either from fellow patients or the medical staff, many of whom were infected themselves.[84]

The great scientific discoveries of the late 19th century marked the beginning of the modern age of medicine, but it took an additional fifty years before effective interventions were developed for the prevention and treatment of infectious diseases. Effective vaccines began to be widely used only in the 1930s (the diphtheria vaccine in the United States) at about the same time the first antibacterial drugs (sulfonamides) appeared, followed by antibiotics several years later. Up until that time, available medical treatment for patients suffering from infectious diseases[s] amounted to palliative care, intended to relieve pain and discomfort. Along with food and rest to aid recovery, that was all medicine had to offer patients.[85] Because of their relatively late arrival on the scene, vaccines and therapeutic drugs were left with just a minor role in the drastic reduction of infectious disease mortality and a secondary role in reducing its morbidity.

An Open Secret: The Real Contribution of Vaccines

Until Thomas McKeown's series of papers were published, historians were of the opinion that the historical decline of infectious disease was due, first and foremost, to the field of medicine. "[McKeown's] work," writes Szreter, "achieved something of a conceptual revolution in the disciplines of history and medicine, overturning a long-standing general orthodoxy regarding the importance of medical science and the medical profession in bringing about the decline in mortality which

---

[s] Diphtheria and tetanus, for which drugs (antitoxins) were developed in the last decade of the 19th century, were the exception. These drugs were based on an antibody compound produced by injecting the toxins of the disease into horses. Hence, their production was limited in scope and their usage dangerous.

accompanied industrialization in Britain. It effectively demonstrated that those advances in the science of medicine which form the basis of today's conventional clinical and hospital teaching and practice, in particular the immuno- and chemotherapies, played only a very minor role in accounting for the historic decline in mortality levels."[86]

McKeown, like Szreter and other researchers, makes a distinction between medical science's contributions in the form of engineering initiatives intended to improve living conditions and fight disease, and the medical interventions that were later introduced.[87] There is no doubt that researchers such as Pasteur and Nicolle and public health officials like Snow and Farr played an important role in understanding the causative agents of infectious disease and in raising public awareness of the importance of sanitation and hygiene.[t] These scientists worked alongside legislators, city officials, engineers, architects, and many others to improve living conditions in cities: building sewer systems, installing running water in homes, providing better nutrition, improving cleanliness, reducing housing density, and so on. While acknowledging medical science's major contributions, researchers have also come to the consensus that McKeown's conclusion that medical interventions played only a marginal role in the battle against infectious disease is well-founded and has proven to be correct.[88]

Presently, more than forty years after the publication of McKeown's research, health authorities around the world are well aware of the key role improvements in sanitation, hygiene, and living standards played in reducing the burden of infectious disease. For example, a celebratory document published by the CDC in the early 21st century (*Ten Great Public Health Achievements in the 20th Century*)[89] dedicates a chapter to the fight

---

[t] However, one cannot attribute the decrease in mortality from measures like construction of major sewer systems in cities, installation of running water in homes, improvements in nutrition, and decreased housing density to the field of medicine alone. "Maintaining public health is the responsibility of the engineer, not the doctor" (*Encyclopedia Britannica*).

against infectious disease. The text notes that the incidence of many infectious diseases has been declining since the beginning of the 20th century thanks to improvements in sanitation and hygiene.[90] A report by the American Institute of Medicine (IOM) states that "the number of infections prevented by immunization is actually quite small compared with the total number of infections prevented by other hygienic interventions such as clean water, food, and living conditions."[91] However, recognition of the primary historical role played by non-vaccine factors in disease prevention is quite rare in CDC publications, and most of the credit, unsurprisingly, goes to vaccines.[u]

Contrary to the scientific consensus on the subject, the conclusion one would draw browsing the websites of government health bodies is that vaccines and vaccines alone were primarily responsible for reducing the mortality and morbidity of infectious disease. One way to create this false impression is by pretending the overall decline in infectious disease was mainly due to the drop in vaccine-preventable diseases. A typical formulation of this notion appears on the US Department of Health website: "Some diseases that once injured or killed thousands of children, have been eliminated completely and others are close to extinction – primarily due to safe and effective vaccines."[92] Similarly, CDC publications tend to focus on the historical decline in the incidence of vaccine-preventable diseases and ignore the decline observed in other infectious diseases.[93] The definitive conclusions generated by the scientific work of McKeown, Szreter, and their colleagues are completely ignored. Thus, the scientific consensus regarding the minor role vaccines played in reducing the burden of infectious disease has become a kind of "open secret" in scientific and medical circles: Everyone knows the truth but nobody cares to share it with the public.

---

[u] Even the *Ten Great Achievements* document mentioned above includes a chapter dedicated to vaccines, and the chapter dealing with the battle against infectious disease also includes a section dedicated to vaccines.

The Rise of Chronic Disease in Children

As previously noted, by the mid-20th century, infectious disease mortality had already been reduced by more than 90% since the start of the century, and morbidity had also decreased considerably. But, unfortunately, at the same time that infectious disease was trending downward, chronic disease was gaining momentum.

Unlike infectious diseases, that usually pass within a few days or weeks, a chronic illness persists for an extended period of time – months, years, or even the duration of a patient's life. As a rule, chronic diseases have no cure and they do not tend to disappear on their own.[94] In addition to the suffering and distress involved in a chronic condition, some patients experience significant limitations in their daily functioning, and many consume medication on a regular basis. Quality of life for the individual may be impaired considerably and the social and economic costs are high.

The United States began conducting periodic health surveys in 1960 that examined various health indicators, including the occurrence of chronic disease in different populations and age groups. The first survey in 1960 found that 1.8% of American children – about one million children – were limited in their major activity due to chronic conditions such as asthma, vision and hearing problems, and mental issues.[v] During the 1960s and 1970s, that rate climbed steadily until it reached 3.8% in 1981 (about two million children).[95] In the 1988 survey the rate rose to 4.1%,[96] in the 1994 survey to 6.5% (about four and a half million children),[97] and in 2010 it had reached 8% (about five and a half million children).[98]

As disturbing as this rise is, a survey conducted in 2007–2008 reported a shockingly high overall incidence of chronic illness in children. The survey, which collected data on a sample of more

---

[v] Major activity was defined as attendance at school or playing with peers (Newacheck 1984, p. 1).

than 90,000 children, found that 43% reported at least one chronic condition, and in about half of those (roughly one-fifth of all children surveyed) the condition was categorized as "moderate" or "severe". Furthermore, about 19% of all American children, almost one in five, were classified as having "special health care needs" and routinely consumed health care services.[99]

Surveys of asthma, autism, and attention deficit hyperactivity disorder (ADHD) found a consistent increase between 2003 and 2012. The rate of asthma increased from 12.5% to 14.6% in this time span (a rise of 18%), the rate of autism increased from 0.5% to 2.3% (a rise of almost 400%), and the rate of ADHD increased from 6.9% to 9.9% (a rise of 44%).[100] Another survey from Harvard University found increases in the incidence of various chronic illnesses from 1988 to 1994, and again in 2000. The rate of asthma patients nearly doubled during that 12-year span – from 1.6 to 1.8 to 2.9 percent. The overall rate of other chronic conditions – including speech, vision and hearing impairments, allergies, epilepsy, and more – rose from 3.1 to 4.1 to 5.0 percent, respectively.[101]

This rise in chronic illness in children has been accompanied by a simultaneous increase in the routine consumption of "chronic" drugs. Medco, a company that purchases medications on behalf of employers and health providers in the United States, published a report based on data from its activity in 2009. The largest company in its field in the US, Medco managed the purchase of medications for about 65 million people (more than 1/5 of the total US population). According to their data, about one in 4 American children (up to age 19) regularly took at least one medication for a chronic condition, and one in 14 took two or more. Topping the list were drugs for asthma, ADHD, depression, and other psychiatric conditions.[102]

In addition to the increase in the use of medications, chronic illness severity was also taking a turn for the worse. A 2010 study found that the rate of hospitalization of children 0–4 years old suffering from "complex chronic conditions" rose by 24% be-

tween 1993 and 2005. The rate of children hospitalized with two
or more concurrent complex conditions increased by 100%
during that same period.[103] A similar study of children up to the
age of 18 found a similar upward trend. Data from this study
show that in 2006 children chronically ill with complex conditions were responsible for about 25% of hospitalization days and
about 40% of total hospitalization costs for children in the
United States. In addition, these children accounted for almost
half of all hospital child deaths.[104]

The huge increase in chronic childhood illness is not exclusive to the United States, of course. In Britain, for example, one
in 11 children has asthma,[105] one in 530 suffers from type 1
diabetes[106] (a disease that was rare in children until the second
half of the 20th century),[107] and one in 14 children under the age
of three has an allergy to one or more foods.[108]

Unlike the United States, Israel does not conduct a comprehensive national survey of chronic health conditions in children.
However, the data that are available indicate that the rate of
chronic illness in Israeli children is rising as well and is not far
behind that of the United States. For example, the incidence of
type 1 diabetes in Israeli children increased by 52% between
1997 and 2010.[109] A 2008 survey of eighth-graders found that
nearly 8% had asthma (almost one in 12 students).[110] A study
examining the data of one of Israel's leading healthcare providers, Maccabi Health Services, found that the percentage of
children diagnosed with ADHD rose from 6.8% in 2005 to 14.4%
in 2014 (one in 7 children).[111] (It should be noted that, despite
these alarmingly high rates, the Ministries of Health and Education in Israel do not maintain accurate data on the number of
school-age children with ADHD.[112]) It is estimated that about
15,000 pupils in Israel suffer from severe food allergies. This high
prevalence prompted the Ministry of Education to publish an
information leaflet stating, among other things, that "any class in
which an allergic student studies will be declared a 'safe environment,' and the entry of allergenic foods will be banned."[113]
Data from Israel's Ministry of Health show that in 2008 1,044

children were hospitalized for allergic reactions to food.[114]

The data on chronic health conditions in children provide only a tiny glimpse into the enormous problem facing health authorities in the 21st century. Contrary to the "our health has never been better" myth promoted by the medical establishment, the data suggest that 21st century children are sicker than ever before and are getting progressively sicker as time goes by.

Chronic Illness vs. Infectious Disease

As we have seen thus far, morbidity trends for infectious and chronic disease are heading in opposite directions. While infectious disease morbidity is on a general downward slope, since the mid-20th century chronic illness has been on a steady, and rather steep, climb. Historically, public health authorities consider fighting infectious disease their primary objective. But in view of the declining threat posed by infectious disease and the corresponding increase in the societal costs of chronic conditions, it seems that a reevaluation of public health priorities is very much in order.

It is difficult to find studies that compare the societal and economic costs of chronic vs. infectious disease, perhaps because there aren't any. As it is a highly complex topic, research questions are difficult to formulate and real answers are difficult to provide. In addition, such research can awaken sleeping giants and provoke opposition among many stakeholders in the public health arena. Nevertheless, the opposing and consistent trends of infectious and chronic morbidity suggest that it is certainly possible that the overall burden of the latter will someday exceed that of the former, if it hasn't already. Indeed, as briefly illustrated below, it's likely that this shift occurred sometime in the previous century.

As you may recall, chronic health conditions, unlike most ordinary childhood infectious diseases, can last for many months, years, and often even for the lifetime of the patient. Most of these conditions cannot be cured with modern medical techniques. Medications and treatments can sometimes alleviate the symptoms of chronic illness, which may help sufferers to cope with its continual challenges. These medical therapies are usually consumed on a daily or weekly basis and tend to be quite costly. Drugs for chronic conditions, especially due to their routine and long-term use, usually come with their own side effects, which have the potential to create new health problems that may require even more medications and treatments. As already mentioned, some chronic health conditions limit patients' daily routine, and sometimes even prevent them from engaging in the main activity appropriate for their age group, like attending school. Some disabilities require personal educational or therapeutic assistance and limit children's ability to learn and function normally, reducing their chances of ever becoming independent and fully functioning members of society. Thus, it is clear that the economic resources required for treating chronic conditions, as well as the costs associated with the loss of patients' future work capacity, are astronomical.[115]

In the United States of today, where one in 7 children has asthma, one in 11 suffers from ADHD, and one in 4 or 5 takes medication regularly, it is plain to see that the burden of chronic illness in childhood is much higher than that of infectious disease. This historic change is hardly novel, it seems, as a comparison of US infectious and chronic morbidity data in 1979 illustrates. That year, reported cumulative incidence for relevant infectious diseases[w] was around 400,000 cases, across all ages.[116] For the sake of argument, we will assume all the cases were in children, and that one in every 20 patients who came down with an infectious disease suffered a subsequent chronic condition.[x]

---

[w] Diseases that are not relevant to children – gonorrhea, syphilis, and rabies (in animals) – were not included in the above figure.

[x] The ratio of one chronic patient to every 20 who fell ill is very high and unrealistic (especially considering that about half of the reported morbidity in the US in 1979 was chickenpox, a mild illness with rare complications). However, we used this ratio to somewhat compensate for the fact that reported morbidity

Under these assumptions, we calculate the number of children who became chronically ill due to infectious disease in the US in 1979 as 20,000. This figure, considerable as it may seem, dwarfs in comparison to the reported number of chronically ill and disabled children in the United States that same year[y] – about two million.[117]

The disparity between the societal burden of chronic and infectious disease morbidity has only grown wider from 1979 to the present. Infectious disease morbidity in children, which was already relatively low, continued to slowly decline. At the same time, the proportion of chronically ill and disabled children, which was already very high in 1979 (3.9%), more than doubled by 2010 (8%). In addition, it should be noted that for every disabled child in 2010, there were two others who routinely took medication for their chronic conditions.[118] These numbers are considerably higher than, for example, the rate of children hospitalized due to an infectious disease during the same period (an average rate of about 1% in ages 0–19).[119]

A State of Emergency

As we have shown, the overall burden of infectious disease has been declining in the Western world for the past 150 years. In our day and age, these diseases constitute only a minor threat to the health of children. They were surpassed, decades ago, by chronic illnesses and conditions, which assumed – or, rather, should have assumed – the role of Public Health Enemy #1. This "changing of the guard" took place, presumably, in the period between the early 1950s and the late 1970s. No one bothered, however, to notify the public about this historic shift.

The health authorities, which are responsible for preventing

---

incidence is presumably much lower than the actual one, since not all cases are reported to medical authorities.

[y] This number is an underestimation in the context of this discussion, as it does not include children who have a chronic illness but are not restricted in their major activity.

infectious and chronic disease alike,[z] should have broken the news and followed through by resetting national public health priorities decades ago. Unfortunately, for their own reasons, public health officials prefer to keep underscoring the threat posed by diseases of the past, while concealing the immense damage inflicted by those of the present and future.

Thus, every two or three years, the public is informed that a new virus (or an old virus in a new guise) has suddenly appeared, threatening to spread rapidly across the world and leave millions dead in its wake. A typical example is the "swine flu" panic that struck the world in the summer of 2009. In April 2009, the CDC and the World Health Organization declared a state of global emergency due to the identification of a new-old strain of influenza (H1N1) in two American children.[120] The entire world was put on high alert, vaccines designed for the new strain were hastily developed by commercial companies, and governments lined up to buy them at a global cost of tens of billions of dollars. By comparison, in the same year, and every year since, approximately one million American children joined the ranks of chronic drug consumers, and, for about 350,000 of them, their chronic illness has limited their daily activities. Despite these astronomical figures, the CDC has not declared a state of emergency regarding the plague of chronic disease that has been "attacking" the United States for decades. Likewise, no alarm bells have been rung by its European counterpart, the European Centre for Disease Prevention and Control (ECDC), nor the World Health Organization, despite a similar trend of chronic morbidity reported in European countries and other industrialized nations.

Browsing the websites of these health organizations, one would never guess that a decades-long epidemic is disabling millions upon millions of children in the industrialized world. Bizarrely, chronic disease does not appear to be a cause for

---

[z] In the United States, the Centers for Disease Prevention and Control (CDC) is responsible for the prevention and control of infectious and chronic disease.

particular concern in the public health sector, as evident by the absence of words such as "crisis" or "emergency" from relevant webpages. Whereas, a mere 84 cases of measles in California in early 2015 were sufficient justification for an immediate press conference in which the CDC urged the entire American public to get vaccinated immediately.[121] One can only speculate on the CDC's response should a measles or influenza epidemic break out, threatening to permanently disable some 350,000 American kids. Presumably, a national state of emergency would have been declared overnight. Yet, as we have seen, such a plague has been ongoing in the United States each and every year for the past 60 years or so, and health authorities do not appear to be the least bit concerned about it.

Counter Arguments

"Thomas McKeown's work has been largely criticized in scientific circles. It cannot be relied upon when it comes to vaccines and the decline of infectious disease." – Indeed, some researchers (such as Szreter, cited in this chapter) disagree with certain aspects of McKeown's interpretation of mortality data in Britain. This criticism seems justified to some extent. However, when it comes to the effect of medication and vaccines on reducing mortality from infectious disease from the mid-19th century onward, the scientific consensus is that McKeown's conclusion – that these medical interventions had but a minute effect – is correct and well-founded.

"The increase in the incidence of chronic conditions in recent decades is not real. Chronic illnesses are mostly caused by genetic factors, and the apparent increase in their incidence is a result of greater awareness and improved diagnostic capabilities. Thus, cases not previously recognized are diagnosed and counted today." – Firstly, a rapid increase in the rate of any chronic disease cannot be caused by a naturally occurring genetic change in the population.[122] The gene pool of a population does not change

quickly enough to cause such a drastic increase in chronic morbidity in only a few decades. Such rapid changes are caused, for
the most part, by changes in lifestyle and living conditions.[123] An
example of such an "environmental" factor's impact on population health is the dramatic decline in infectious disease mortality
beginning in the last third of the 19th century that was caused
by improvements in urban living conditions.

Second, the claim that most of the increase is due to improved diagnosis of chronic illness is untenable and not
supported by science. Mild cases of previously undiagnosed
conditions are presumably being diagnosed now, thanks to
greater awareness and improvements in diagnostic methods and
tools. These cases can explain a small portion of the recorded
increase at most.[124] Moreover, it is hard to believe that severe
chronic illness, which has also been consistently and continuously increasing over the years, eluded the diagnosis of past medical
professionals. It is unlikely that cases of regressive autism, for
example, were not detected by parents and doctors 30 or 40 years
ago. It is even harder to accept that past doctors failed to correctly diagnose, in significant numbers, chronic illnesses such as
diabetes, asthma, eczema, acute food allergy, and others that
have also become much more common in recent decades and
whose root causes are physiological in nature, with pronounced
and easily recognizable symptoms.

Another point worth making is that attributing the increase
in chronic morbidity in children to "better diagnosis" serves the
health establishment's interests and should, therefore, be taken
with a grain of salt. If this increase is real, then it can only be
regarded as a colossal fiasco on the part of health authorities and
the officials in charge of public health. Alternatively, if the
increase in chronic conditions' incidence were not real (or we
could be convinced that it isn't), but just an artifact of improved
diagnostic methods, then the tables would be turned: The authorities and the medical establishment would not be at fault
and, rather, should be praised for their efforts to improve diagnostic tools and raise public awareness of chronic conditions.

Despite the authorities' clear interest in funding research to establish the "better diagnosis" claim, the scientific evidence accumulated on the subject is far from convincing.

Either way, it is important to emphasize that the real cause of chronic illness is irrelevant to the main point of this chapter: Chronic morbidity significantly exceeds infectious disease morbidity and has for decades, and that fact should have modified Western public health priorities a long time ago.

"The increase in chronic morbidity in recent generations is due to gradual developments in medicine that have led to the survival of 'weak' children who previously died of infectious diseases (which have all but disappeared, thanks to vaccines). These children, who would have died at a young age in the past, are at a higher risk of chronic illness and thus have artificially raised the incidence of chronic conditions in past decades." – See answer to the previous claim. In addition, as we have seen, vaccines are responsible for only a minimal reduction in infectious disease mortality. The number of deaths presumably saved by vaccines pales in comparison to the rise in chronic morbidity incidence. This is easily observed if one looks at the relevant data from the 1980s to the present. While infectious disease mortality in children has been very low and relatively stable for the past 30–40 years, chronic morbidity in children has more than doubled, with many millions of children in just the United States becoming chronically ill during that period. This fact alone negates the above claim.

Also, in addition to raising child survival rates, improvements in medicine work to reduce the proportion of "weak" children in the population as well. For example, prenatal screening has reduced the number of babies born with various birth defects, and thanks to advanced medical treatments preterm infants now suffer much less than before from chronic morbidity.[125]

"Indeed, most of the major infectious diseases of the past were effectively eradicated even before the introduction of vaccines. Still, even in the 21st century, there are infectious diseases that

affect millions of children, and vaccines are our most effective tool for combating them." – The veracity of this claim should be evaluated by studies that accurately weigh the net benefits of vaccines (see chapter 6). In any case, it is irrelevant to the main points made in this chapter, which examines the myth that vaccines are primarily responsible for the disappearance of the dreadful infectious diseases of the late 19th and early 20th centuries. The historical record clearly shows that this myth is fallacious, and therefore it is incumbent upon scientific and medical bodies to disseminate well-founded, accurate, and complete information regarding this issue.

"Vaccines have significantly reduced the mortality rates of their respective diseases." – Indeed, the data show that at least some vaccines (diphtheria, pertussis, and measles) reduced mortality rates once they were widely used. However, the hard scientific evidence proves that most of the reduction in infectious disease mortality in the Western world was either unrelated to vaccines (for diseases which had no vaccine) or occurred before the introduction of vaccines (for diseases which did have vaccines). In addition, the declines in mortality rates for the major vaccine-preventable diseases mentioned above would probably have continued even in the absence of their vaccines. Vaccines, according to the scientific consensus, have made only a marginal historical contribution to mortality reduction from infectious disease.

"Most of the decline in infectious disease mortality in the 20th century is attributed to improvements in medicine: drugs, vaccines, modern hospitals, better medical care, and the like." – This claim is patently incorrect. The scientific consensus among researchers, backed up by irrefutable evidence, is that the vast majority of the decline was achieved even before the widespread use of medical interventions such as medications and vaccines that could positively affect infectious disease mortality.

Summary

The rapid growth of large cities during the 19th century generated favorable conditions for the spread of infectious diseases. Filthy streets, inadequate sewage treatment, poor living conditions, lack of fresh, healthy and varied food, a general unawareness of the role of hygiene in curbing the spread of infectious disease – all of these degraded city residents' overall health and weakened their immunity to infectious disease. Epidemics that hit urban populations in the mid-19th century were followed by civil reforms aimed at improving living conditions and public health. Centralized sewage management systems began to appear in the last third of the century. Improvements were made to the supply of drinking water, and running water was gradually introduced into homes. At the same time, the nutritional content of the food city residents ate improved dramatically due to new technologies in transportation that enabled delivery of fresh food from afar throughout the year. Following the great discoveries of microbiology in the late 19th century, the role of hygiene in preventing the spread of disease became widely recognized. This newly formed awareness, along with a gradual improvement in living conditions (more spacious living, better storage of food at home, etc.) also contributed to reduction of infectious disease morbidity.

These improvements in living conditions led to a dramatic decrease in infectious disease mortality between the mid-19th and mid-20th centuries, as well as a sharp decline in morbidity to the point that some were virtually eliminated. Effective medical drugs and vaccines, however, only became available in the 1930s and 1940s, after most of the reduction in infectious disease mortality had already been realized. Historically, vaccination contributed marginally to reductions in the mortality of a small number of diseases, which were trending downward anyway in a decline that would probably have continued (albeit at a slower pace) even without vaccines. In terms of reducing morbidity, vaccines have made a more significant, though not major, contribution. Incidence of some of the worst diseases of the 19th century has declined greatly, and some have disappeared altogether, for reasons unrelated to vaccines. Incidence of several major diseases (specifically, diphtheria, pertussis, and measles) greatly decreased thanks to vaccines that were introduced in the mid-20th century.

Concurrent with the gradual disappearance of the intimidating infectious diseases of the past, chronic illnesses began appearing in the industrialized countries of the 20th century at ever-increasing rates. A consistent rise in the incidence of chronic illness in children has been documented in the United States since 1960, and continues to this day, with chronic conditions that were once rare becoming alarmingly common. In the 21st century, when one in 12 American children is disabled by chronic illness, and one in 4 takes medication for a chronic condition (with similar numbers reported in other Western countries), the "silent epidemic" has become a major threat to children's health and a huge burden on the economy.

Although they are well aware that the bulk of the reduction in the burden of infectious disease cannot be attributed to vaccines, and that extensive research literature and rock-solid scientific evidence have proven that fact, health authorities around the world continue to promote the largely false "vaccines eradicated the great diseases of yore" myth. At the same time, they feed the public another misleading myth – "our health has never been better" – while ignoring the surge of chronic morbidity that has plagued the Western world since at least the mid-20th century. This huge wave of morbidity continues to gain momentum even now, physically disabling an ever-increasing proportion of the population, especially children, and rendering them dependent on medication for daily functioning.

The same medical establishment that takes (largely undeserved) credit for the successful battle against infectious disease should rightfully assume responsibility for its five decades of failure to curb, or even slow, the spread of chronic disease in the children of industrialized nations.

9

HERD IMMUNITY

Of the founding myths of vaccination, herd immunity is perhaps the medical establishment's most important and essential one. Vaccination policies in countries all over the world are based, both ethically and practically, on the supposition that vaccines provide herd immunity. This supposition is the main justification for the vaccine mandates that some countries have imposed.

What exactly is this herd immunity that we attribute to vaccines? What conditions are required for its existence? Which vaccines provide it? And is it either a moral or practical justification for vaccine mandates? This chapter will provide answers to all of these questions.

What is Herd Immunity?

Before explaining the concept of *herd immunity*, we first need to clarify the meaning of the term *immunity*. In the context of infectious disease prevention, immunity has two primary meanings: (a) protection against getting ill and (b) protection against infection with the disease pathogen (causative agent). These two are not the same thing. To understand this better, let us consider a hypothetical example.

Suppose that John was exposed on a number of occasions to a

certain disease pathogen but remained healthy throughout, without ever showing any disease symptoms. Since John didn't get sick, we could say that John has immunity to that particular disease. But even though John himself did not become ill, he was infected by the disease pathogen (a bacterium, for this example) and became its carrier for a while. During that time he could have infected anyone with whom he had been in close contact. Thus, even though John is immune to the disease itself, he is not immune to being infected by the bacterium and spreading it to other people.

Mark, like John, did not get sick despite being repeatedly exposed to the bacterium. But unlike John, Mark wasn't infected by the disease pathogen and did not become a carrier. He is immune to both the disease and infection by the disease pathogen. Although Mark was exposed to the bacterium, he does not spread it around. Thus, his immunity protects his contacts from potential infection. Because he doesn't carry the pathogen, in addition to being protected from disease himself Mark also contributes to curbing dissemination of the disease, thereby reducing the overall level of morbidity in the population.

Herd immunity, then, exists when a large proportion of individuals in a population, like Mark, are immune to being infected by a particular disease pathogen. In this scenario, the pathogen has difficulty moving from one human host to another, and disease distribution never gains momentum. Over time it might even disappear completely.[1] Thus, if all of John's family, friends, and acquaintances were immune to infection by our example bacterium, then even though he himself somehow got infected, he would be very unlikely to transmit it to others because the pathogen would not encounter a non-immune person to jump to. Thus, the chain of infection would be broken.

Herd immunity in a population, then, depends on the immunity of large numbers of individuals to infection by a disease pathogen. As barriers against the spread of the disease pathogen, these immune individuals provide indirect protection for those in their vicinity who are not immune to the disease.[2] A population's high level of immunity against infection may even prevent entry and spread of an external pathogen. Thus, if most of the population were protected against infection by a certain virus, a tourist who entered the country carrying the virus would not be likely to cause a widespread outbreak of the disease. The virus would not be able to find enough non-immune individuals to keep the infection chain going.[3]

Natural Immunity

The discussion thus far has used the term *immunity* without specifying how that immunity was acquired. At the individual level immunity to disease may be acquired naturally or artificially (through vaccination). Natural immunity to disease and/or infection can develop through exposure to the disease's causative agent[a] or, in the specific case of young infants, through receiving maternal antibodies during pregnancy and lactation. In most cases, after people are exposed to a disease pathogen, whether or not they exhibit symptoms, they develop long-term immunity to the disease, including protection against future infection.[4] However, this immunity may come at the price of coming down with the disease and all that can entail. Maternal antibodies provide infants with some degree of immunity, but that usually wears off within several months, after which the child is no longer protected from infection.[5]

Natural immunity cannot in itself lead to the eradication of diseases.[b] Even when those who fall ill (or are exposed to the pathogen) gain lifelong immunity from both disease and infec-

---

[a] Natural immunity is not attainable for all infectious diseases. Influenza infection, for example, does not provide long-term immunity (see discussion later in the chapter).

[b] As we saw in the previous chapter, however, other factors such as improved nutrition, better hygiene, and steps that blocked the chain of infection (e.g., patient isolation) certainly led to dramatic decreases in incidence and severity of various infectious diseases, and even de facto elimination of some (for example, cholera in the Western world). In addition, natural immunity can eradicate disease in an isolated area, such as an island.

tion, new children are continually being born, adding to the pool of susceptible individuals. These non-immune persons can be exposed to the disease pathogen at some point in their lives and become infected (and possibly ill). If they then pass it on to other non-immune people, the cycle continues. In this way the pathogen continues to circulate in the population, moving from one host to another, ad infinitum.[c]

This dynamic also explains the outbreak pattern typical of common childhood diseases such as measles or pertussis (whooping cough). In the period preceding the introduction of their respective vaccines, these diseases were characterized by major outbreaks every few years, after which there would be several years of relative quiet. In those years of low disease activity, the pool of non-immune children in the population gradually increased, until, at some point, the scales would tip and an epidemic wave would occur, when most of the children who had not already had the disease would be infected. These children then developed their own natural immunity against future infection. After a while the wave of illness would dissipate, but the disease pathogen would continue to circulate in the population, albeit less conspicuously, for the next several years. During this period, children born since the last epidemic wave would be added to the pool of the non-immune. At some point, a new outbreak would erupt, and many of those non-immune children would be infected, thereby gaining immunity to the pathogen – and so on and so forth.[6]

Herd Immunity and Disease Eradication

As we have seen, natural immunity alone cannot eradicate an infectious disease in most circumstances. Conversely, a vaccine could potentially do so, but in addition to preventing illness, it

---

[c] This is a simplistic discussion of the issue intended to illustrate the principle. Various diseases have appeared and disappeared throughout history spontaneously; the reasons for this are not fully understood in many cases.

would also have to prevent, or at least significantly reduce, the spread of the pathogen in the population. In other words, it should be capable of conferring herd immunity.

For a vaccine to generate herd immunity, it must protect against infection with the disease pathogen so that the vaccinated cannot infect the unvaccinated. Correspondingly, a vaccine that does not protect against infection and transmission of a pathogen cannot confer herd immunity – and cannot eradicate the disease. If a significant barrier to pathogen spread doesn't exist, cases of illness are likely to occur. Thus, a vaccine that effectively prevents illness (but not infection) may reduce the level of morbidity, but it cannot eliminate it altogether.[7]

A perfect example of the above is tetanus. The tetanus bacterium lives in soil and is not transmitted from person to person. The vaccine does nothing to limit the pathogen's prevalence and does not prevent exposure to it.[8] Therefore, as the tetanus vaccine is not 100% effective in preventing disease and tetanus vaccine coverage is not complete,[9] a few cases are likely to occur every year even in highly vaccinated countries, as is indeed the case.[10]

On the other hand, a vaccine that provided permanent protection against infection with the pathogen could theoretically lead to the eradication of the disease, even with incomplete (yet high) vaccine coverage and vaccine efficacy of less than a hundred percent.[11] Erection of a high enough barrier against the spread of the pathogen in the population should lead to a gradual decrease in morbidity and potentially even, provided suitable conditions, to complete elimination of the disease.[d]

Herd Immunity and Vaccination Policy

One of the major considerations that influence public health

---

[d] One such condition is that humans must be the sole host for the disease pathogen. Tetanus, as mentioned above, cannot be eradicated by vaccination because the tetanus bacterium does not rely on humans to survive.

policy is the balance between the expected benefit from a certain measure and the measure's potential impingement on individual freedom. For example, there is a broad scientific consensus that the consumption of soft drinks has detrimental effects on health; therefore, from a health perspective it would be quite reasonable to completely ban their sale. However, the expected health benefits of such a ban must be weighed against people's right to consume what they wish, regardless of the health risks.

Another consideration, in this context, is the extent to which an action taken by an individual affects the health of others. The more an action's consequences are limited to the individual doing the action and the less it affects others, the more that prohibiting the action would be viewed as a violation of personal freedom – and vice versa.

A typical example of this idea is smoking. As long as smoking's negative health effects were believed to be limited to the smoker, severe restrictions on smoking were harder to justify, as they were perceived as a disproportionate violation of the individual's freedom of choice. When the detrimental health effects of "passive smoking" (simply being around smokers) became known, however, many countries enacted laws restricting smoking in public spaces based on the premise that smokers have the right to harm themselves, but not to put others at risk.

In light of the above discussion, it is easy to see why the assertion that vaccines also protect the unvaccinated by providing herd immunity is so important to most countries' national vaccination policies. If the benefits of vaccines were limited to the vaccinated (preventing them from getting ill), then choosing not to vaccinate would be essentially equivalent to consuming sugary beverages or smoking in private. In which case, each person (or legal guardian in the case of children) should have the right to decide for themselves whether to receive any or all recommended vaccines. But if vaccines provided protection to both the vaccinated and the unvaccinated, then mandating them in the name of the public good would not be that farfetched, despite the restriction of individuals' freedom.

Today, health authorities around the world operate on the assumption that vaccines provide herd immunity, and thus it is in the public interest, as well as morally just, for vaccination to be managed and promoted by the government.[12] As such, health authorities in many countries have assumed responsibility for vaccination by establishing national childhood vaccine programs, purchasing vaccines with government funds, marketing and distributing vaccines, educating the public on the importance of vaccination, and taking other measures to ensure high vaccination rates.

In addition, the indirect protection attributed to vaccines serves as the authorities' principal justification for forcing the public to vaccinate.[13] Since the benefit inherent in doing so goes beyond the vaccinated individual, they argue, it is not unreasonable for the public interest to prevail over individual rights. Therefore, vaccination should be mandatory.[14] These considerations are not purely theoretical – mandatory vaccination already exists in countries such as the United States,[e] France, and Italy.[15] In other countries, including Israel, vaccine proponents frequently call for mandates when outbreaks occur or vaccination rates fall below a certain threshold.[16]

The Moral Basis for Mandatory Vaccination

As stated above, the notion that it is acceptable, under certain circumstances, to force a person to be vaccinated (or to vaccinate their children) rests almost entirely on the concept of herd immunity. In the absence of a greater societal benefit, it would be even more unreasonable to require the injection of foreign substances into one's body than it would be to ban the consumption of soft drinks. However, since vaccination presumably confers benefits that go beyond that of the vaccinated individual,

---

[e] In the US vaccination laws vary by state. All 50 states have school vaccination requirements; however, which particular vaccines are required varies somewhat from state to state.

a moral argument can be made for mandating vaccination.

Even if mandating vaccines seems morally justified by the concept of herd immunity, despite conflicting sharply with the principle of individual freedom, is there sufficient scientific evidence to support such a measure?

It would seem appropriate to set the evidentiary bar particularly high to justify such an invasive practice, with both individual and societal benefits being undeniable. Unlike banning smoking in public places – which everyone agrees provides only benefit and no harm to physical health (no one has yet been severely harmed by *not* smoking) – the vaccination issue is more complex. Though some vaccines have a proven track record of reducing disease incidence, they also have side effects, sometimes serious ones, which must be incorporated into any cost–benefit analysis. To substantiate the claim that vaccines are both personally and societally beneficial, their disease-reduction capabilities need to be weighed against their side effects. In more precise terms, the benefits of vaccines (reduction in infectious disease and disease-related hospitalization days, medications, and lost workdays) should be compared to their direct costs (the price of the vaccines themselves and costs involved in their distribution) plus their indirect costs (medical treatment for their side effects, loss of parental workdays, loss of future earnings, and so on). Only such a comprehensive and detailed analysis can provide a solid evidentiary basis for the claim that the individual and societal benefits of vaccines outweigh their harms.

Unfortunately, such an analysis has never been done.

As demonstrated in the first part of this book, the true rate of vaccine side effects is systematically concealed by vaccine manufacturers and health authorities. Recall from chapter 1 that the true extent of the side effects of a new vaccine is obscured during its pre-licensing clinical trials by testing it against another vaccine or some bioactive vaccine-like compound. Thus, for example, the Prevnar vaccine was tested in a clinical trial against a control group that received a different vaccine (an experimental meningococcal vaccine). The trial demonstrated that the vaccine was effective in preventing invasive pneumococcal disease: Among the 19,000 infants who were vaccinated with Prevnar, there were 18 fewer cases than expected. But in the same trial, nearly 1,200 of the Prevnar-vaccinated infants had to visit the emergency room, and more than 500 of them had to be hospitalized.[17] It is difficult to say how many of these incidents were caused by the Prevnar vaccine since the control group received a different vaccine (with an unknown safety profile) and both groups were given DTaP vaccines as well. Still, at the very least, the trial results raise the serious possibility that the vaccine's side effects far outweigh its benefits.

As we've seen, the true rates of common short-term vaccine side effects are unknown. Similarly, reliable data on the long-term side effects of vaccines are also scarce. As discussed in the previous chapter, chronic morbidity in children has been rising steadily since the middle of the 20th century in step with the increase in vaccine use. However, any impact vaccines have had on this dramatic increase is unknown, as their effect on chronic illness (and overall health) in children has never been properly studied. Health authorities do not perform – or, more precisely, refuse to perform – the necessary studies required to answer this crucial question (see chapter 6).

Without reliable data on the indirect costs of vaccines, no valid cost–benefit analysis can be performed, and it is impossible to determine whether their benefits outweigh their risks – or the other way around. As it stands today, with no solid scientific evidence of the net benefit of vaccination – either personal or societal – there is no moral justification for vaccine mandates. Universally imposing a medical intervention that carries serious risks should be inconceivable without first providing conclusive proof of its net benefit to both the individual and the society.

Theoretical Model and Practical Application

We have shown that the public health benefit attributed to vaccines – herd immunity – cannot in and of itself tip the scales in favor of mandating vaccination due to the lack of reliable information on vaccines' true costs. Now, let's look at some of the science behind herd immunity – how credible and convincing is it? If we somehow miraculously came up with reliable information on vaccine costs, would there be enough scientific evidence of herd immunity to justify mandates?

The basic premise of herd immunity makes a lot of sense: The more roadblocks an infectious disease pathogen encounters, the less likely it is to move through a population, causing disease. In fact, humanity has been aware of this principle for the past 150 years or so and has since applied it in a variety of effective ways – through treatment of sewage, encouragement of personal hygiene, isolation of infectious patients, and more. By the same token, if a particular vaccine built a personal barrier against disease transmission, and a sufficiently high proportion of the population were vaccinated, the spread of the disease would be halted, morbidity would decline to a very a low level, and outbreaks would become rare. The herd immunity threshold, the proportion of the population that needs to be vaccinated to achieve this effect, is the magic number – the Holy Grail – of vaccine research, and a great deal of effort goes into building complex mathematical models to calculate it for every vaccine.[18] Reaching these herd immunity thresholds in the first place, and maintaining them once reached, is one of the primary goals of the agencies that promote vaccination. These magic herd-immunity-threshold numbers often affect operational decisions – such as whether to add a booster dose for a particular vaccine, launch a campaign to increase vaccination rates, or add a new vaccine to the schedule.

Despite their importance to vaccine policy, herd-immunity-threshold computations are based on a rather sketchy theoretical scientific foundation. Simplistic mathematical models are used, applying crude assumptions that fail to emulate the complex real-world interplay of vaccine and disease in a population. Thus, for example, most models assume that individuals are either fully protected or completely unprotected from disease and fully protected or completely unprotected from infection, that the protection level is uniform in all individuals across a population or subpopulation, and a slew of other unrealistic assumptions.[19] Complicating the modeling even further, vaccine-induced immunity is not identical for all vaccines, it can be partial, and it often wanes over time.[20]

Attempts by researchers to refine these models to better simulate reality have not been successful. As a result, herd immunity threshold estimations for individual vaccines vary according to the calculation model applied and the specific assumptions used. Thus, different studies set the vaccine coverage rate required for the elimination of measles somewhere between 55 and 96 percent,[21] and for diphtheria between 50 and 90 percent.[22] The threshold required for a sustained reduction in congenital defects due to rubella is between 50 and 80 percent.[23] The herd immunity threshold, the authors of the relevant chapter in the canonical textbook *Vaccines* conclude, is merely a "crude estimate" that serves as a "rough guideline" in predicting the impact that a particular vaccination strategy may have and provides only "hints" as to the potential eradication of a disease.[24]

Thus, the herd immunity threshold – the magic vaccination rate that's supposed to ensure the elimination of a particular disease – is not an accurate numerical value based on robust scientific data and meticulous calculation; it is a "crude estimate" based on simplistic models, fed by arbitrary and unrealistic assumptions.

Herd Immunity and Routine Vaccinations

As was explained above, vaccines do not necessarily confer herd immunity. The *Vaccines* textbook explains: "If a vaccine were to protect only against disease, and not at all against infection, then it would have no influence on infection transmission in the community and there would be no indirect protection (vaccination of one person would have no influence on any others in the community). It would be possible to reduce disease with such a vaccine but not to eradicate the infection."[25] In other words, vaccines that do not prevent infection with the disease pathogen cannot confer herd immunity.

Health authorities make frequent and broad use of the term *herd immunity* to denote the indirect protection provided by vaccines. Their formal publications, however, rarely, if ever, mention that such immunity is theoretically possible for some vaccines, but not for others. We will use the rest of the chapter, then, to examine the scientific evidence for herd immunity for each of the routine childhood vaccines.

Tetanus Vaccine

Tetanus is caused by a toxin secreted by the bacterium *Clostridium tetani*. The bacterium lives in the digestive tract of various animals and is excreted in their feces. It can also survive in soil for many years in the form of a spore. If a dormant spore somehow makes it into the human body – typically through an open wound or incision – it can "wake up", revert back into a bacterium, and begin to multiply rapidly. During its multiplication process in the body, the bacterium secretes the toxin that causes tetanus, which if not treated promptly and properly, can be fatal.

Unlike many other infectious diseases, tetanus is not transmitted directly from person to person. The bacterium, as mentioned above, penetrates the human body through a wound and is not excreted from the body in a way that might normally lead to the infection of another person.[26]

Tetanus was more common in the distant past, when most of the population lived in rural areas, and later on, when horses became the main means of transportation in large cities of the pre-modern era. In addition, tetanus was common among wounded soldiers on battlefields, which were often saturated with horse feces. Incidence of tetanus in industrialized countries began declining steadily in in the early 20th century. Several factors contributed to this: mass migration to cities, the departure of horses from city streets, the replacement of horses with machines in agriculture, better treatment of wounds, and the use of antibiotics. In the US in 1947, a year before the tetanus vaccine came into wide use, morbidity was already quite low at 0.39 cases per 100,000.[27] This rate continued to decline gradually after the vaccine was introduced.

The tetanus vaccine protects against the toxin secreted by the bacterium, not the bacterium itself. Thus, it does not prevent the bacterium or spores from entering and multiplying in the body. When the bacterium enters the body, the antibodies stimulated by the vaccine neutralize the toxin it releases into the bloodstream. This, plus the fact that the tetanus bacterium normally lives in soil, means that the vaccine is not a barrier to infection with the bacterium and hence does not confer herd immunity.[28]

Polio Vaccine

Polio will be covered in depth in chapter 10, which includes a detailed review of herd immunity and polio vaccines – the Salk vaccine (or IPV, the inactivated polio vaccine) and the Sabin vaccine (OPV, oral polio vaccine). The main points of that discussion are presented below.

The institutional narrative on polio is riddled with gaps, contradictions, and unexplained facts. Similarly, the scientific debate on whether polio vaccines confer herd immunity is largely based on conjecture intended to bridge the gap between theory and reality. For example, researchers are incapable of providing an evidence-based explanation for the disappearance of poliovirus from the US as early as 1970, even though the OPV vaccination rate was only at around 65 percent in children, and much lower in adults. Did the poliovirus actually disappear from the United States? And if so, did it disappear because Sabin's vaccine generated herd immunity? Did the vaccine's attenuated poliovirus, excreted in the stools of the vaccinated, seize the ecological niche that was formerly inhabited by the wild poliovirus and thus push it out of the country? The paucity of evidence on this topic precludes researchers from providing compelling answers to these important questions.[29]

Another key question concerns the disappearance of polio (and the poliovirus) from countries such as Sweden, Finland, and the Netherlands, which made exclusive use of the Salk vaccine. As will be detailed in chapter 10, Salk's inactivated vaccine is supposed to prevent polio paralysis by stimulating antibodies that prevent the virus from traveling through the bloodstream to the nervous system. But the vaccine doesn't stop poliovirus transmission, as explained by prominent polio researcher, Yale professor of epidemiology and pediatrics, Dorothy Horstmann: "The extent to which the inactivated vaccine has suppressed the circulation of wild polioviruses [...] is not well documented [...] This is not surprising, for although the vaccine induces antibody formation, it does not provide a significant barrier to intestinal infection with either wild or vaccine strains."[30] Thus, the Salk vaccine, by design, is not supposed to confer protection against contagion and therefore cannot prevent dissemination of the poliovirus in the population. How, then, did the poliovirus disappear from countries that used only the Salk vaccine? Polio experts have no convincing answers to this question. On the contrary, some experts go so far as to speculate that the alleged disappearance of poliovirus from Sweden, Finland, and the Netherlands is proof that the Salk vaccine does indeed prevent the spread of the virus (that is, confers herd immunity).[31] However, they cannot provide solid evidence to back their claims.

Since scientific discussion of herd immunity and polio vaccines is rather murky, for the sake of this discussion we will settle for the scientific consensus.

Regarding the Salk vaccine (IPV), the World Health Organization asserts that it is incapable of producing substantial herd immunity. A WHO official document states that the vaccine "induces only very low-level immunity to poliovirus inside the gut. As a result, it [...] only marginally reduces the spread of wild poliovirus. In a person immunized with IPV, wild virus can still multiply inside the intestines and be shed in the stool. Because of this, IPV could not possibly be used to eradicate polio."[32]

The scientific consensus maintains that the Sabin vaccine (OPV), however, does prevent infection with the virus and is a barrier to the spread of the poliovirus in the population.[33] In addition, it is believed to contribute further to indirect protection and herd immunity because vaccinated people excrete the weakened vaccine virus in their stools for several weeks following vaccination. Those who come in contact with feces of a vaccinated person may then be infected with the weakened virus and gain future protection from polio.[34]

The Sabin polio vaccine, the one that can affect herd immunity according to the WHO, has not been used in North American or Western European countries for more than ten years.[35] These countries do not seem to see a need to prevent poliovirus transmission in the 21st century and are content with the personal protection provided by the Salk vaccine.

Pertussis (Whooping Cough) Vaccine

Pertussis is one of the three major infectious diseases whose morbidity significantly declined thanks to a vaccine. The pertussis vaccine, widely used in the United States since 1948, has long been considered one of the main pillars of the vaccination program. Although the vaccine has been in general use for the past seventy years, the way in which it curbs the spread of the pertussis bacterium (*Bordetella pertussis*) has almost never been studied, and experiments testing its ability to prevent human infection and person-to-person transmission have never been performed.[36]

Despite the lack of scientific evidence, or perhaps because of it, the medical profession has always considered the pertussis vaccine capable of generating herd immunity, with the potential to eradicate the disease.[37] In recent years, with a steep rise observed in pertussis morbidity in most Western countries, health officials have repeatedly emphasized vaccination's key role in limiting disease distribution and protecting vulnerable populations (particularly newborns and the elderly). Their recommendations are obviously based on the assumption that vaccinated people prevent the spread of the pertussis bacterium, thereby protecting their contacts from contracting the disease.

The unexpected resurgence of pertussis morbidity in Western countries in the first decade of the 21st century led three researchers from the FDA's Center for Biologics Evaluation and Research (CBER) to conduct, for the very first time, an experiment to test the indirect protection that the vaccine was assumed to confer.[38] Warfel and colleagues published their surprising outcomes in the American National Academy of Sciences' journal in 2014. In the experiment, the researchers compared the response of pertussis-vaccinated baboons to that of baboons who contracted the disease naturally. Baboons were chosen as test animals because when infected with the pertussis bacterium they exhibit symptoms and a clinical disease course similar to pertussis in humans. In addition, like humans, an infected baboon carries the pertussis bacterium in its throat for several weeks and can transmit it to other baboons in its vicinity.[39]

The researchers divided the baboons into four trial groups: Group A was vaccinated with the current, acellular, pertussis vaccine (DTaP) according to the US vaccination schedule – at two, four, and six months of age. Group B was vaccinated with the former, whole-cell, pertussis vaccine (DTP) on a similar schedule. Group C baboons were not vaccinated and were not exposed to the pertussis bacterium. Baboons in group D were also not vaccinated, but they were exposed to the pertussis bacterium in a way that mimicked natural infection, contracted the disease, and recovered.

At seven months of age, the researchers exposed all the baboons to the pertussis bacterium and examined their response. The vaccinated baboons as well as those previously infected (groups A, B, and D) showed no symptoms of illness, which indicated that both previous pertussis illness and receipt of either vaccine provided protection from the disease. The baboons from group C, who were not vaccinated and had not previously contracted pertussis, got sick and carried the bacterium in their respiratory tract for about 30 days. In contrast, baboons that had not been vaccinated but had been infected in the past (group D), had complete protection against re-exposure – tests showed they didn't carry the bacterium at any time.

So far, all was as expected.

When the researchers examined the vaccinated baboons, however, they discovered something totally unexpected. Group A baboons, which were vaccinated with the current pertussis vaccine and later exposed to the bacterium, carried the bacterium for 35 days following exposure (five days longer than the unvaccinated baboons of group C). Those vaccinated with the old vaccine (group B) carried the bacterium for 18 days – a shorter, but still significant length of time.

Following that surprising outcome, the researchers sought to further test whether a vaccinated baboon that was colonized by the bacterium could infect other baboons. Two baboons vaccinated with the current vaccine (group A) were exposed to the pertussis bacterium and placed in separate cages. Twenty-four hours later an unvaccinated baboon that had never contracted pertussis before was placed in each of the cages. Several days later tests indicated that the "naïve" baboons had been infected with the bacterium by their vaccinated cage-mates. Group D baboons, who had had pertussis in the past, were placed in similar conditions with very different results. Not only were they not re-infected, they also did not infect other baboons placed in their cages.[40]

In a subsequent experiment, an unvaccinated baboon was infected with the pertussis bacterium and then placed in a cage with one unvaccinated and two DTaP-vaccinated baboons (current vaccine). All of the animals ended up being infected with the bacterium.[41] "[T]he key finding of this study," the researchers conclude, "[is that acellular pertussis] vaccines do not prevent infection or transmission of [the bacterium]."[42] This finding was reconfirmed by the same research team in a study the following year.[43]

The results of Warfel and colleagues' "baboon study" contradict previous scientific understanding of the protection provided
by the pertussis vaccine. Until Warfel 2014 it was widely believed that the vaccine protected the individual from being
infected by the bacterium and passing it on to others. In fact,
some official pertussis vaccination guidelines are directly derived
from this assumption. Now, the Warfel study results were suggesting the opposite: Even if they do not come down with
pertussis, the vaccinated can carry the bacterium and infect
others for weeks after exposure (possibly even longer than the
unvaccinated).[44] [f] The current pertussis vaccine, then, does not
prevent infection or transmission of the bacterium, and therefore
does not confer herd immunity. Warfel and colleagues were well
aware of the implications of their study results, writing, "To
protect the most vulnerable members of the population and
achieve optimal herd immunity it will be necessary to develop a
vaccination strategy that effectively blocks pertussis infection
and transmission."[45] Or, put more concretely, "[it] will require
the development of improved vaccines."[46]

Despite the fact that Warfel 2014's findings nullified some
recommendations pertaining to pertussis vaccination from health
authorities around the world by highlighting the shortcomings
of the pertussis vaccine and its role in the recent surge in pertussis morbidity, they did not surprise those who had been
following pertussis research for the last few decades. Prior

---

[f] Recall that in Warfel 2014 baboons vaccinated with the current (acellular)
vaccine carried the bacterium five days longer than their unvaccinated counterparts (35 days versus 30). However, it is difficult to infer from this outcome who
actually contributes more to the spread of the pertussis bacterium in the human
population – the vaccinated or the unvaccinated. On the one hand, the study
results suggest that the vaccinated carry the bacterium longer, which gives them
more opportunities to infect others. In addition, they typically display no disease
symptoms, which means they and their contacts are less likely to take the
necessary precautions to reduce transmission. On the other hand, the unvaccinated usually develop the typical symptoms of the disease, including the classic
cough that in itself contributes to the spread of the bacterium (although taking
antibiotics kills the pertussis bacterium and limits its spread).

studies had already suggested that the pertussis vaccine does not generate herd immunity, and other studies reinforced the notion by demonstrating that natural disease conferred individual immunity superior to that of the vaccine. For example, Fine and Clarkson examined outbreak patterns of pertussis in the UK in the 1980s and found that the interval between outbreaks did not change significantly after the introduction of the vaccine. The two researchers interpreted this as a sign that the vaccine reduces morbidity but does not prevent the spread of the bacterium.[47] Studies in the 1990s reported cases in which those vaccinated with the whole-cell pertussis vaccine became infected with the bacterium and transmitted it to others, even though they did not get sick (making them asymptomatic carriers).[48] James Cherry and colleagues found (2004) that the pertussis vaccine does not elicit an antibody to a toxin called ACT, which is secreted by the pertussis bacterium and is known to play a key role in the disease build-up process. Contracting pertussis, on the other hand, does generate ACT antibodies in unvaccinated individuals. All of these findings are consistent with the results of Warfel 2014, which showed that pertussis vaccination does not provide resistance to future infection, while the natural disease does.[49]

Several months after the publication of Warfel 2014, William Smallridge and colleagues from the University of Pennsylvania reported similar results in lab mice. The Pennsylvania team followed Warfel's example, but replaced the baboons with mice. "We were surprised to determine," the researchers wrote, "that an acellular vaccine previously found to affect pathology and colonization of the lungs was ineffective at inhibiting shedding and transmission."[50] (In layman's terms: The vaccine prevents the bacterium from reaching the lungs to cause disease but does not prevent infection and transmission to others.) The significance of these findings is evident: "...These results suggest that the resurgence of B. pertussis [the pertussis bacterium] could be due to two deficiencies of the acellular vaccines: failure to protect the vaccinated individual from infection, only blunting the severity of disease, and failure to prevent the transmission of B. pertussis."[51] And lastly, they note, "Current vaccines do not effectively prevent transmission of Bordetella and thus fail to confer the full benefits of herd immunity in reducing clinical cases [i.e., morbidity]."[52]

It is worth noting at this point that the groundbreaking findings of these 2014 studies, in addition to elucidating the limitations of the pertussis vaccine, also illustrate the wide gap between the way vaccine science is portrayed by the medical establishment and its reality. From the 1930s, when the pertussis vaccine was first developed, until 2014, medical scientists and officials held firm to a misconception about its ability to generate herd immunity and derived vaccination guidelines and recommendations from it. One could, perhaps, argue for leniency in the case of the old (whole-cell) pertussis vaccine, which was developed in the first half of the previous century at a time when vaccine science was still in its infancy.[53] But the new (acellular) vaccine was developed in the late 1980s, when vaccine manufacturers, scientists, and health authorities had vast resources and sophisticated scientific tools at their disposal. No fewer than nine different acellular pertussis vaccines made it to the clinical trial phase in the early 1990s,[54] and none were tested for its ability to prevent the spread of the bacterium.

Thus, while spokespeople for the medical establishment continually assure the public that vaccination policies and guidelines are based on broad and well-founded scientific knowledge, in practice – as was highlighted by the Warfel and Smallridge studies – they often rely on incomplete and/or sketchy science. For an example one need look no further than the CDC's recommendation (adopted by numerous international health agencies) of the "cocooning" method to protect newborns and young infants from pertussis. "Cocooning" requires that members of an infant's immediate family (including parents, grandparents, and siblings) be vaccinated shortly before the infant's birth, assuming they will then serve as a protective shield against infection with the pertussis bacterium.[55] This guideline, which is currently practiced in many industrialized countries, was established despite the absence of solid evidence that the vaccine provided such protection. In addition, it is one of the guidelines that the Warfel 2014 study clearly negates. As the researchers point out, "Our data [...] suggest that cocooning is unlikely to be an effective strategy to reduce the burden of pertussis in infants."[56] In fact, the study results suggest that vaccinating family members for pertussis just might increase the risk of infants' infection, instead of lowering it (see the previous footnote).

The scientific evidence clearly shows that health authorities' long-time working assumption that the pertussis vaccine provides herd protection was mistaken and has led to decades of dissemination of misinformation, as well as guidelines that may have increased, rather than decreased, pertussis morbidity. The vaccine industry and health authorities, however, express neither regret nor remorse, or even acknowledge their past errors. Adding insult to injury, the medical establishment has yet to share the dramatic new evidence and its practical implications with the public. At the time of writing – almost eight years after the publication of the Warfel 2014 study – medical authorities are still withholding the fact that cutting-edge science indicates that the pertussis vaccine does not confer herd immunity.[57] They even continue to recommend cocooning,[58] despite the scientific evidence indicating that it does not prevent pertussis in young infants.[59]

Diphtheria Vaccine

Diphtheria is caused by a toxin secreted by the diphtheria bacterium (*Corynebacterium diphtheriae*). There are different strains of the bacterium, some of which secrete the toxin while others do not. Only the toxin-secreting strains cause the classic symptom of the growth of a thick membrane over the patient's throat, a dangerous condition that can lead to death. Furthermore, even these strains cannot secrete the toxin if patients are not deficient in iron.[60] The toxin-free strains cause milder disease.[61] The rate of severe morbidity and complications varies from outbreak to outbreak – the reason for this variance is unknown.[62] The exact mode of transmission of the bacterium is also unknown.[63]

The diphtheria vaccine was developed in the 1920s and began to be used routinely in the US in the late 1940s, as a component of the diphtheria-tetanus-pertussis (DTP) vaccine. Like the tetanus vaccine, the diphtheria vaccine does not protect against infection with the bacterium, but rather against the toxin it may secrete. The toxin is weakened using formaldehyde during the vaccine's production process. The resulting toxoid is no longer harmful, but when it is injected (with an aluminum adjuvant to boost its effect) it causes the human immune system to generate antibodies that protect against future exposure to the toxin.[64] Neither the efficacy nor the safety of the vaccine has ever been tested in a clinical trial; however, observational studies have reported disease prevention effectiveness ranging from 55 to 90 percent,[65] with even better protection against severe illness and death.[66]

The diphtheria vaccine is a prophylactic (preventive) treatment. People who are already ill, whether vaccinated or not, are treated with a passive vaccine (antitoxin). The passive vaccine is a serum extracted from animals, usually horses, who have developed resistance to the diphtheria toxin and whose blood, then, contains antibodies against it.[67] Injecting the serum into a diphtheria patient neutralizes the toxin circulating in the blood. At the same time, the patient is placed in isolation and treated with antibiotics in order to kill the diphtheria bacteria, thus ending production of the toxin as well as impeding transmission of the disease to others. (Before antibiotics were introduced as part of the standard treatment for diphtheria, many patients carried the bacterium for many weeks, making it difficult to stop the spread of the disease.[68]) In addition to treating the patient, any immediate contacts and members of the community found to be carrying the bacterium are also treated with antibiotics and kept in isolation in order to keep the disease from spreading. Vaccine booster doses are administered "as needed".[69]

Until the 1970s, it was widely believed that the diphtheria

vaccine protected against clinical disease but not against infection, because its action was directed only against the toxin secreted by the bacterium rather than the bacterium itself.[70] The handful of studies that examined the issue in the early 20th century found no difference in the risk of bacterial infection between the vaccinated and the unvaccinated, as did later studies.[71] In recent years, however, weak efforts have been made to attribute herd immunity to the diphtheria vaccine. This claim is presented, among others, in the canonical textbook *Vaccines*, which asserts that patients with active illness spread the bacterium more than asymptomatic carriers, and therefore, the reduction of morbidity due to the vaccine "may have been an important contributor to the disappearance of diphtheria in vaccinated populations."[72] The assertion that the diphtheria vaccine provides herd immunity by reducing morbidity conflicts with the traditional view which holds that a vaccine confers herd immunity by preventing the vaccinated from contracting the disease pathogen. In addition, the assertion that a drastic reduction in morbidity could lead to elimination of the bacterium rests on the assumption that diphtheria patients are the primary source of bacterial transmission. But is that really true? Is there sufficient scientific evidence to say that diphtheria patients are the main spreaders of the bacterium?

A 1925 study in Baltimore, Maryland, did find that a typical diphtheria patient spread the disease at a much higher rate than a healthy carrier of the bacterium. In the study, Doull and Lara calculated that diphtheria patients infected family members at a rate ten times higher than healthy carriers of the bacterium. [g] [73] Despite the fact that diphtheria patients appeared to be much more contagious than carriers at the individual level, at the population level the situation was quite different, as the researchers note. In the pre-antibiotic era, the number of diphtheria carriers in the population was presumably much

---

[g] The researchers assumed that an in-family infection occurred when one family member became ill within 30 days of another becoming ill.

higher than the number of diphtheria patients, so it was quite likely that the former were primarily responsible for spreading the disease. Carriers also come in contact with many more people, as, unlike patients, they are not restricted in their movement.[74] Supportive evidence for this supposition was found in another Baltimore study that examined the possible source of infection in diphtheria patients. Of the approximately 500 patients studied, the researchers found possible links to other patients for only 20% of the cases. The rest were attributed to infection from healthy carriers.[75] "It seems impossible to explain the general distribution of diphtheria and the usual absence of traceable lines of contact from clinical cases," conclude Doull and Lara, "on any other hypothesis except that infection is spread largely by carriers."[76]

Nearly half a century later, Dr. Louis Miller and colleagues from the CDC's Epidemiology program reached similar conclusions following two diphtheria outbreaks they studied in the late 1960s. During an outbreak at a school in the city of Elgin, Texas, among the 306 students and faculty members, they found 104 diphtheria carriers. Only 15 of them contracted the disease. Furthermore, no difference in the proportion of bacterial carriers was found between the vaccinated and non-vaccinated.[77] The researchers, who conducted a thorough search of the medical literature regarding the epidemiology of the disease, cite Doull and Lara's study as evidence of the importance of carriers in spreading diphtheria, adding that "recent epidemics in Austin and Elgin Texas, provided ample evidence that carriers continue to play a very important role in the transmission of diphtheria."[78] "However," they add, "diphtheria outbreaks have been described in populations with as much as 94% of the people being previously immunized. These outbreaks, the known importance of carriers in the spread of diphtheria, and the demonstrated failure of toxoid to prevent the carrier state lead us to conclude that the concept of herd immunity is not applicable in the prevention of diphtheria."[79]

Studies conducted in the Soviet Union in the second half of

the 20th century led researchers from the Epidemiological Center of the Soviet Ministry of Health to draw conclusions similar to those of their American counterparts. One study found that toxin-secreting diphtheria strains circulated in schools for many months even though the vaccination rate, as one might expect in the Soviet Union, was 100%, while no cases of illness were recorded. Another study found toxin-secreting bacteria in several Soviet provinces, although the child vaccination rate exceeded 97%. "The experience in Russia and elsewhere," the researchers conclude, "suggests that circulation is likely to persist in areas of lesser economic development even with good overall vaccination levels."[80]

Thus, the mild assertion made in *Vaccines* – that diphtheria vaccine should be credited with the disappearance of the disease – contradicts studies conducted by researchers from American and Soviet health agencies' that reached the opposite conclusion.

How, then, can one explain the disappearance of the disease from the Western world despite a relatively low level of population immunity to the disease (as reported by serologic studies)?[h] [81] A perusal of the relevant scientific literature fails to find an unequivocal answer to this question, in part due to the scarcity of research on the subject. The rate of diphtheria bacterial carriers in the population is virtually unstudied,[82] and the current level of disease immunity in the population, especially in adults, is unknown.[83] There is, however, at least one promising line of inquiry, if and when someone wishes to look into the matter.

As already noted, the diphtheria vaccine began to be widely used in Western countries in the 1940s, coinciding with the period in which antibiotics became the primary treatment

---

[h] Another attempt to explain the phenomenon was made by Pappenheimer (appears, for example, in Chen 1985, p. 4). Pappenheimer's hypothesis rests on evolutionary considerations concerning the relationship between the diphtheria toxin, the gene that triggers it, and the human body. Pappenheimer's hypothesis, too, has no solid epidemiological backing. For that reason, as well as space considerations, this chapter does not address it.

against bacterial infection. Antibiotics cannot cure diphtheria, as they are not effective against the toxin secreted by the bacterium,[84] but they can limit its spread, as demonstrated in a 1947 study.[85] A combined treatment of isolation and antibiotics for both diphtheria patients and bacterial carriers has been the medically accepted treatment for decades[86] and is still considered standard protocol today. Upon detection of a diphtheria patient, medical personnel locate their immediate contacts, vaccinate those that are not fully vaccinated and identify carriers of the bacterium. Carriers receive antibiotic treatment and remain in isolation for several days until laboratory tests show that the bacterium has cleared their bodies.[87]

The combination of isolation and antibiotics was introduced in order to stop the spread of the bacterium and prevent outbreaks of the disease. But does it also have a positive long-term effect of lowering diphtheria morbidity? It is hard to say, as no relevant studies have ever been conducted. Nevertheless, it would be interesting to research the effect applying (or not applying) this standard diphtheria protocol had in two countries – Romania and the Soviet Union – whose patterns of diphtheria morbidity are mentioned as supporting evidence for vaccine-induced herd immunity in the scientific literature.

Diphtheria morbidity decreased dramatically in Romania during the 1960s and 1970s, following an increase in the country's vaccination rate. But that wasn't the whole story. Tests conducted by Romanian researchers found that the percentage of toxin-secreting strains also fell sharply in that time period (from 86% in the 1960s to 5% in the 1970s). CDC's Dr. Robert Chen attributes this decrease to the hypothetical herd immunity provided by the vaccine, as the rate of morbidity decline exceeded the population's vaccination rate.[88] But was this sharp decline in the prevalence of toxic strains due to the vaccine? Another possibility is that the combined treatment of isolation and antibiotics, applied in Romania during the period in question,[89] is what led, or at least contributed heavily, to the decrease in the prevalence of toxic strains. This possibility is no less plausible, and perhaps even more so, than the hypothesis attributing herd protection to the vaccine.

The diphtheria epidemic that plagued former Soviet nations in the mid-1990s adds another interesting perspective to this subject. The institutional explanation for the outbreak is that vaccination coverage dropped significantly following the collapse of the Soviet Union, which led to re-emergence of the disease in Russia and other former Soviet countries.[i] This is considered by some to be evidence of a herd immunity effect from the vaccine. However, this account is not entirely consistent with the facts. Unlike Western countries, the Soviet Union has never been completely free of diphtheria.[90] In the 1950s, high morbidity was recorded in various areas despite vaccination coverage of over 80%. Following the enforcement of a strict national vaccination policy, morbidity decreased and reached an all-time low in the mid-1970s, but the end of the decade saw a continuous rise spanning several years.[91] "The Soviet and Russian experience," write Svetlana Markina and colleagues at the Russian National Institute of Microbiology and Epidemiology, "has been that of persistent circulation of toxigenic strains of [diphtheria bacterium] and at least two resurgences of diphtheria despite fairly high levels of vaccine coverage among most childhood age groups."[92]

Another important point concerns the difference between Soviet and Romanian approaches to the treatment of diphtheria. In the Soviet Union, unlike in Romania, antibiotics were not given to contacts of diphtheria patients. The prevailing medical opinion was that antibiotics had a negative effect on intestinal bacteria, and it was advisable to avoid their widespread use in treating diphtheria.[93] Soviet health-system personnel imple-

---

[i] A comprehensive discussion of the events of the 1990s ex-Soviet diphtheria outbreak and its causes goes beyond the scope of this chapter. The disintegration of the former Soviet Union was accompanied by numerous social and economic changes that presumably had an impact on the eruption of the diphtheria epidemic, as noted, for example, by Charles Vitek and Melinda Wharton of the CDC (1998).

mented a policy of early detection and treatment of patients through the nationwide network of clinics and laboratories, while avoiding the use of antibiotics as a preventative measure.[94] This policy was still in effect during the epidemic of the 1990s, when prophylactic antibiotics were not provided to carriers or immediate contacts of diphtheria patients.[95] Even after the epidemic subsided, pathogenic diphtheria strains continued to circulate among the Russian population, Markina and colleagues write, "and interruption of circulation in most areas is unlikely in the near future."[96] Thus, the Soviet experience demonstrates that a high level of vaccination, in the absence of antibiotic treatment for carriers and contacts of patients, does not inhibit the spread of the bacterium in the population and, hence, does not generate herd immunity either.

Because diphtheria no longer poses a significant threat to public health in industrialized countries, and hasn't for decades, scientific interest in the disease has waned. As a result, new studies on the vaccine's herd immunity capabilities are not likely in the foreseeable future. Although the vaccine has been widely used for the past 70 years, the case for a herd-immunity effect is still quite weak, as findings from several countries indicate the opposite. In the absence of robust scientific evidence, there is no justification for claiming that the diphtheria vaccine provides herd immunity or for using such a claim to set public health policy.

Influenza Vaccine

The influenza (flu) virus has an unusual trait that distinguishes it from most other pathogens: It is constantly evolving.[j] The virus undergoes frequent changes that force the human immune system to repeatedly re-adapt to it. Coming down with influenza confers future protection against the virus that is currently

---

[j] Type A influenza viruses are responsible for most cases of the disease. Type B viruses do not change frequently.

circulating, but it does not guarantee protection from next winter's version, which may have mutated to the extent that it can evade early detection by the immune system.[97]

This feature of the influenza virus is the reason why influenza morbidity doesn't guarantee future immunity and why, unlike many other infectious diseases, it is not specific to children. Typical pathogens of childhood diseases do not change significantly over time and therefore a bout of illness at a young age usually generates an immune response that provides disease protection for many years, or even for a lifetime. The influenza virus, on the other hand, changes frequently; thus, the disease can be contracted many times during one's life.

Because it can be contracted many times and at different ages, it is particularly challenging to achieve herd immunity for influenza. A one-off jab will not do the trick. The population would need to be re-vaccinated every year with a vaccine tailored to the common influenza strains of that particular season. Because health authorities frequently do not accurately predict which strains will circulate the next winter, vaccine effectiveness is usually not very high. And when the strains included in the vaccine differ markedly from those common in the population, as happens every few years, its effectiveness can even reach zero.[98]

The medical establishment is well aware that the vaccine cannot generate herd immunity. As the influenza chapter in *Vaccines* notes, studies conducted to date have failed to convincingly demonstrate that influenza vaccination of the entire population or specific subpopulations results in protection for the unvaccinated.[99] (These studies are also quite complicated to perform due to frequent changes in circulating influenza strains, seasonal fluctuations in morbidity, relatively low vaccine coverage, and other factors.)[100]

In conclusion, the influenza vaccine does not confer significant herd protection due to frequent and impossible-to-predict changes in circulating strains, which entails annual re-formulation of the vaccine in anticipation of next season's dominant strains. This results in a vaccine that is partially effective, at best, and occasionally utterly ineffective.

Hepatitis A Vaccine

The hepatitis A virus is transmitted from person to person through the fecal–oral route. Once it enters the body, the virus settles in the liver, where it replicates, potentially causing inflammation and disease. The early symptoms of hepatitis A – fatigue, stomachache, and vomiting – are similar to other forms of hepatitis. In some cases, jaundice will develop. The disease has no specific treatment, and patients receive only supportive care. Complications are rare, and so is mortality. But recovery time in adults can be relatively long – up to several months. Unlike hepatitis B, there is no chronic carriage of the virus. Infection grants immunity for life.[101]

The hepatitis A virus is common in geographical areas where sanitary conditions are poor and crowding is high. In developing countries, most children are infected with the virus in infancy but do not exhibit disease symptoms. By adolescence, virtually everyone has been infected. In industrialized countries, the prevalence of the virus is low, and the average age of infection is higher.[102] Most virus transmission occurs from person to person, mainly within the family. Young children are a major vehicle of transmission. Since their hygiene habits are typically less developed, the rate of infection among children is relatively high. In addition, infection at a young age does not usually manifest in symptomatic disease, so carriers are not identified and transmission-preventive measures are seldom applied.[103]

The hepatitis A vaccine was approved for use in 1999. The vaccine is routinely given to children in the second year of life. In the United States, the inclusion of the vaccine in the childhood schedule has significantly reduced the incidence of the disease, from about 10 cases per 100,000 before the vaccine to less than 1 in 100,000 after it.[104] Israel, which was the first nation to add the vaccine to its national childhood vaccination program

(1999), also recorded a dramatic morbidity drop, from about 35 cases per 100,000 to about 1 per 100,000.[105] Epidemiological studies indicate that a significant proportion of this decline is attributed to a herd immunity effect of the vaccine.[106] Because young children are the major source of infection, curbing the spread of the virus in this age group contributes to reducing its prevalence throughout the entire population.

So, it turns out the hepatitis A vaccine does confer herd immunity. But it's imperative to clarify, who benefits from it.

Up to 90% of children infected with the hepatitis A virus before the age of five develop no disease symptoms, while gaining full immunity for the rest of their lives. In those who present symptoms, the illness is typically mild and jaundice rarely develops. Mortality is almost zero. In contrast, nearly all adults infected with the virus for the first time get ill, and most develop jaundice. Recovery from the disease can take several months. The mortality rate is still low but increases with age.[107]

It is evident, therefore, that hepatitis A is a mild disease in children, often imperceptible, and more severe in adults (although uncommon). Young children infected with the virus become immune for life, without risking any potential side effects from the vaccine. Hence, vaccination of toddlers mainly serves a small portion of the adult population, by reducing its risk of disease. Toddlers are generally considered to be a susceptible subpopulation, whose health should be protected by the rest of society. When it comes to the hepatitis A vaccine, however, toddlers serve as human shields for their parents, grandparents, and the rest of the adult population.

Hepatitis B Vaccine

Infection with the hepatitis B virus can also cause hepatitis, which manifests itself in a variety of symptoms, the most prominent of which is the yellowing of the skin and pupils. Most patients recover, with the virus clearing the body and antibodies remaining in the bloodstream to protect from future infection. In about 5% of the patients, the "chronic carriers", the virus remains in the body indefinitely. Chronic carriers are at high risk for serious, life-threatening illnesses, such as cirrhosis of the liver and liver cancer.[108]

Unlike classic childhood diseases such as chickenpox, measles, or pertussis, transmission of hepatitis B does not occur in ordinary daily encounters. A measles or chickenpox patient who enters a crowded room is likely to infect at least some of the people there. A hepatitis B carrier, however, does not pose a significant risk in a similar situation since the hepatitis B virus is not passed through air, food, or water.[109] Infection only occurs when body fluids (particularly blood) or mucous membranes of a healthy individual are exposed to those of a hepatitis B carrier. However, superficial contact with saliva, tears, sweat, urine, or stools does not cause infection.[110] The vast majority of infections occur through sexual contact, the use of dirty hypodermic needles (in medical procedures or narcotic drug injections), a carrier mother giving birth, or exposure to others' bodily fluids through non-sexual contact (more on the last two below).[111]

The risk of infection is obviously affected by the total number of carriers in the population. According to official data, the prevalence of chronic hepatitis B virus carriers in the West is quite low – less than two percent[112] – but it is actually less than one percent in most Western countries. In the US, for example, carriers are estimated at 0.3 percent of the population (less than one in every 300 people).[113] An estimated 0.5 percent of pregnant women are carriers (one in every 200 women).[114] The annual disease mortality rate associated with the hepatitis B virus is quite low as well – about 0.5 per 100,000.[115] In the UK, the prevalence of chronic carriers is similar to that of the US (estimated at 0.1 to 0.5 percent of the population).[116] In Israel the Ministry of Health does not track carriers[117] but various studies have found rates between 1 and 2 percent. Among women of childbearing age in the Jewish sector, the carrier rate is estimated to be 0.7 percent.[118]

This combination of low carrier prevalence and the infrequency of conditions that favor infection mean that natural hepatitis B outbreaks are extremely rare in industrialized countries. Large outbreaks described in the scientific literature have resulted, for the most part, from improper medical procedures, most notably vaccination. The first hepatitis B outbreak ever was recorded in 1883, during a smallpox vaccination campaign at a shipyard in Bremen, Germany.[119] The largest documented outbreak – 28,585 patients and 62 deaths – occurred among World War II American soldiers who were given a yellow fever vaccine that happened to be contaminated with the hepatitis B virus.[120]

Unlike the pertussis and diphtheria vaccines, which do not prevent infection with the disease pathogen or its transmission to others, the medical literature indicates that the hepatitis B vaccine provides good protection against contracting the virus. As such, the vaccine contributes to curbing the spread of the virus and ostensibly generates a herd protection effect. However, recall that distribution of the virus through the population is limited by the relatively uncommon circumstances it requires to move from one person to another. The question that needs to be examined, therefore, is what benefit does the vaccine provide for the general population and, in particular, for the infants and children being vaccinated?[k]

Of the common sources of hepatitis B infection described above – sexual contact, contaminated needles, birth from a carrier mother, and daily contact with a carrier – only the last two are relevant for infants and children. Infection from a carrier mother is most likely at birth – the virus rarely infects

---

[k] As discussed previously, an evaluation of the net benefit of a vaccine must also include the "costs" associated with side effects. This is particularly important for the hepatitis B vaccine, which is given to infants on the day they are born and again at one month of age. Like other routine vaccines, the safety of the hepatitis B vaccine has never been properly tested in a clinical trial. Additionally, it seems that the medical establishment does not attach much importance to ensuring the safety of the vaccine. For example, the chapter devoted to the hepatitis B vaccine in *Vaccines* (Plotkin 2013), which consists of 30 pages, devotes only one paragraph (about 1/6 of a page) to the subject of the vaccine's safety, and cites only 7 relevant references (of the 650 cited in the chapter).

the uterus and does not pass in breastfeeding.[121] A child living with a carrier could theoretically be infected by careless use of a razor or toothbrush or contact between the child's blood and a bleeding wound of the carrier.[122] For infants under one year of age, the risk of becoming a chronic carrier if an accidental infection actually occurs is very high (about 90%) but decreases sharply thereafter (about 30% in children aged one to four, and about 5% in adults).[123] In addition, young children infected with the virus usually do not exhibit disease symptoms and are not identified as carriers, which, in theory at least, increases the risk of infecting other children.

According to *Vaccines*, in areas of the world where the hepatitis B virus is common, most cases of infection occur during infancy or early childhood[124] (this is due, among other things, to reuse of hypodermic needles during vaccination campaigns in developing countries).[125] However, in the Western world the situation is radically different. Risk groups for hepatitis B infection primarily consist of adults – people who have frequent casual sex, dialysis patients, prison inmates, narcotic drug users, professionals at high risk of direct exposure to blood (emergency room nurses and physicians, paramedics), residents of mental institutions, and travelers to areas where the virus is common. Only one of the groups known to be at risk of hepatitis B infection includes children: "Family members of chronic carriers".[126]

As already mentioned, the prevalence of hepatitis B chronic carriers in Western countries is around 1% of the population or less. What, then, is the risk of contracting hepatitis B for the 99% of children who do not live with a chronic carrier, and thus do not belong to any of the risk groups mentioned above?

The answer is that the risk is probably extremely low, but no one really knows for sure. In an official document describing the recommendation to vaccinate all US infants on the day they are born against hepatitis B, the CDC does not cite any relevant data or mention a study that examined the issue.[127] The textbook *Vaccines*, which provides a plethora of statistics on the risk of infection for the various risk groups mentioned above, does not specify a number or reference data as to the risk of infection for a child in a family with no carriers. The authors of the chapter are content with laconically stating that such infection "typically occurs [in] child-care centers and schools", but they do not provide any statistical evidence to back their claim.[128] (Later, they apparently contradict themselves by noting that teachers and child day-care personnel are not at increased risk of contracting the hepatitis B virus.)[129]

It isn't difficult to comprehend why the authors of the chapter, hepatitis B experts, and avid supporters of vaccination, try to create the impression that infants in day care and schoolchildren are at risk of contracting the virus. This issue is vital to the rationale behind the decision to vaccinate all newborns and infants even when their mothers do not carry the virus. The more infants and children are exposed to hepatitis B infection in educational settings, the greater the potential benefit of vaccinating them in infancy. Likewise, should this risk turn out to be negligible, so, too, would the potential benefit of this policy. But as we have seen, this policy is not based on data, let alone accurate and reliable data. In practice, despite the many millions of carriers in the Western world, the scientific literature documents only a handful of times when a child was infected in a school setting, and even in those few the circumstances were ambiguous, at best.[130]

What, then, can we infer from all of the above regarding the hepatitis B vaccine and herd immunity? Vaccinated children who are at risk of contracting the virus – that is, they live with chronic carriers – provide their family and contacts with herd protection. The vaccine protects them from infection and thus reduces the risk of viral spread. For the remaining 99% of children, who are not members of any risk group, any herd immunity provided by the vaccine is irrelevant. These children already possess better herd protection than the vaccine can provide: They belong to a family with no carriers. The risk of hepatitis B infection for these children, as inferred from the lack of relevant evidence in the scientific literature, is close to zero.

The risk of such a child infecting another, particularly in the first year of life, is even slimmer.[1]

To sum up: The hepatitis B vaccine protects against infection and provides herd immunity. However, as far as 99% of the child population in Western countries is concerned, that herd immunity is irrelevant, as their risk of contracting the virus is essentially zero anyway.

Rotavirus Vaccine

The rotavirus causes diarrhea and vomiting in infants, occasionally with fever. In severe cases the loss of fluids can lead to dehydration that may require hospitalization. Because the symptoms are not specific to the rotavirus, a lab test, rather than a clinical diagnosis, is required for a definite diagnosis of the disease. Rotavirus infection is common in the first two years of life. Breastfeeding provides protection against illness: Infants up to the age of three months usually do not get sick, most likely due to the passage of maternal antibodies during pregnancy and lactation.[131] Older children, teens, and adults are not at risk for severe illness.[132]

The rotavirus is transmitted from person to person mainly through the fecal–oral route, directly or through contact with objects, but also through contaminated food or water.[m] It is replicated in the intestines and excreted in large amounts in the stools from two days before the onset of symptoms until ten days after.[133] Natural infection with the virus confers only partial immunity from future infection (about 40%), but higher immunity to another bout of disease. The first illness event is usually more significant than those that follow, if any.[134]

The CDC doesn't mandate reporting of rotavirus disease.

---

[1] As such, there is no medical or scientific merit for restricting admission to educational institutions on the basis of hepatitis B vaccination.

[m] This point is in dispute between the CDC (whose position is cited above) and the book *Vaccines* (Plotkin 2013, p. 672), which states that "little is known about the exact mode of transmission of rotavirus."

However, they estimate that before the vaccine nearly all children (95%) were infected with the virus by the age of five. This finding is similar in both industrialized and developing countries, which seems to indicate that better sanitation and hygiene do not play a significant role in inhibiting the spread of the virus.[135] The rotavirus is the leading cause of gastroenteritis and related hospitalizations in the United States. It is estimated that about 1 in 70 infants is hospitalized due to a rotavirus illness and 1 in 66,000 to 200,000 dies from the disease.[136] The mortality rate is also very low in the UK – about 3 deaths a year – with other contributing causes in almost all of them.[137] In Israel, rotavirus mortality is "very rare".[138]

The first rotavirus vaccine – RotaShield – was added to the US routine schedule in 1998, but was removed a year later when it was found to cause a life-threatening condition called intussusception. In 2005, Merck's Rotateq vaccine was introduced in the US and two years later GSK's Rotarix vaccine was also approved for use. Many countries have added these vaccines to their vaccination programs and have considerably reduced the incidence of gastrointestinal diseases caused by rotavirus.[139] The vaccine was less successful in developing countries in which it was introduced.[140]

Although its efficacy in preventing disease has been demonstrated in clinical trials, the rotavirus vaccine was not expected to generate herd protection as well. Natural infection with rotavirus does not confer full immunity to future infection, and the prevailing opinion was that the vaccine should not be expected to surpass the natural disease in this respect. The vaccine was thought to prevent morbidity in those vaccinated, but not to curb the spread of the virus.[141]

This assumption was questioned after numerous studies conducted in different countries about 3–4 years after the vaccine's launch examined its effectiveness and found larger decreases in morbidity than expected.[142] According to these studies, rotavirus-induced disease has decreased significantly not only in vaccinated children, but also in children too young or too old to be vaccinated, which suggests the vaccine provides herd immunity. The authors of a 2012 review of the subject note that there are two possible explanations for this phenomenon: a) The vaccine inhibits the spread of the virus; or b) the attenuated vaccine virus, secreted by vaccinated infants, infects unvaccinated children and protects them from disease.[143] Although the initial findings seem promising, the authors write, they should be taken with a grain of salt: "The evidence regarding herd immunity associated with rotavirus vaccines is of poor quality because this effect was not anticipated and studies were not specifically designed to detect it [...] Every study reviewed has significant potential flaws in relation to herd immunity and thus should be interpreted with caution."[144] In addition, in some studies the herd protection effect wasn't detected.[145]

A later review, this one in 2015, was the first to try to quantitatively assess the level of herd immunity provided by the vaccine.[146] After a review of the scientific literature and careful screening of irrelevant or low-quality studies, fifteen adequate studies remained. However, these studies also lacked essential data and obliged the researchers to base their calculations on some arbitrary assumptions[147] which led to unreasonable results that the researchers found difficult to explain.[148] For example, almost all the outcomes reported in Latin American countries indicated a decrease in overall morbidity and hospitalizations from diarrhea that was above and beyond the maximum theoretical rate that could be attributed to the rotavirus vaccine.[149] In addition, no correlation was found between the vaccination rate and the extent of the herd protection effect attributed to the vaccine.[150] "There is evidence that rotavirus vaccination confers a herd immunity effect [...]," the authors conclude, but "more studies are needed to better examine herd immunity effects in high mortality regions."[151]

Thus, at the time of writing, there is some epidemiological evidence to suggest that the rotavirus vaccine might confer herd immunity. However, the evidence accumulated thus far is not clear or consistent enough to provide unequivocal proof of a herd protection effect for the vaccine. Another limitation is that there are no biological studies confirming the existence of a vaccine-induced herd protection.

Pneumococcal Vaccine

Humans are the only natural hosts for the pneumococcal bacterium. The bacterium is carried in the nose and throat and is transmitted from person to person by droplets from sneezing and coughing. At any given time, between 5 and 70 percent of the population carry the bacterium in their throat without exhibiting any symptoms (asymptomatic carriers). This number varies depending on age, geographic area, and other parameters. There are over 90 different serotypes of the bacterium but only a handful is responsible for most of the morbidity.[n] The bacterial serotypes vary in their ability to cause disease (pathogenicity), their effect on different age groups, the length of time they are carried in the throat, and the level of immunity this carriage generates.[152] The numerous serotypes of the bacterium are constantly circulating in the population, transmitted from person to person (particularly young children).[153] Serotype distribution varies according to geographical area. Some of the serotypes have developed resistance to antibiotics.[154]

As noted above, a large portion of the healthy population carries the bacterium in their throat without ever getting sick. However, sometimes the bacterium migrates from the throat to other parts of the body and causes disease – to the middle ear (ear infection), sinuses (sinusitis), or lungs (pneumonia). In addition, the bacterium can cause meningitis or sepsis. Risk factors include overcrowding, age of less than two years, winter season, flu infection, and a weakened immune system.[155]

Before the vaccine there were about 17,000 cases per year of pneumococcal disease in children under the age of five in the US, including about 700 cases of meningitis and 200 deaths. The

---

[n] About 10 serotypes cause 62% of global pneumococcal disease.

pneumococcal bacterium is the primary cause of ear infections and was estimated to be responsible for around 15 million resulting doctor visits a year. Most of the morbidity was in children aged 6 to 11 months (235 per 100,000). In Europe, morbidity was significantly lower than in the United States: 36 per 100,000 children aged 6–11 months in the UK, and 45 per 100,000 in Finland.[156] In Israel, there were about 30–40 annual cases of pneumococcal meningitis in the pre-vaccine years, and about 2 deaths a year.[157]

A pneumococcal vaccine was added to the US childhood routine schedule in 2000 (in Israel in 2009). The vaccine (*Prevnar*) protected against 7 serotypes of the bacterium. In 2010 it was replaced by a newer version (*Prevnar-13*) protecting against 13 serotypes. It is estimated that the vaccine has significantly reduced the incidence of invasive pneumococcal disease (IPD) in the US (specifically, a reduction of about 80% in children under the age of five). Although the vaccine confers almost full protection against disease caused by the serotypes in the vaccine, serotypes that are not included in the vaccine have partially replaced the vaccine serotypes and slowed the decrease in morbidity somewhat.[158]

In addition to the large drop in IPD incidence in children after the introduction of Prevnar in the early 2000s, a significant decrease in morbidity in (unvaccinated) adults was also observed, suggesting that the vaccine provided a herd protection effect.[159] But how was this effect achieved?

Studies in children in different countries have consistently found that the proportion of pneumococcal carriers in the population did not change significantly in the period after the introduction of Prevnar. However, the composition of the serotypes carried by children has changed dramatically: The vaccine serotypes have almost completely disappeared and have been replaced by non-vaccine serotypes (a phenomenon known as *serotype replacement*). The accepted assumption is, therefore, that the decline in IPD morbidity in the unvaccinated (i.e., the herd protection effect) was not caused by a reduction in the prevalence of the bacterium but because of the reduced *patho-genicity* (ability to cause disease) of the serotypes that replaced the vaccine serotypes.[160] Thus, the vaccine presumably generates herd immunity by reducing the prevalence of the more pathogenic pneumococcal serotypes, but at the same time increases the prevalence of other serotypes that can also cause disease.[161]

Indeed, a few years after the introduction of Prevnar, the US and Europe began reporting rising rates of pneumococcal disease due to non-vaccine serotypes.[162] This rise, recorded in children and adults alike, somewhat diminished the initial effect of the vaccine, leading to its replacement in the US in 2010 with the Prevnar-13 vaccine, which protects against six additional serotypes (the same serotypes that became common after the introduction of Prevnar).[163] In the UK serotype replacement led health authorities to replace Prevnar with a vaccine covering additional serotypes just three years after its introduction.[164] In Israel Prevnar was replaced by Prevnar-13 after just one year.[165]

Recent studies, conducted in a number of Western countries, which examined the effect of replacing Prevnar with Prevnar-13 have found that this move has not fundamentally affected the underlying issue. The United States saw a large (and rapid) decline in child IPD morbidity from the serotypes included in the new vaccine, as well as a significant reduction in the incidence of IPD in adults from the same serotypes, which led to a decrease of about 12–32% in the overall incidence of IPD. This decrease is attributed to the herd protection effect of the vaccine.[166] In Europe, however, the results were not as good. In Italy, the introduction of Prevnar-13 did not lead to a reduction in the rate of IPD in adults. In Sweden, there were no significant changes in IPD morbidity in adults or children under 2 years of age. The UK and Denmark had modest declines in IPD morbidity in adults.[167] This relative failure was due to the fact that Prevnar-13, like its predecessor Prevnar, did not significantly reduce the rate of carriers in the population; it just changed the distribution of serotypes. The vaccine serotypes have almost completely disappeared and been replaced by other, less common, serotypes which have since become prevalent.[168] This serotype replacement limited the herd protection effect of Prevnar-13 even more than its predecessor.[169] Although the vaccine had some effect in this regard, the overall burden of pneumococcal diseases remained high.[170] Other studies found that the protection provided by the vaccine wanes over time and may prove insufficient to prevent carriage of vaccine serotypes and transmission to other people.[171]

In conclusion, the pneumococcal vaccine generates herd protection against the serotypes included in the vaccine but does not reduce the overall spread of the bacterium, as other serotypes fill the niche evacuated by vaccine serotypes. The reduction in the incidence of pneumococcal disease since the introduction of the vaccine is probably due to the fact that, so far, the replacement serotypes have been less pathogenic, but there is no certainty that will continue in the future. The vaccine has led to comprehensive changes in the distribution of bacterial serotypes, and the dynamics of these changes, which also vary from region to region and from population to population, are unpredictable.[172] Thus, for example, the introduction of Prevnar vaccines in Sweden has increased the diversity of the pneumococcal bacteria prevalent in the population.[173]

So, the pneumococcal vaccine provides a limited herd protection against the bacterial serotypes included in the vaccine, but it is unable to provide a wall-to-wall protection, one that can significantly reduce the spread of the bacterium in the population. Because the vaccine covers only 13 of the more than 90 pathogenic pneumococcal bacteria serotypes and the maximum number of vaccine serotypes is limited by technical constraints,[174] it is unlikely this problem will be solved in the near future.

Hib Vaccine

There are several types of the *Haemophilus influenzae* bacterium. Type b has been the most common and the one causing most of the illness associated with the bacterium. Haemophilus influenzae type b (or Hib) is restricted to humans. It cannot survive in the environment or on objects. Although solid evidence is lacking, it is assumed to be transmitted through droplets of fluid from the nose and throat, presumably following close and continuous contact.[175] On entering the body, the bacterium settles in the nose and throat and may stay there for several months without causing illness. Maternal antibodies passed during pregnancy and lactation provide short-term protection against disease. In the pre-vaccine era the bacterium could be found in 1–3 percent of children at any given time. Morbidity was low in the first months of life and peaked at 6–7 months of age. By the age of five, most children had developed immunity to the bacterium.[176]

As noted above, most cases of Hib colonization in the body do not cause disease.[177] For unknown reasons, it sometimes moves from the nasopharynx to the bloodstream and from there to other parts of the body, most often to the membranes that cover the brain (meninges). Bacterial proliferation in the bloodstream can cause a number of diseases, including meningitis, epiglottitis, pneumonia, and arthritis. Meningitis, the most common of these, accounts for 50–65 percent of Hib invasive disease and can cause neurological damage (15–30% of cases) or death (2–5% of cases). Hib disease usually requires hospitalization. After the bacterium is detected in the lab, the patient is treated with a third-generation antibiotic drug because some of the strains have developed resistance to antibiotics.[178]

Diseases caused by the Hib bacterium were not reported in the US until 1991 (the first Hib vaccine was introduced several years earlier). It is estimated that in the pre-vaccine era there were about 20,000 cases of disease each year, most of them in children under five.[179] In Israel, in the 13 years before the vaccine was added to the schedule, between 70 and 110 annual cases of meningitis caused by the Hib bacterium were recorded, with about 1 death every two years (7 deaths in the entire period).[180]

In the United States, a 99 percent reduction in the incidence of Hib diseases was recorded following the introduction of the vaccine, most notably in children. Most of the child morbidity in the post-vaccine era is in infants too young to be vaccinated and children who are either partially vaccinated or not vaccinated. Vaccine efficacy is estimated at 95% or more.[181] The vaccine was introduced in Israel in 1994, and the incidence of Hib-induced meningitis in the following decade fell to about 5–10 cases per year, with zero deaths.[182] The reduction in Hib morbidity was accompanied by a less pronounced increase in the incidence of disease from other *Haemophilus influenzae* serotypes.[183]

Although not previously anticipated, several years after the vaccine was added to the routine schedule, it was found to generate herd protection. Evidence for the presence of a herd immunity effect was obtained from large-scale epidemiological studies,[184] controlled studies of specific groups,[185] and biological studies demonstrating the efficacy of the vaccine in protecting against infection and bacterial carriage.[186]

Varicella (Chickenpox) Vaccine

Varicella is most common in early childhood. Its typical symptoms are fever and the eruption of itchy blisters – usually several hundred – on the body. The disease lasts about a week and is considered mild. Its complications are rare, the most common of which is bacterial infection caused by contaminated blisters (usually after being scratched by the patient). Aspirin-based fever reducers should be avoided due to the risk of severe liver and brain damage from Reye's syndrome.[187] Disease onset in adults is more severe, and the complication rate is significantly higher than in children.[188] The exact mode of infection is unknown, but it is believed that virus particles detach from the wounds on the patient's skin and are transmitted through the air (and probably also through direct contact).[189] In about 70% of patients, the varicella virus remains in the body even after recovery, and under certain conditions may cause shingles.°

Before the vaccine was added to the US routine schedule in 1995, varicella was a very common disease and nearly everyone contracted it before the fourth decade of life. Most people got it before they started school. It is estimated that about 4 million cases occurred annually, with around 12,000 hospitalizations and 125 deaths.[p] These numbers seem quite high, but adjusted for the entire population they amount to 4.5 hospitalizations and 0.05 deaths per 100,000.[190] Another fact testifying to the mildness of the disease is that it wasn't reportable.[191]

Reporting isn't required for varicella in the UK, even now.[192] Unlike the US, the vaccine is not routinely given to infants or children there, but only to those who are in close contact with people with compromised immune systems (health care workers and family members).[193] In Israel, the disease has been reportable since 1978. The mortality rate recorded in the 1980s (2 deaths throughout the decade) and the 1990s (11 total deaths) was even lower than in the United States.[194] A vaccine for the disease was added to the routine program in 2008.

A sharp decline in varicella morbidity and resulting complications was recorded in the US following the introduction of the vaccine. A large drop was also recorded in cohorts that were not vaccinated, particularly infants under one year, and this decrease is perceived as indicative of the herd protection provided by the vaccine.[195] It is assumed that prevention of disease by the vaccine inhibits the transmission of the virus, which is mainly spread by the blisters that erupt on the skin during illness.

The US was the first country to include the vaccine in its childhood vaccination program. Other Western countries such as Canada, Germany, Israel, Greece, Spain, and Italy followed suit.[196] However, at the time of writing, many other Western

---

° Shingles is quite common even among vaccinated people, whether due to the vaccine virus or the natural virus. (Plotkin 2013, p. 854).

[p] That is, 1 in 333 patients was hospitalized, and 1 in 32,000 died. The mortality rate in adults was twice as high as in children.

countries have chosen not to use the vaccine. In Norway, Sweden, France, Portugal, Denmark, Belgium, the Netherlands, Austria, and New Zealand, the vaccine is not given at all, and in Australia and Switzerland it is only recommended for children over 10 years of age.[197] Presumably contributing to the reluctance to use the vaccine more broadly are studies that found that the savings from a reduction in chickenpox cases do not offset the cost of the vaccine[198] and concerns that this reduction of varicella in children will lead to an increase in shingles in adults.[199]

In summary, the varicella vaccine has greatly reduced the incidence of the disease, presumably at least in part thanks to the herd immunity it provides. Despite this, many countries have chosen not to include it in their vaccine programs, which implies that these countries do not regard the disease as a significant burden on public health.

Rubella Vaccine

Rubella morbidity is characterized by low fever and fatigue, typically followed by eruption of a reddish rash that begins on the face and neck area and subsequently spreads to other body parts. The disease is considered mild in children, and its complications are rare (in adults the complications are more frequent). About 50% of those infected with the rubella virus have no symptoms. The disease is considered to be moderately infectious. The virus is transmitted from person to person through droplets secreted from the nose and throat of patients or asymptomatic carriers. There is no chronic carriage of rubella virus. Because there are many diseases that cause a rubella-like rash, a clinical diagnosis of the disease by a physician is not considered reliable and a lab test is required for definitive identification.[200]

Rubella disease itself does not constitute a substantial threat to the health of a population, especially in children. The greater risk arises when it is contracted by women in the first 15–20 weeks of pregnancy, when it can infect the fetus. This condition is called *congenital rubella syndrome* (CRS), and it can cause miscarriage, fetal death, premature birth, and congenital defects such as deafness, visual impairments, heart problems, neurological problems, and more.[201]

In the pre-vaccine era, rubella was not a reportable disease. Hence, data on pre-vaccine rubella morbidity, as well as the more dangerous congenital rubella syndrome (CRS), is scarce. In the US, rubella reporting became mandatory in 1966.[q] In 1969, about 57,600 cases were reported (58 cases per 100,000). A year later, the rubella morbidity level remained unchanged and the number of CRS cases – which had reached a record level since reporting began several years earlier – stood at 67 (a rate of about 1 in 45,000 births).[202] [203] For comparison, in Sweden between 1975 and 1985, an average of 2 CRS cases were recorded annually.[204] In Israel, CRS has never been a reportable disease.[205]

The rubella vaccine was added to the US recommended schedule in 1969. Although the vaccine was never tested in a randomized controlled clinical trial, evidence of its efficacy abounds.[206] No major outbreak of rubella has been recorded in the United States in the post-vaccine period.[207] Studies have found that a single vaccine dose provides protection for many years, and probably for life.[r] [208]

The main reason for including the rubella vaccine in the vaccine program is to prevent CRS in fetuses. A secondary goal is to prevent rare complications of the disease in adults.[209] To prevent CRS, two main strategies were devised. The first is vaccination of

---

[q] Probably as a result of a large and unprecedented epidemic that occurred in the United States in 1963–4, in which about 12 million cases of rubella and 30,000 cases of CRS were reported.

[r] Despite this, the vaccination programs of many countries, including the United States and Israel, stipulate that children be vaccinated twice, as rubella is a component of the MMR. According to the CDC (Pink Book 2011, p. 9 [283]), a single vaccine dose is sufficient for the vaccinee to be considered protected from rubella.

pre-adolescent girls and young women.[s] The second is general
vaccination of infants in the second year of life (with another
dose at 5–6 years of age). Vaccination of girls and young women
has been found to reduce the rate of CRS, but it has no effect on
the spread of the rubella virus. Thus, it does not significantly
reduce rubella morbidity in the population. Vaccination of
infants reduces the spread of the virus in the population, and
therefore also reduces the occurrence of both rubella and CRS.
This strategy could potentially lead to the complete elimination
of the disease in the future. Both strategies may be combined in
order to achieve more rapid results.[210]

Sweden, which adopted the combined strategy, has vaccinated 18-month-old infants and 12-year-old girls with the MMR
since 1982. The last case of CRS was recorded in the country in
1985 (after an average of two cases per year in the previous ten
years).[211] A similar outcome was obtained in Finland after the
MMR vaccine was given to 18-month-olds and 6-year-olds. The
last CRS case was in 1985, and rubella morbidity disappeared in
the mid-1990s.[212] The UK began vaccinating girls in 1970. Rubella morbidity dropped only slightly, but CRS cases dropped by 75
percent. Then in 1988, the UK began giving infants the MMR
vaccine, and within a few years cases of rubella and CRS were
greatly reduced.[213] In Canada, some provinces chose to vaccinate
infants, while others selectively vaccinated girls before they
entered school. Rubella morbidity decreased in infant-vaccinated
provinces only, but the CRS rate decreased in all of them. Subsequently, all provinces switched to infant vaccination, and from
2000 on there has been almost no rubella in Canada.[214]

The success of the rubella vaccine (as part of the MMR) in
almost completely eliminating the disease in many countries
provides supporting evidence that it reduces the spread of the
virus in the population and, therefore, confers herd immunity.

---

[s] Only girls or women who have not been previously infected with rubella
should be selectively vaccinated, but since a clinical diagnosis of rubella is not
certain, it is better to perform a laboratory test to verify previous illness.

Mumps Vaccine

Mumps is considered a mild childhood disease.[215] The disease's most prominent symptom is swelling of the glands in the area between the cheek and the ear on one or both sides of the face. The disease is caused by the mumps virus, and is transmitted by droplets of fluid secreted from the nose or throat traveling through air or through direct contact. A large quantity of virus is produced for several days before symptoms appear, making it difficult to prevent infection through isolation of patients. Mumps is considered medium-level infective, similar to rubella and influenza, but less than measles and varicella. The virus lives only in humans, and chronic carriage does not exist.

Mumps was very common among preschoolers and elementary schoolchildren and was clinically diagnosed by the typical swelling of the cheeks. No symptoms appear in about 20 percent of cases, and 40 to 50 percent of patients exhibit flu-like symptoms such as fever, weakness, and headache. The disease tends to be more severe in adults. Inflammation of the testicles can occur in up to a third of adult male patients. The inflammation causes infertility only rarely but can impair sperm count. In women, up to about a third may experience mastitis (breast inflammation). The virus crosses the placenta and can sometimes cause miscarriage or fetal death. It has not been found to cause congenital defects. About 5 percent of patients experience inflammation of the meninges (meningitis), but this is usually mild and passes within 3–4 days. Temporary deafness is a relatively common complication, but permanent deafness is rare (about 1 in 20,000 patients).[216] Death is rare: In the US, only 8 mumps deaths were reported in 1975 (after the vaccine was introduced, but before it was recommended for routine use). In Israel, only one mumps death was reported in the decade before the vaccine was introduced.[217]

The mumps vaccine was licensed in the United States in 1967. In 1971 the MMR vaccine was released, and in 1977 it began to be widely used following the CDC's recommendation.[218]

Although actual vaccine effectiveness was found to be slightly lower than that reported in its clinical trials,[219] mumps morbidity in the US dropped 98 percent after it was introduced.[220] However, the immunity conferred by the vaccine appears to somewhat wane with age. Local mumps outbreaks in well-vaccinated populations are occasionally recorded in the US, particularly among young adults spending time in close quarters (military units, colleges and universities, and sports teams).[221]

Despite outbreaks in vaccinated populations, indicative of the incomplete protection afforded by the vaccine, US mumps morbidity remained very low compared to the pre-vaccine period.[222] Similar results were recorded in other industrialized countries where a mumps vaccine was added to the routine vaccination program.[223] (An exception is Japan, where the vaccine is not included in the recommended routine schedule, and less than a quarter of children are vaccinated against mumps).[224]

In conclusion, the drastic decrease in mumps morbidity after the introduction of the vaccine – above and beyond the expected effect of its efficacy and vaccination rate – indicates that the vaccine confers herd immunity.[225]

Measles Vaccine

Measles is a highly contagious disease. Prior to vaccination, almost all children contracted measles by age 15 and measles outbreaks erupted every two or three years.[226] The measles virus settles in the nose and throat and can be transmitted to another person through droplets, whether through the air or direct contact. The virus could be transmitted anytime from four days before the onset of the typical rash up to four days after.[227] In addition to the rash, the disease is characterized by fatigue, fever (potentially high), and cough. Clinical diagnosis of measles is not always accurate, and it is sometimes difficult to distinguish it from diseases that cause similar rashes. Diagnosis can be confirmed with a laboratory test.[228] A bout of measles is assumed to confer lifelong immunity.[229]

About 500,000 measles cases were reported annually in the United States in the late 1950s. However, since almost everyone contracted the disease, the real incidence was closer to four million annually, which implies that about 7 out of 8 measles cases were not reported.[230] Thus, measles mortality during this period, about 500 cases per year, translates to a rate of one death for every 8,000 patients, rather than one per 1,000, as is cited in various official publications.[231] In the three years preceding the introduction of the vaccine (1969), the UK had an average of 77 deaths per year, which is roughly one death per 11,000 patients.[t] [232] In Israel in the mid-1960s, about 30 measles deaths a year were reported, which corresponds to a rate of about 1 in 2,000 children.[u] [233] Yet, as noted in chapter 8, measles mortality was steadily declining in the second half of the 20th century. In the Netherlands, for example, measles mortality continued to fall and reached almost zero even before the vaccine was introduced in 1976 (about a decade after the US, the UK, and Israel).[234]

As with "official" measles mortality rates, official statistics for its main complications should also be taken with a grain of salt: ear infection (8% of patients), stomachache (8%), pneumonia (3%), and encephalitis (one in 1500 patients).[235] These rates are calculated from the number of reported cases, which includes only a fraction of the actual number of cases. Subsequent development of subacute sclerosing panencephalitis (SSPE), a serious but rare complication, has been reported at a rate of about one in 100,000 measles patients (although the measles outbreak in the United States in 1989–91 recorded a rate of 22 per 100,000).[236] In developing countries the complication rate for measles is higher, probably due to poor nutrition (mainly vitamin A deficiency) combined with a younger average age at onset.[237]

---

[t] In Britain (England + Wales), an annual average of 77 measles deaths were recorded between 1966 and 1968 (the vaccine was introduced in 1969). The average size of the cohort in those years was about 834,000 children. Assuming that everyone had measles, there was one death for every 10,831 children.

[u] In Israel, an average of 33 measles deaths and about 66,000 births were recorded in the three years prior to the introduction of the vaccine (1967).

The measles vaccine was first used in the US in 1963 and from 1977 onward was provided as a component of the MMR vaccine. Its efficacy is estimated at 90–95 percent. The minimum age for vaccination is 12 months, as maternal antibodies passed to the fetus during pregnancy impair vaccine efficacy in younger infants.[238] Although the level of vaccine-generated antibodies wanes over the years, the protection conferred by the vaccine is considered to last a lifetime. Testifying to this is the fact that measles morbidity has remained at very low levels in the post-vaccine era.[239]

The measles vaccine confers herd protection by reducing the spread of the virus among the vaccinated and unvaccinated. The vaccination coverage threshold required for herd immunity is estimated at 92 to 95 percent. In industrialized countries it has been found that one vaccine dose is sufficient to significantly reduce measles morbidity, but two doses are required to stop the spread of the virus.[240]

Routine Vaccines and Herd Immunity: A Summary

Table 9-1 below presents the vaccines of the US childhood routine schedule and summarizes the relevant information regarding herd immunity for each. Of the 14 vaccines, only 5 (one-third) can be said to definitely provide relevant herd protection for children, as is detailed below.[v] [241]

Table 9-1: Herd immunity of Vaccines of the US Routine Schedule

Vaccine / Disease	Herd Immunity	Description	Disease Pre-vaccine Incidence	Severity
Tetanus	—	The bacterium lives in animal feces and soil. The vaccine targets the	Very rare	Lethal

[v] A similar list is provided by Dr. Stanley Plotkin, editor of the book *Vaccines*, in an article published in 2008 (see reference).

		toxin rather than the bacterium and therefore cannot prevent trans-mission.		
Inactivated Polio (Salk)	—	The vaccine does not prevent replication of the virus in the gut and its excretion in the feces.	Low	Severe
Pertussis	—	The current (acellular) vaccine does not prevent infection with the bacterium or transmission to others.	High	Medium
Diphtheria	—	The vaccine works against the toxin, not the bacterium, and therefore does not prevent infection and transmission. There is no solid evidence for herd protection.	High	Severe
Influenza	—	Vaccine efficacy is moderate to low. The virus is constantly evolving; therefore a new vaccine must be formulated every year, targeting the strains that are expected to be common in the coming winter season.	High	Medium–high
Hepatitis A	—	The disease is very mild in children, and infection with the virus provides lifelong immunity. Children receive no benefit from the herd protection provided by the vaccine.	Low	Very mild in children (moderate in adults)
Hepatitis B	—	The vaccine is redun-dant for about 99% of	Low	Moderate

		children. The herd protection it provides is relevant only to children living with a chronic carrier of the disease.		
Rotavirus	–	The disease itself does not fully prevent future infection or morbidity. There is some evidence for the existence of a herd protection effect for the vaccine, but the body of research on the subject is preliminary and definitive conclusions cannot be drawn.	Very high	Mild– moderate
Pneumo- coccal	+/-	The vaccine provides partial herd protection – only against the serotypes it contains. It does not reduce the rate of bacterial carriers in the population due to the phenomenon of serotype replacement.	Low	Moderate
Hib	+	There is epidemiological and biological evidence of vaccine-induced herd immunity.	Low	Moderate
Varicella (Chicken- pox)	+	The vaccine appears to provide herd protection, but it is not routinely given in some industrial- ized countries.	Very high	Mild
Rubella	+	The vaccine appears to have nearly extin- guished the spread of the virus in the popula- tion.	Low	Very mild in children (serious in fetuses)
Mumps	+	The vaccine almost completely eliminated morbidity (despite	High	Mild

		sporadic outbreaks in adults reported from time to time).		
Measles	+	The vaccine almost completely eliminated the disease.	Very high	Mild

The tetanus and diphtheria vaccines do not affect the infective bacteria, just the toxins they secrete, and therefore do not prevent spread of the diseases. The pertussis and inactivated polio vaccines do not prevent infection with the pathogen or transmission to another person.

The influenza virus constantly mutates, and the vaccine, therefore, does not provide long-term protection against infection. Hepatitis A is a mild disease in children. Getting sick confers lifelong protection, so the herd immunity induced by the vaccine is redundant for children. Similarly, the herd protection provided by the hepatitis B vaccine is irrelevant for the vast majority of children, who do not live in a household with a chronic carrier of the virus. Rotavirus disease does not induce complete immunity to virus re-infection, and therefore it is unlikely that the vaccine could provide such protection. Current research into potential herd immunity provided by the vaccine is not well-established and cannot provide an unequivocal answer regarding the issue.

The pneumococcal vaccine provides herd protection against the serotypes it contains but not against the dozens of bacterial serotypes it does not contain. Because of this the vaccine does not reduce the rate of carriers of the bacterium in the population, and this limits its efficacy in preventing disease.

The last five vaccines in the table confer some level of herd immunity: The four components of the MMRV vaccine (measles, mumps, rubella, and varicella), and the Hib vaccine. A consistent and long-term morbidity decline was recorded for these diseases following the introduction of their respective vaccines, as well as similar reductions in the distribution of the disease pathogens.

Counter Arguments

"Your unvaccinated child is a threat to my vaccinated (or not-yet-vaccinated) child!" – Vaccines have serious side effects, the extent of which is unknown. As long as there are no reliable studies that unequivocally prove that the benefit of a vaccine outweighs its harm, there is no moral basis to require a parent to vaccinate their children. Even if we set aside the issue of vaccines' unknown safety profiles and consider only their efficacies, only about a third of routine vaccines provide herd immunity that is relevant and beneficial to children. It is also worth noting that vaccinated children are purportedly protected by their vaccination and should not get sick. If the vaccine fails to confer protection from disease (or even infection) for a particular child, that child, despite being vaccinated, could potentially be infected with the pathogen and infect others – the same as an unvaccinated child. In that case, the vaccinated child and the unvaccinated child pose the same risk to one another.

"Your unvaccinated child risks individuals who are immunocompromised and cannot get vaccinated!" – See answer to previous question. In addition, the immunocompromised must take measures to avoid exposure to countless disease agents. Only a tiny fraction of these pathogens are blocked by vaccines.

"Even if vaccines have no societal benefit, parents must vaccinate their children to provide them with personal protection from illness, just as they must put their child in a car seat." – If car seats were (not) tested for safety the way vaccines are (not), and if children were occasionally injured or killed by a car seat for no apparent reason, people would think twice before putting their children in them.

In the absence of proven societal benefits for a vaccine, anyone who wishes to enforce vaccination must clear a very high evidentiary bar. Health authorities must provide highly reliable and unequivocal proof that the benefit of the vaccine significantly outweighs its potential harm. Without such proof there is no moral justification for restricting parents' freedom to decide how to best protect their children's health. Even if a vaccine were to have a net positive effect on a population level, that doesn't mean that it would on an individual level.

"Hepatitis A vaccine: Without a vaccine, people who did not contract the disease in childhood might come down with it as adults, which is usually more severe. Hence, it is imperative to vaccinate children." – This claim poses a moral question for which the answer is not clear-cut: Should infants be required to be vaccinated for a very mild disease, thus depriving them of the probability of lifelong immunity and forcing them to assume the unknown risk of side effects just to protect a relatively small number of adults from getting sick? Whatever the answer, an alternative worth considering is to vaccinate young adults who have not yet developed hepatitis A antibodies.

"Diphtheria vaccine: The bacterium multiplies and spreads itself effectively thanks to toxin secretion that damages the tissues and creates a convenient environment for the bacteria to thrive. Therefore, if vaccine antibodies target the toxin, it is much more difficult for the bacterium to thrive and spread itself, thus creating a herd protection effect." – This claim was first made by Pappenheimer in the 1970s, but remains a hypothesis and nothing more, as he did not provide solid backing evidence. Pappenheimer's work in this field was not followed up by other researchers, perhaps due to declining interest in the study of diphtheria.

"Pertussis vaccine: The disease is mainly spread by patients who transmit the bacterium by coughing. The vaccine provides herd protection by reducing the number of coughing patients, thus significantly decreasing the spread of the bacterium." – This claim makes some sense, but it is not backed by proper evidence. Keep in mind that asymptomatic carriers of the pertussis bacterium can spread it very effectively, as they are not aware of their status due to the absence of a cough (or other disease symptoms), thus are unlikely, along with their contacts, to take preventive measures.[242] At the time of writing, data on the relative contributions of people who exhibit pertussis symptoms and asymptomatic carriers to pertussis transmission is lacking, so the answer to this question remains up in the air.

"Pertussis vaccine: The experience gained in Sweden since the introduction of the acellular vaccine in 1996 shows that the vaccine confers herd immunity." – Sweden removed the whole-cell pertussis vaccine (DTP) from its program in 1979, due to diminished efficacy and rising safety concerns.[243] Seventeen years later (1996), pertussis vaccination in the newer, acellular form was re-introduced into the routine program. Swedish studies examining national pertussis morbidity data have found a reduction in incidence even in unvaccinated populations, especially in adults and infants under three months of age who are too young to be vaccinated. This decline, the researchers conclude, demonstrates that the pertussis vaccine provides herd immunity.[244]

The researchers' pronounced optimism notwithstanding,[w] [245] a careful examination of their work raises a number of reservations: The data on which the researchers based their conclusions are not unequivocal, and it's questionable how well they represent the situation in Sweden. In addition, generalizing from the Swedish data to other countries is inappropriate, and – most importantly – the Swedish researchers' conclusions contradict the preponderance of scientific evidence accumulated on the subject.

Sweden's coverage rate of pertussis vaccination in the late 1990s was almost complete – around 98–99 percent of infants

---

[w] This optimism is likely due, at least in part, to the fact that the lead researcher who authored the papers in question, Rose-Marie Carlsson, headed the pertussis vaccine surveillance project in Sweden, a project funded by GSK and Sanofi-Pasteur, manufacturers of pertussis vaccines.

were vaccinated with the recommended three doses in their first year of life.[246] Despite the high vaccination rate, the first seven years of follow-up (1998–2005) saw an increase in pertussis incidence in infants too young to be vaccinated.[247] In the next two years (2006–2007) this upward trend reversed, but the decline was halted in 2008 and the rate remained fairly constant for the final four years of the study's period. These data do not necessarily suggest a herd protection effect for the vaccine, and certainly do not prove one.[x] In addition, pertussis-related infant mortality in the decade following vaccine introduction was higher than in the preceding decade (8 cases versus 3), and the researchers seem unable to reconcile these numbers with their herd immunity supposition.[248]

The Swedish data, from which the researchers inferred a herd protection effect for the vaccine, are based on a passive surveillance system set up specifically to monitor the incidence of pertussis following the re-entry of the vaccine. A passive system typically records only about 10% of actual morbidity cases, as the researchers note,[249] and thus a significant reporting bias in the study's data cannot be ruled out.

Either way, it is difficult to generalize from the vaccination experience of one country to the pertussis epidemiology of another, the researchers point out, due to differences in vaccine policy, surveillance systems employed, vaccine coverage, and more.[250] Indeed, other industrialized countries — the US, Canada, Australia, the UK, Ireland, and Spain — have seen significant increases in pertussis since switching to the acellular vaccine, despite high vaccination rates. In the United States, in particular, pertussis morbidity in 2012 equaled that of the early 1950s.[251] In the Netherlands, the vaccine did not reduce the spread of the bacterium in adolescents and adults.[252]

Thus, contrasting with the Swedish epidemiological data that

---

[x] For example, the rate of vaccine coverage for the entire population, which increases with every new vaccinated cohort, was supposed to gradually reduce the incidence of pertussis in young infants even after 2008.

may be interpreted as supporting a herd protection effect of the vaccine, there are data from other countries that suggest the opposite. In addition, the outcomes of biological studies (including experiments in baboons and mice), the failure of the cocooning technique to prevent illness in young infants, various mathematical models,[253] and epidemiological studies that documented pertussis in populations with near universal vaccination coverage – all point to the fact that the pertussis vaccine does not prevent transmission, nor does it confer herd immunity.

Summary

The societal benefit attributed to vaccines is primarily based on the concept of herd immunity, that is, the assumption that, in addition to themselves, the vaccinated also protect the unvaccinated. A herd immunity effect is achieved when a high proportion of individuals in a population are protected against infection by a particular disease pathogen. Vaccines can potentially provide herd protection, but in order to do so they must provide protection not only from the disease, but also from being infected by the pathogen and transmitting it to others.

Health authorities and other stakeholders are promoting the false impression that all vaccines, by virtue of being vaccines, provide herd immunity. The reality, however, is quite different: Of the 14 vaccines on the US childhood routine schedule, only 5 clear the herd immunity bar by targeting diseases for which herd immunity is relevant for children and being capable of actually delivering it. For the other 9 vaccines, either the vaccine does not generate herd immunity, or the protection it provides for infants and children is partial or irrelevant.

The herd immunity myth, with its implicit assumption that all vaccines offer social benefit, perfectly suits the agenda of vaccine marketers: It glorifies the supposed benefit of vaccines and nurtures a public discourse that exerts social pressure on parents to vaccinate their children. If a child's vaccination is assumed to contribute to the protection of those around them, then refusing vaccination would appear to endanger that child as well as their classmates, family, and friends. Thus, unvaccinated children are presented as "hitchhikers" who benefit from the herd protection provided to them courtesy of vaccinated children. This harsh accusation is often directed at parents who choose not to vaccinate their children and puts pressure on them to align with formal vaccination guidelines.

In addition, the myth of herd immunity provides health authorities the legitimacy and justification they need to impose vaccine mandates. The assumption underlying forced vaccination is that the social benefits conferred by vaccines outweigh people's right to decide whether to inject government-recommended substances into their bodies. Violation of such a fundamental human right as sovereignty over one's own physical body requires particularly strong evidence of the benefit inherent in such a measure. In the present case, solid evidence must be provided that the benefits of vaccines, both individually and cumulatively, substantially outweigh their harm. Unfortunately, a true cost-benefit analysis for vaccines cannot be performed at present because the cost side is unknown. The full magnitude of vaccination's side effects (both short and long term), as well as the personal and societal costs involved, cannot be determined from the available science and data, as the first part of the book demonstrates.

Presently, in the absence of solid evidence for a positive net benefit for individual vaccines, as well as the totality of childhood vaccination programs, there is no moral justification for mandating vaccination, or enforcing it in any other way. Imposing medical interventions on the public – in the absence of robust and conclusive proof of their benefit – is patently unacceptable in a democratic society.

10

THE MYSTERIES OF POLIO

The epic tale of science's victory over polio – more than any other account of a fight against disease, even the fable-like story of Edward Jenner and his smallpox vaccine – is the foundational myth of vaccination. In the industrialized world, the horrible scars smallpox left on its victims' faces can only be seen in yellowing photographs taken more than a hundred years ago; whereas, children who were paralyzed by polio in the 1950s – whether they ended up using a wheelchair, crutches, or leg brace to move about – are a living and chilling testament to the ravages of the disease that terrorized the entire Western world hardly three generations ago.

It wasn't only the death and paralysis polio left in its wake which terrorized the public. As far as they knew, the causative virus was sly and stealthy, capable of penetrating all conventional defense lines – even complete isolation! – to spell death or paralysis for people who were perfectly healthy just days before. When the disease made its sudden appearance, not even the world's best doctors could stop it or slow its course. The best medical science could do was to provide paralyzed patients with supportive care in the hope that they would somehow find the strength to prevail.

Polio outbreaks began appearing in the Western world in the late 19th century and gained momentum in the first half of the

20th century. At the same time modern science was winning the battle against infectious disease, dramatically reducing both the death toll and the suffering caused by scourges such as tuberculosis, cholera, typhoid, scarlet fever, and pertussis. Against this backdrop of science's growing confidence in its ability to eradicate diseases that had plagued humanity throughout history, polio was a glaring exception. Despite the huge sums of money invested in polio research in the first half of the 20th century, scientists and physicians weren't able to develop any effective means of curbing its spread or minimizing its harms. This decades-long failure of public health authorities to control polio epidemics contributed to a growing sense of helplessness and trepidation among the public.

Finally, science prevailed: In the mid-1950s with polio epidemics at an all-time high, Dr. Jonas Salk appeared. Clad in white with a miracle potion in his sack, Salk was the modern-day savior everyone was waiting for. Salk's polio vaccine, first used in the United States in 1955, then shortly thereafter throughout the Western world, wiped out the disease within a few years, and later pushed the poliovirus to the brink of extinction. This victory in the fight against polio put Salk and his vaccine in the limelight. He became an instant larger-than-life figure; images of the dedicated scientist clad in a white lab coat adorned the front pages of newspapers all over the globe. Everyone stood in line to shower him with praise, honors, and prizes. Parents flooded him with thank-you letters, and children fantasized about being like Salk "when they grew up". Thus, the polio vaccine became an emblem of humanity's victory in its epic battle against the mighty forces of nature.

The heroic story of polio and the vaccine was cemented in our collective consciousness as the scientific miracle that brought an end to the accursed disease. And thus it became the cornerstone of vaccine mythology in the modern age and an enduring asset of Western culture, immediately claiming a prominent position in science lore. For those seeking to glorify vaccines, it was a godsend, the perfect narrative. The apparent success of the polio vaccine paved the way for the many vaccines that followed. Even today, that same combination of fear of polio and faith in its "lifesaving" vaccine – a chord first struck in stories we heard as children in school – is used as an effective public relations tool to convince parents of the importance of vaccination.

Much like other science myths, the polio myth weaves historical facts into a beautiful tapestry destined to increase public support of the medical establishment's vaccination agenda. But this highly tailored and curated version of history brazenly omits myriad events and facts that are inconsistent with the heroic tale of "the dreadful paralytic disease that was vanquished by the vaccine."

This chapter, then, will examine those pieces of history left out of the official story, the institutional narrative promoted by health authorities. In addition, we present an alternative version of the story of polio, one that better fits the historical facts and offers plausible answers to intriguing questions that remain unanswered to this day.

Polio's Story: The Concise Institutional Version

The story of polio is repeated, almost uniformly, in numerous medical and scientific publications. The following is a summary of the accepted "official" account of polio history:

Polio is caused by the poliovirus, a member of the enterovirus family.[a] The virus typically enters the body through the mouth and makes its way to the gastrointestinal tract (the gut), where it multiplies rapidly. From the gut, the virus sometimes passes into the bloodstream, and from there it may, in some cases, invade the central nervous system and damage the nerve cells responsible for motion. Injury to the nerve cells most often manifests in a specific type of paralysis – medically termed acute flaccid paraly-

---

[a] Enteroviruses are viruses that mostly multiply in the gut and are transmitted through feces.

sis[b] – of one or more limbs. The course of the disease is quite rapid – about ten days elapse between the entry of the virus into the body and the onset of paralysis. In a small proportion of cases, the muscles that activate the respiratory system are also damaged, and the patient may die of suffocation. Not all people infected with the poliovirus will be paralyzed. Most will not even get sick, while others may come down with a flu-like illness. Only about one in 150 or 200 infections result in paralysis (and some of those spontaneously recover). Transmission occurs mainly through the fecal–oral route: The virus is excreted in the feces for several weeks following contagion, and hand contact with the feces may spread the virus, which thus may infect other people orally. The infected person then excretes the virus in their feces, and so on.[c] The poliovirus causes disease only in humans, and the human race is its only natural host. Because of this, it is possible to completely eliminate the disease by globally eradicating the virus.[1]

Polio has been with the human race for thousands of years. A pharaonic stele from 1500 BCE depicting a young man leaning on a crutch, one leg appearing withered and shrunken, is considered the oldest evidence for the disease.[2] The first medical description of a polio case appears in a book by the English physician Michael Underwood published in 1789.[3] Underwood described a combination of symptoms that have since become the hallmark of the disease: acute fever followed shortly by weakness in one or more limbs. The disease was limited to infants and young children, he added, and it wasn't uncommon, though there is no mention of outbreaks. The cause of the disease, he further noted, was unknown.

Over the next hundred years additional reports of cases of

---

[b] Acute flaccid paralysis (AFP) is a condition characterized by muscle weakness of rapid onset. Unlike other paralysis syndromes, the muscles are relaxed or soft (hence the term *flaccid*), as opposed to being rigid.

[c] A less common transmission route, according to medical authorities, is through contact with droplets of throat secretions (saliva, phlegm) from a person carrying the virus.

flaccid paralysis appeared in the medical literature, especially in children, and the disease became known as "infantile paralysis". Jakob Heine, a German orthopedist, published an essay on the disease in 1840, noting that its characteristic paralysis was caused by a spinal cord injury. Fifteen years later, a French doctor, Duchenne, discovered that nerve damage was evident in the anterior horns of the gray matter in the spinal cord (which gave the disease its name, *poliomyelitis*[d]). The cause of the disease remained unidentified.

Polio did not garner any special attention by the medical profession in the 19th century. Only sporadic reports of paralysis appeared in the medical literature, and no disease outbreaks were recorded.[e] However, that changed abruptly for no apparent reason toward the end of the century, when outbreaks began occurring in Europe and the United States. In 1890, Karl-Oskar Medin, a Swedish pediatrician, published a description of 44 cases of paralysis recorded in Stockholm in the summer of 1887, and American physician Charles Caverly reported an outbreak of 132 cases in the state of Vermont in 1894. These reports heralded polio's transformation from relatively obscure disease to a relevant and ongoing threat to public health in the Western world. In the late 19th and early 20th centuries, polio outbreaks occurred with increasing frequency, with the number of victims steadily rising, the largest of which took place in New York City in 1916 with about 9,000 cases of paralysis. Polio epidemics came and went during the first half of the 20th century, with no clear or predictable pattern. Their intensity further increased in the second half of the 1940s, after World War II, and reached a peak in the early 1950s. Surprisingly – and confusingly for researchers – the polio epidemics of the first half of the 20th century were confined to industrialized nations. No outbreaks were recorded

---

[d] In Greek, poliós means *gray* and myelós is *marrow* (of the spinal cord). The suffix *itis* indicates inflammation. This chapter will use the abbreviated name of *polio*.

[e] An outbreak is defined as a number of cases of disease that appear in temporal and geographical proximity to one another.

in developing countries during this period, just a small number of isolated cases.

Researchers linked polio paralysis to damage to the gray matter of the spinal cord in the mid-19th century, but the cause of both the illness and the nerve damage remained mysterious. In 1908 the mystery was solved when Karl Landsteiner, an Austrian biologist, was able to isolate the virus that causes the disease (named after the disease, it was called the poliovirus). Landsteiner's groundbreaking research marked the beginning of a long journey, involving thousands of researchers and scientists, which ended with the development of the vaccine.[4] Led by the National Foundation for Infantile Paralysis,[f] a charitable organization founded in the 1930s by US President Franklin Delano Roosevelt, who was himself paralyzed by polio, huge sums were invested in studying the disease. That extensive research effort resulted in Jonas Salk's injected vaccine and Albert Sabin's oral vaccine.[g] These vaccines, now routinely administered to infants all over the world, led to the disappearance of the disease from industrialized countries in the 1960s and 1970s, and to a dramatic reduction in morbidity in developing nations in the early 21st century. Today, the World Health Organization is striving to eradicate the disease through intensive vaccination campaigns in the developing world.

Unsolved Mysteries

The official version of polio history, summarized above, has successfully convinced the public that polio was comprehensively and thoroughly studied for over a hundred years, and that science has a very good grasp of its various characteristics – case

---

[f] The National Foundation for Infantile Paralysis (NFIP), later known as the March of Dimes, was an American charity that raised donations to fund polio research as well as the treatment of polio patients.

[g] Salk's inactivated polio vaccine (IPV) is given by injection. Sabin's oral polio vaccine (OPV) is given by mouth drops. In this chapter the terms "Salk vaccine" and "Sabin vaccine" will be mostly used.

diagnosis, outbreak patterns, transmission modes, how the virus causes paralysis, means of prevention, and more. But this conviction, as we shall see later in the chapter, is largely inconsistent with the facts. In reality, there are giant knowledge gaps in science's understanding of polio, and the official story fails to explain many of the prominent and essential pieces of its history.

Public discussion of these knowledge gaps is virtually nonexistent today and was very limited even in the first half of the 20th century, when polio epidemics were common in industrialized countries. For the most part, conversation regarding the unresolved mysteries of the disease was restricted to scientific circles, far from the public eye. Scientists and physicians of the period were well aware that their understanding of polio was sketchy at best. For example, Dr. Archibald Hoyne, a professor of pediatrics at the Chicago Medical School and an attending physician at two Chicago hospitals, begins his 1951 article, titled "Poliomyelitis Problems", with the following statement: "Notwithstanding the intensive studies of investigators, very little information of practical value has been added to our knowledge of poliomyelitis during the past forty years."[5] Writing two years earlier (1949) in the journal *Pediatrics*, Shaw and Thelander of the San Francisco Children's Hospital note that "Every aspect of poliomyelitis has been subjected to intensive study during the last two or three decades, in spite of which the clinician has not been presented with any inescapably sound doctrine regarding its epidemiology and transmission, its precise pathogenesis, or the details of diagnosis and treatment."[6] Dr. Albert Sabin himself, inventor of the oral polio vaccine and one of the most prominent researchers of the disease, published a transcript of a lecture he gave on the epidemiology of polio in 1951. The paper concludes with a quote from Sigmund Freud, indicative of Sabin's mindset regarding the matter at hand: "Even lectures I have given up, in order not to be forced to tell something that I only hope to learn some day."[7]

Thus, in the early 1950s, after an intensive research effort of more than 40 years, science could not provide convincing, evidence-based explanations for most features of polio. Thousands of researchers working tirelessly for decades had failed to come up with solid answers to basic questions:

❖ Why did polio outbreaks begin appearing in the late 19th century?

❖ Why were the polio epidemics in the late-19th and early-20th centuries limited to industrialized countries?

❖ Why did morbidity increase during the summer and early autumn?

❖ Why did polio spread and intensify during the same historical period when infectious disease was in rapid decline?

❖ Why could researchers identify no contact with another infected person for most polio victims?

❖ Why does the poliovirus (rarely) attack the central nervous system?

❖ Why is it not possible to infect laboratory animals with the disease orally, the pathway through which humans are supposedly infected?

These questions, and many others, remained largely unanswered in 1955, when large-scale dissemination of Salk's polio vaccine began in the United States. The apparent rapid success of the Salk vaccine (and later Sabin's as well) in eliminating polio from Western countries rendered the unsolved mysteries inconsequential. Having lost the battle against polio for more than half a century, health authorities could finally breathe a sigh of relief. The doubts, apparent contradictions, and open questions – all were swept under the enormous rug of the vaccine's meteoric success. Polio history was re-weaved into the familiar heroic fabric, leaving out the many inconvenient threads that conflict with the "science vanquishes polio" narrative.

Concurrent with the rapid decrease in polio incidence in industrialized countries in the 1960s and 1970s, polio research also waned. Since the disease had all but disappeared, "thanks to the vaccines", solving no-longer-relevant scientific riddles seemed unnecessary. But polio was in no hurry to exit the stage of history. At the same time it was departing from industrialized countries, it began appearing in increasing numbers in the developing world. Thus, after a hiatus of about twenty years, polio research regained momentum, driven by a global eradication initiative set forth by the World Health Organization. But even though modern polio research makes use of the most advanced tools and techniques available to science, it still hasn't found satisfactory answers to the old riddles. Dr. Julie Pfeiffer, from the Department of Microbiology at the University of Texas Southwestern Medical Center, writes in 2010: "Why did certain people develop paralysis? How does the virus move from the gut to the CNS? What limits viral trafficking to the CNS in the vast majority of infected individuals? Despite over 100 years of poliovirus research, many of these questions remain unanswered."[8] Dr. Neal Nathanson of the University of Pennsylvania School of Medicine, a respected veteran polio researcher, summarizes some of the open questions regarding the epidemiology of the disease in a 1979 paper. The title of the article – "The Epidemiology of Poliomyelitis: Enigmas Surrounding Its Appearance, Epidemicity, and Disappearance" – testifies to its content.[9] In a more recent paper (2010), Nathanson still fails to provide compelling answers to the mysteries of the past.[10] In fact, as becomes clear later in the chapter, not only have these mysteries not been solved, they have become even more puzzling over time.

Polio Takes the Stage

Polio is one of a handful of diseases that have become a major threat to public health during modern times, and its appearance on the stage of history is well documented.[11] As we have seen, early case descriptions of polio began to appear in the medical literature toward the end of the 18th century. Isolated cases of paralysis were occasionally documented in the following hundred years or so. The first polio outbreaks – of dozens of cases or more – were reported in Sweden and the United States near the end of the 19th century. Within twenty years, polio outbreaks had also been recorded in England, Austria, Germany, Norway, New Zealand, and Canada.[12] This sudden, almost simultaneous, emergence of polio outbreaks in Europe and North America in the late 19th century has been puzzling polio epidemiologists for more than a hundred years.[13]

The distinctive typical course of the disease – a healthy toddler experiences paralysis in one or more limbs a few days after a short bout of high fever – left experts little doubt that polio's emergence in epidemic form was indeed a new phenomenon. "The disease's striking presentation," Nathanson writes in 2010, "would have made outbreaks conspicuous. However, few if any cases were reported until late in the 19th century."[14] Dr. Albert Sabin, who devoted much of his time to the study of the epidemiology of polio, writes in 1947: "The bulk of the evidence suggests that the epidemic outbursts, of the type which have occurred especially in the United States and a few other countries in the past thirty to forty years, are events that could not readily have been missed in the past."[15]

Thus, the first major question that polio epidemiologists were trying to answer concerned the sudden emergence of the disease:

❖ Why did polio outbreaks first appear in the late 19th century?

When polio spread to other countries, researchers noticed an unexpected phenomenon: Outbreaks were mostly restricted to industrialized countries. Dr. Dorothy Horstmann, a veteran polio researcher at Yale University School of Medicine, describes the early 20th-century polio outbreaks in a 1985 paper: "Epidemics emerged only in economically advanced countries of the world while in the underdeveloped areas the disease remained endemic."[16] Sabin, in a 1947 article, summarizes the scientific knowledge accumulated on the subject over the previous sixty years and asks: "...why does [paralytic poliomyelitis] seem to be affecting more and more the countries in which sanitation and hygiene, along with the general standard of living, are presumably making the greatest advances, while other large parts of the world [...] are still relatively unaffected?"[17] He cites Africa and China as areas where polio outbreaks have never been reported,[18] although Western doctors lived in both areas for many years and would probably have reported paralysis epidemics among the locals if there were any.[19] Dr. Archibald Hoyne also writes in 1951 that Chinese doctors told him they had never seen polio cases in their country.[20]

Moreover, when rare polio outbreaks were reported in non-industrialized countries, the illness was largely limited to foreign nationals from industrialized countries and only sporadically affected local residents. Sabin points out that while American soldiers stationed in the Philippines after World War II contracted polio in large numbers, there were no outbreaks of the disease in the local population.[21] Similar figures were recorded among American soldiers stationed in the Middle East, China, and Japan during World War II.[22] In the Middle East, for example, dozens of cases of death and paralysis were reported in American and British soldiers, while morbidity among the locals was relatively low (and zero in local adults). Notably, the incidence of polio among American soldiers stationed in the Middle East was ten times higher than among their counterparts who remained in the mainland United States.[23]

Sabin proceeds to describe his own personal experience of the polio outbreak of the previous year, in Tientsin, China. While four US Marines stationed in the city died and one was severely paralyzed, no evidence of polio was found in the local population. A British doctor, practicing for 25 years in Tientsin, informed Sabin that while he occasionally sees paralytic polio cases among the children of the city's foreign colony, it is rare in local children.[24] Dr. John Paul of the Yale University School of

Medicine, one of polio's most prominent epidemiologists, investigated polio incidence in the Moroccan city of Casablanca with Dorothy Horstmann. The two found that between 1947 and 1953 the incidence of polio among the European population in the city was about twenty times higher than that of the local population.[25] Dr. Douglas McAlpine, an expert in diseases of the nervous system and a special adviser to the British Army in World War II, found a large disparity in polio morbidity between officers in the British Army and soldiers, and an even larger one between those groups and the local population. The incidence of polio among British officers stationed in India between 1942 and 1944 was about 120 per 100,000, five times higher than that of British soldiers in India, and 120 times higher than the rate of local Indian soldiers.[26] In the British troops stationed in North Africa and Italy in those years, the incidence among officers was nine times higher than that of soldiers.[27] In addition, polio morbidity among British soldiers in India and the Middle East was ten and four times higher (respectively) than among soldiers who served in Britain.[28]

Thus, the notable disparities in polio morbidity in industrialized and developing countries, between foreign residents and soldiers and the local population, and between soldiers of different ranks, presented researchers with a number of additional puzzles:

❖ Why did polio epidemics of the first half of the 20th century strike industrialized countries, while almost no outbreaks were reported in developing countries?

❖ Why was considerable polio morbidity observed in Western residents of various developing countries, while only sporadic cases, if any at all, were recorded among the locals?

❖ Why was polio incidence in American and British soldiers stationed in different parts of the world during and after World War II much higher – ten times or more – than in their comrades serving at home?

❖ Why was the incidence of polio among British officers in India, North Africa, and Italy during World War II five to ten times higher than among the enlisted men?

These are fundamental issues that any scientist seeking to formulate a comprehensive and cohesive explanation of the epidemiology of polio must address. To this day, as we shall see shortly, the official polio story provides no satisfactory answers for these essential questions.

The "Improved Hygiene" Theory of Polio

A dramatic decline in the mortality and morbidity of most infectious diseases was recorded in industrialized countries in the period from 1850 to 1950. As shown in chapter 8, the main reasons for this reduction were gradual improvements in sanitation, personal hygiene, and nutrition. Such improvements included construction of centralized sewage systems, modern plumbing installation in homes, increased availability of fresh food, and emphasis on bathing and cleanliness. Peculiarly, though, while infectious disease in general was trending dramatically downward, polio was doing the opposite, steadily gaining momentum.

Researchers who investigated the first polio outbreaks struggled to explain its sudden emergence. Even after Landsteiner's discovery in 1908, when it became widely accepted in scientific circles that polio was caused by a virus, no plausible explanation was formulated for the marked change in incidence observed over the previous decades. It was only in the late 1940s, after much information had accumulated on various aspects of the disease, that an explanation for its abnormal outbreak patterns emerged. This theory was intended to provide convincing answers to the riddles posed by polio's unique epidemiological traits.

The theory formulated by 1940s researchers, which can be summarized as "too much hygiene", was rooted in the fact that polio morbidity rose in parallel with the improvement in living conditions in Western countries. Dr. Hart Van Riper, Medical Director of the National Foundation for Infantile Paralysis, writes in 1947: "The period of evolution from sporadic to epidemic poliomyelitis corresponds roughly with the institution of widespread measures for improved sanitation." Until that time, Van Riper explains, polio was rare because of the "frequent exposures of the young infant to virus during the time when he still retains a high [level] of passive immunity from his mother." Thus, infants since antiquity were fortunate to develop immunity to the disease, while rarely suffering its paralyzing effects. "This theory," he continues, "might explain the infrequent cases of poliomyelitis in young children as they occurred in the early history of the disease in Europe and the United States. But, in regions where epidemics predominate, people are exposed to the virus less frequently and at a later period in life, when they have lost all or most of the passive immunity acquired from the mother. Thus there results a greater chance for the development of [paralytic] disease among older age groups rather than an increased resistance."[29]

It is worth noting that Van Riper chooses his words carefully, recognizing that the proposed explanation is lacking solid evidence, and largely constructs a broad and vague story that only coarsely fits the historical data. Nevertheless, over the years, in the absence of a better explanation, the "Improved Hygiene" theory [h] became one of the main pillars of the institutional story

---

[h] The polio-related concept of "too much hygiene" wasn't specifically named in the 1940s. In this chapter we will refer to it as the *Improved Hygiene Theory*. Apparently, it was a precursor of the *Hygiene Hypothesis* proposed by Strachan in 1989. According to this theory, the increase in allergic and autoimmune diseases in the West, and more recently in developing countries, is attributed to the reduced exposure of infants to bacteria and viruses in the first years of life, due to "excessive" hygiene.

of polio. Sabin, for example, reinforces Van Riper's observations, writing in 1951: "In general, the poorer the population, [and] its standard of living and sanitation, the more extensively is polio-myelitis virus disseminated among them and the lower is the incidence of paralytic poliomyelitis [...]"[30] Dr. Stanley Plotkin's canonical book *Vaccines* also cites the concept of Improved Hygiene as "the generally accepted explanation, supported by numerous studies" for the sudden emergence of polio in Western countries.[31] Neal Nathanson, who was a young polio researcher in the 1950s, repeats Van Riper's main points and adds a more comprehensive and detailed formulation of the theory in a paper published sixty years later (2010). In the period before the first polio outbreaks, he explains, sanitation was bad and the po-liovirus so prevalent that most of the population became infected during infancy. Infants received antibodies against the poliovirus during pregnancy and early breastfeeding from their mothers. Then, when the children later contracted the virus, which settled in the digestive tract, antibody levels were still very high. Thus, in the uncommon event that the virus made its way from the gut to the bloodstream, it was neutralized by the maternal antibodies and prevented from entering the central nervous system where it could potentially cause paralysis. The end result, Nathanson writes, was that infants developed their own im-munity to the poliovirus while they were protected by the maternal antibodies in their blood. With the improvement in personal hygiene and sanitation in industrialized countries, the poliovirus became less common, which meant that many chil-dren did not become infected until they were more than a year old, long after any maternal antibodies had disappeared. Thus, not having developed their own immunity and devoid of their mothers' antibodies, these children were now at higher risk of paralysis from passage of the virus from the gut to the blood, and from there to the nervous system.[32]

The Improved Hygiene theory purportedly provided answers

to most of the unsolved riddles of polio epidemiology. It ostensibly explained why the disease broke out in the late 19th century (*answer:* during this period there was a significant improvement in sanitation and hygiene in the West and the virus became less common); why it initially emerged only in Western countries (*answer:* improvements in sanitation and hygiene had not yet been implemented in the developing world); why Western residents (and soldiers) living in pre-industrial countries contracted polio in relatively large numbers compared to locals (*answer:* unlike locals, who contracted the virus in infancy, Westerners first encountered it at a later age and were at a higher risk of paralysis); and even why soldiers serving in pre-industrial countries contracted polio in higher numbers compared to their comrades stationed at home (*answer:* poliovirus was more prevalent in countries with poor sanitation). Although it was only partly based on scientific evidence and some of its assumptions were never proven while others were inconsistent with the data,[33] the Improved Hygiene theory became the formal, officially sanctioned explanation for the "odd" outbreak patterns of polio.[34]

The Improved Hygiene Theory vs. Reality

Studies conducted in the United States in the 1950s found that about 90% of American mothers passed poliovirus antibodies to their babies in the first months of life. According to the Improved Hygiene theory, maternal antibodies were supposed to wane and disappear in the first year, exposing American infants to polio's harms thereafter. And, indeed, studies showed that the level of polio antibodies in infants' blood dropped rapidly: At three months of age over 50% of infants were no longer adequately protected, and at six months of age this number rose to almost 100%.[35] These findings apparently confirmed the theory: Mid-20th century American infants, raised in a clean environment, were not exposed to the poliovirus and thus did not develop proper gut immunity while protected by their mothers' antibodies. Hence, when encountering the poliovirus at a later age, they were at a relatively high risk of contracting the disease.

However, contrary to the underlying suppositions of the Improved Hygiene theory, similar findings were obtained in countries where sanitary conditions were very different from those in the United States. Sabin himself investigated the issue in 1951 and found that the level of poliovirus antibodies in infants aged 6–12 months was very low not only in the US, but also in countries where no polio outbreaks had ever been recorded (Japan, Korea) and in countries where sanitation and hygiene were particularly poor (Egypt). According to the theory, infants in these countries were supposed to be exposed to the poliovirus in early infancy and gain immunity for the rest of their lives as a result. But the low level of polio antibodies found in their children's blood indicated that this did not happen. These findings led Sabin to categorically state that "the hypothesis of extensive immunization as a result of [...] subclinical infection among certain population groups during the first year of life therefore became untenable."[36] In doing so, Sabin effectively dismisses the entire Improved Hygiene theory.

Thus, the biological mechanism proposed by the Improved Hygiene theory for the sudden emergence of polio is not consistent with the scientific evidence.

But wait, there's more.

When looking at the Improved Hygiene theory from an epidemiological perspective, an even more serious problem emerges: The theory's fundamental premise, that there is a correlation between polio incidence and the level of sanitation and hygiene, is patently false. This hypothesis was initially formulated in the United States in the post-WWII period, when polio seemed to be more prevalent in affluent suburbs while sparing somewhat the more densely populated, inner-city neighborhoods (the opposite of typical outbreak patterns for infectious diseases).[37] The theory allegedly provided an explanation for the mysterious appearance of the disease in industrialized countries and its relative absence from developing countries. But this presumed link between polio morbidity and the level of sanitation and hygiene is based on a narrow slice of polio's historical record and doesn't fit the majority of evidence accumulated on the subject.

Naomi Rogers, an American historian, researched the early history of polio in the United States. The title of her book[38] – *Dirt and Disease: Polio Before FDR*[i] – concisely depicts the image of polio in the early 20th century: a disease of uncleanliness. Rogers writes that during this early period polio was considered a disease linked to "immigrants and urban slums".[39] She describes a scene from a propaganda film called *Fighting Infantile Paralysis* that was released in 1917, a year after the great polio epidemic that struck the east coast of the United States. The film, produced with the help of the Rockefeller Institute, the leading US polio research center, conveys how the disease was perceived by the medical establishment of the era. One scene, described by Rogers, shows a typical New York residential neighborhood, believed to be the ideal breeding ground for the disease: "Narrow streets lined with dirty and unsanitary pushcarts, the latter filled with fly-specked cakes and candy and decaying fruit... all are touched by many hands before they are finally eaten; there are uncovered garbage cans near which cats and children play and squabble over crusts of bread and other tid-bits."[40]

This cinematic depiction reflected the events of the previous year in New York (1916), when the city was hit by the largest polio epidemic recorded to date. The first cases occurred in *Pigtown*, a slum populated by Italian immigrants, whose name

---

[i] The reference is to the period up to 1921, the year that future president Franklin Delano Roosevelt was paralyzed.

was presumably a testament to its living conditions.[41] *The New York Times*, in its July 1st 1916 issue, reports on the early stage of the epidemic: "Italians living in crowded tenements have been the chief sufferers... The infected area contains many old tenements, and garbage and ashes are deposited in the halls. It is reported that these areas are infested with cats, and the garbage and ash piles draw flies. With the co-operation of the various [municipal] departments these areas are being cleaned up."[42] However, by the end of the summer, Rogers notes, when the epidemic waned and morbidity data was collected, New York public health officials were surprised to learn that polio had struck similarly in all sections of the population: "both rich and poor, long-time residents as well as recent immigrants."[43]

Polio's reputation in the early 20th century as a disease that thrived in conditions of poor sanitation and hygiene stemmed from the fact that it was classified as an infectious disease. Experience gained during the 19th century indicated that infectious diseases tend to break out in conditions of poverty and filth. This presumably explains the beliefs of the New York City public health authorities in 1916 and the propaganda film that was aired a year later, but it was clearly wrong. As Rogers points out, "economic or sanitary conditions seemed to make little difference; rich or poor, clean or dirty, no child seemed immune."[44]

In fact, the disassociation between living standards and polio morbidity observed in New York in 1916 was consistently reported by researchers since polio's early days in the United States. Dr. Charles Caverly, president of Vermont's State Board of Health, wrote a report on the polio epidemic in the state's Rutland County in 1894, the first major outbreak reported in the United States. Caverly, who closely examined each of the 132 cases, found that the disease affected all classes to a similar degree. "General sanitary conditions," Caverly sums up, "did not seem to have any influence on the epidemic."[45] Dr. Robert Lovett, a renowned orthopedist and polio expert (who was called upon to treat future President Roosevelt when he was paralyzed in 1921), submitted a summary report to the Massachusetts State Board of Health in 1908 regarding the state's polio outbreak the previous year. He describes the living conditions of the victims as follows: "One hundred and fifteen lived in detached houses; 110 in tenements [...]. Sanitary conditions were described as exceptionally good in 21. Good, in 123. Fair, in 55. Poor or bad, in 23 [...] house was screened in 133 cases, and not screened or insufficiently so in 80." Like Caverly before him, Lovett cannot identify a correlation between the onset of the disease and living conditions and concludes "Analyzing these data for what they are worth, it would seem that it was not an affection confined to the lower classes."[46] Dr. Herbert Emerson, Massachusetts' State Inspector of Health, published a 1908 report on polio cases in the state. "Sanitary conditions," Emerson notes in the report, "were found to be excellent in 4 cases, good in 17, fair in 31 and bad in 17 [...] 23 houses had water closets connected with the sewer and 46 had earth closets; the sink water from 30 houses was carried into the sewer and in 39 cases it was disposed of in various ways on the land nearby or in pipes to the nearest brook, pond, etc."[47] Dr. Milton Rosenau briefly reviews the early polio outbreaks in his book *Preventive Medicine and Hygiene* (1918) and writes, "It is important to note that social and hygienic conditions apparently have no influence whatever in determining the infection. All classes are affected in about equal proportion."[48]

It is evident from the above reports that the Improved Hygiene theory's underlying assumptions directly conflict with the circumstances of early polio outbreaks. The researchers who constructed the theory were probably heavily influenced by the epidemics of the "middle period" (from the end of WWII to the early 1960s), which were more intense in middle-class neighborhoods, and chose to ignore epidemiological data from the early period. This dogmatic approach probably also led researchers to disregard more recent data that contradicted the institutional story. For example, a study conducted by John Paul in Egypt in the late 1940s, found a relatively high level of polio in and around Cairo. Paul's calculations suggested that disease incidence among children in Cairo and nearby villages was similar to the average US incidence of the previous 15 years.[49] According to the Improved Hygiene theory, similar morbidity levels would be expected for similar levels of sanitation and hygiene. Thus, if the theory were correct, Paul's results would imply that living standards were similar in and around Cairo in the 1940s to those in the United States at the time, which seems implausible.

Morbidity patterns in the young state of Israel provide another good example of the disparity between polio epidemiological theory and the historical record. Until 1949, polio incidence in Israel was quite low at about 1-2 cases per 100,000 people.[50] However, from 1949 onward epidemics occurred in consecutive years, with peak morbidity rising a hundred-fold compared to pre-1949 levels (150 per 100,000 in 1950).[51] What could have caused this huge and unexpected increase in morbidity? In a 2008 paper on the epidemiology of polio in Israel, Dr. Tiberio Swartz of the Israeli Ministry of Health, the leading expert on the history of polio in Israel, struggles to provide an explanation for this phenomenon. Although he subscribes to the Improved Hygiene concept,[52] Swartz cannot reconcile actual 1950s data with the theory's predictions. For example, morbidity among immigrants in 1950, most of whom came from African and Middle-Eastern countries where sanitation conditions were much worse than Israel's, was twice as high as that of longtime residents.[53] Despite a marked difference in living standards, polio incidence was similar for children living on kibbutzim and those living in immigrant transit camps, and the incidence in these two groups was twice as high as that of the urban population.[54] Another interesting fact is that morbidity in the non-Jewish population, whose standard of living was inferior, was significantly lower than that of the Jewish population in the period 1949–1954 but unexplainably eclipsed it in 1955.

Thus, despite Swartz's best efforts, the Improved Hygiene theory fails to explain the sudden emergence of polio in epidemic proportions in Israel in 1949 or its morbidity patterns in subsequent years. Swartz cannot identify any significant change in sanitation and hygiene conditions that occurred in Israel in the late-1940s that could explain the massive rise in polio incidence.[55] The prominent change that did occur – the great waves of immigration, mostly from Africa and the Middle East, which began in 1949 and lasted several years – should have pushed polio incidence down, if anything. The newcomers arrived from countries with poorer living conditions and should have had better immunity compared to veteran Israelis.

Improved Hygiene and Polio in the Third World

Polio began to wane in industrialized countries in the early 1960s and all but disappeared in the late 1970s. However, even as it was making its way out of newspapers and into history books in the First World, it unexpectedly re-emerged in the Third at rates similar to those of the peak epidemic years of the 1950s in the United States.[56] At the end of the 20th century, the official story of the epidemiology of the disease was turned on its head. Polio was once again linked to poor sanitary conditions and hygiene, this time in countries such as India, Afghanistan, Pakistan, Nigeria, and Somalia. Thus, the World Health Organization's Roland Sutter and his colleagues, authors of the oral polio vaccine chapter in Stanley Plotkin's *Vaccines*, state that "Lower socioeconomic status has been shown to be a risk for paralytic poliomyelitis in developing countries, probably because children belonging to the lower socioeconomic group experience more intense exposure to poliovirus."[57] Similarly, an Australian Ministry of Health document asserts that "The risk of [poliovirus] infection is directly correlated with poor hygiene and poor sanitation and overcrowding, [...]. This is a major health problem in the developing world causing mortality and morbidity among thousands of children annually."[58] Senior officials at the WHO's Global Polio Eradication Initiative (GPEI) report on the status of the eradication operation in India in *Science* magazine (2006): "High population densities and poor sanitation therefore appear to explain the persistence of polio. These factors act to facilitate the transmission not only of poliovirus but also of other enteroviruses and diarrhea [...]"[59] These statements, however, completely contradict the tenets of the Improved Hygiene theory, which asserts that conditions of overcrowding and poor hygiene lead to better polio immunity and low morbidity.

Thus, the wheel had turned once more, and polio epidemiology was back at its starting point. Polio was commonly associated with dirt and lack of sanitation in the early days and later linked to "too much hygiene" (1940s and 1950s), only to return to its origins in the late-20th century as a disease ostensibly caused by poor living conditions. Thus, the institutionally endorsed version of the polio story magically has it both ways: Polio epidemics in industrialized countries resulted from "excessive" hygiene, while those in developing countries were due to poor hygiene.

This inherent contradiction has not been resolved to this day. Nathanson, for example, completely ignores it in his 2010 article on the epidemiology of polio. Horstmann, for her part, acknowledges that the later polio surge in developing countries "proved false" the assertion that wide dissemination of the poliovirus leads to early-life exposure and ensuing lifelong immunity to the paralytic disease.[60] Nevertheless, even she seems oblivious to the far-reaching implications of this insight. If polio immunity is not acquired in early infancy when living conditions are poor, then the Improved Hygiene theory instantly collapses, along with the formal, accepted explanation for the emergence of polio epidem-

ics in the West in the late-19th century. The fundamental contradiction inherent in the institutional account of polio
epidemiology is nicely exemplified by Horstmann in the paper
cited above. While she acknowledges that widespread polio
morbidity in developing countries demonstrates that poor sanitary conditions do not confer polio immunity in early age, she
argues the exact opposite when she explains the reasons for the
disease's emergence in late-19th century: "Improved sanitary
environment in industrialized countries," Horstmann writes,
"protected young children from early exposure to the virus [...].
In contrast, in the underdeveloped, largely tropical countries of
the world where the sanitary environment remains poor, infection and immunity develop in the first few years of life."[61] Thus,
according to Horstmann, the central supposition of the Improved
Hygiene theory – that poor sanitation and hygiene facilitate
transmission of the poliovirus and the acquisition of immunity in
infancy – is both correct and incorrect at the same time.

As alluded to earlier, Horstmann is by no means alone in her
bizarre acceptance of this logical inconsistency: No explanation
for this glaring contradiction can be found in the medical literature, nor in health agency publications, nor in the rather
extensive popular literature on polio. The institutional story of
polio, based as it is on the supposition that polio epidemics
appeared because of improving living conditions, simply cannot
provide a plausible explanation for the abnormal outbreak
patterns of the disease.

Polio-like Illnesses

Contrary, perhaps, to prevailing public perception, the flaccid
paralysis characteristic of polio is not caused by the poliovirus
alone. Citing historical case reports by Underwood, Heine,
Medin, and others and retrospectively attributing them to "polio" conveys the impression that nothing else could have caused

such flaccid paralysis. But the reality is that polio-like paralysis has long been known to be caused by myriad illnesses and conditions.

Dr. Ralph Scobey, a New York State physician, scanned the medical literature from the 18th century onwards and found case, and even outbreak, reports of polio-like paralytic illnesses under no less than 200 different names.[62] In a 41-page paper he published in 1950, Scobey lists the names of these conditions,[j] along with numerous medical citations proving his claims. This great assortment of paralytic diseases was attributed to numerous and varied types of "poisoning", including bacterial contamination of food and water, insecticide spraying of vegetables and fruits, toxic fruits and vegetables due to drought, contamination of water by toxic chemicals, and more. In a 1953 paper, Scobey adds examples from the medical literature of polio-like morbidity following infectious diseases (influenza, diphtheria, smallpox, measles) and vaccines (for pertussis, smallpox, and rabies).[63]

In a 1984 paper, Dr. James Gear, a polio expert at the National Institute for Virology in South Africa, cites additional causes of polio-like paralysis: spinal cord infection due to injury, the bites of venomous reptiles (snakes, scorpions, and spiders) and ticks, parasitic worms, and more.[64] Gear, like Scobey, also describes cases of paralysis resulting from sprayed food and water and infectious diseases (rabies, mumps, herpes). In addition, he lists a number of mysterious "polio" outbreaks in the first half of the 20th century – in South Africa, Iceland, Los Angeles, and London – for which no causative agent was found.[65] Guillain-Barré syndrome, a paralytic disease with symptoms very similar to polio's, is also discussed at length. Guillain-Barré's cause has

---

[j] A small sample from this list: intermittent fever, epidemic fever, arachnitis, reflex paralysis, rheumatic paralysis, palsy, spastic spinal paralysis, spinal atrophy, summer fever, teething paralysis...

not yet been identified with certainty.[k]

Given the plethora of diseases, syndromes, and conditions which can cause polio-like paralysis, it shouldn't be surprising that polio diagnosis, even in the 20th century, was largely inconsistent and unreliable. When non-paralytic cases of poliovirus infection were included under the definition of the disease, it become even more challenging. For example, in a 1934 paper reporting the events of the polio epidemic in Los Angeles, Dr. Meals and colleagues from the Los Angeles County Hospital, note that many patients initially diagnosed with polio, actually had other diseases. According to their calculation, 57 different diseases were mistakenly diagnosed as polio.[66] In an addendum to the Meals paper, Dr. Archibald Hoyne of the University Hospital of Chicago adds his recollections of polio outbreaks in Chicago in 1916 and 1917, during which "almost every conceivable disease and condition was reported by physicians as poliomyelitis."[67] In a 1951 paper, Hoyne lists about 25 such diseases, noting that "it is frequently stated that no two cases of poliomyelitis are exactly alike."[68] Dr. Douglas McAlpine and colleagues from the Department of Nervous Diseases at Middlesex Hospital, England, report that out of 104 "polio" patients referred to their department in the summer of 1947, the diagnosis was actually confirmed in only 60 cases.[69] In view of the relative novelty of polio, and considering that physicians were not provided with specific diagnostic guidelines,[70] it is understandable that misdiagnosis was so common.

The reputation that polio gained following the great epidemics of the early 20th century meant that nearly every case of flaccid paralysis was diagnosed as "polio". This dynamic was exemplified by a number of "milk-borne polio" outbreaks reported in the medical literature in the first third of the century.

---

[k] Guillain-Barré syndrome is one of the diseases associated with the modern category of polio-like diseases – AFP (acute flaccid paralysis).

Dr. John Dingman, a physician from Spring Valley, New York, reported six cases of polio in children from three boarding schools in the city in 1916.[71] All cases occurred within a few days of each other and all of the sick children, according to Dingman's investigation, consumed milk from the same provider. Other children who stayed in the same residences but drank milk from other providers were not harmed. Dingman also found that in the residences where the children got sick, the milk had not been boiled before it was consumed. In private homes that received milk (from the first provider) that was boiled before it was consumed, no cases of illness were reported. His conclusion was that the paralysis was caused by the poliovirus contaminating the milk during its production process.

A similar "polio" outbreak was reported by Dr. Knapp, the health inspector in Cortland City, New York.[72] During a ten-day period in December 1925, eight cases were reported in the city. The eight victims lived in different areas of the city and had no direct contact. A vigorous investigation by Knapp and colleagues revealed that all eight had consumed milk originating from a specific distributor (who handled only 4% of the city's milk supply). In addition, a boy who worked at the dairy that supplied most of that distributor's milk, contracted polio shortly before the outbreak. The geographic distance between the patients, the almost simultaneous onset of the illness, and the consumption of milk from a common source led Knapp to assume that the disease was transmitted through milk.

Dr. Lloyd Aycock, an expert in preventive medicine and hygiene at Harvard Medical School and one of Knapp's colleagues for the aforementioned study, reported an epidemic in the English city of Broadstairs in October 1926. The epidemic lasted about two weeks, during which polio affected 73 patients, 43 of whom were paralyzed. Most of the patients lived in a number of boarding schools located outside Broadstairs, and the rest lived in the city. No contact was found between the boarding schools' patients and those living in the city. Only two polio cases had been reported in Broadstairs in the previous five years, and none in neighboring cities. Aycock notes that since most of the cases occurred almost simultaneously, the source of the infection was likely common. The investigation he conducted revealed that of the 43 paralytic cases, 35 had consumed milk from a specific distributor, with the other 8 getting their milk from a second distributor who had bought some of his milk from the first distributor.

Another polio outbreak linked to contaminated milk was reported by Dr. Edward Rosenow of the Mayo Clinic.[73] During the outbreak, which occurred at a college in the central US and lasted six days in October 1930, two students died and six others were paralyzed. The investigation did not find a direct connection between the patients, and no other cases were reported in or around the city. Rosenow writes that the illness disappeared as quickly as it appeared after the college dining halls stopped serving the unpasteurized milk and cream produced by the college dairy.

It is worth noting that the investigators in each of the four outbreaks reviewed above determined the illness to be polio, even though the poliovirus was never isolated from patients nor otherwise identified in any of them. Moreover, each outbreak was short-lived and confined to a small geographical area, despite the fact that no special measures were taken to curb disease spread. This pattern is atypical of viral diseases, such as influenza or chickenpox, where the virus is transmitted from person to person at ever-increasing distances from the focus of the outbreak. This classic viral pattern, while not observed in the milk-borne outbreaks, was observed in some of the polio epidemics of the early 20th century, giving polio its reputation as "highly contagious".[74]

An Alternative Explanation: Pesticides

Sporadic cases, and even small outbreaks, of polio-like illnesses have been reported since the end of the 18th century. However, there is no denying that late in the 19th century some fundamental change occurred in the Western way of life which led to larger and more frequent outbreaks of paralysis, initially reported in Sweden and the United States, and later in other industrialized nations. The official story holds that improvements in sanitation and hygiene led to a dramatic increase in polio morbidity, but, as we have seen, this version of events doesn't match the historical record. Was there another alteration in the late 19th-century way of life that could better explain the sudden emergence of polio epidemics in the Western world?

In the mid-18th century two German chemists invented a new green dye that later became known as *Paris green*. Paris green was a toxic substance, a mixture of copper and arsenic, mainly used in the textile and wallpaper industry.[1] During the 19th century, it became very popular in Europe and the United States, and was produced by nearly every dye manufacturer of the period.[75] Although arsenic was already known to be a deadly poison, Paris green was considered safe to use. Many household products – children's toys, candy wrappers, playing cards, rugs and wallpapers, decorations, and more[76] – were dyed the fashionable green color, and toxic arsenic fumes were daily inhaled by household inhabitants. Arsenic was also used as an ingredient in numerous medical drugs. Fowler's Solution, for example, was a popular drug containing a large amount of arsenic that was prescribed by doctors for a wide range of ailments – headache, eczema, psoriasis, asthma, whooping cough, bronchitis, cancer, and many others.[77]

---

[1] Paris green was based on an earlier dye called *Scheele's Green*, also made of copper and arsenic, invented in Sweden in 1742 by the chemist Carl Wilhelm Scheele.

As the use of arsenic increased, doctors' reports of arsenic poisoning began appearing in the medical literature. Some poisonings were due to single exposures to large amounts of the substance, while others were due to continuous exposure to smaller amounts. Dr. James Putnam, a professor of neurology at Harvard University, collaborated with other Boston doctors to raise awareness of the dangers of using arsenic in the home.[78] In an article published in 1891, Putnam describes 12 cases of arsenic poisoning.[79] In order to estimate the degree of arsenic exposure in the general population, Putnam sent urine samples from 150 of his patients for laboratory testing. The analysis, performed by an experienced Harvard chemist, found that about 30 percent of the samples contained some level of arsenic. "These results conclusively show," Putnam writes, "that the community is exposed to arsenical contamination on a very large scale."[80]

In the late 19th century, on top of its numerous uses in household products and medicines, Paris green became a popular pesticide as well. In 1867, an anonymous American farmer sprayed his potato bushes with the green compound in an attempt to protect them from the devastating Colorado potato beetle. News of Paris green's resounding success in controlling the beetle quickly traveled far and wide, and American farmers began applying it to other crops as well. By 1880, Paris green was widely used throughout all of North America,[81] opening the door to the use of synthetic chemicals in agricultural pest control. The increasing use of pesticides in agriculture initiated an upsurge of inventions and improvements in spraying technology. New mechanical sprayers and various accessories made spraying an effective and affordable pest-control technique. At the same time, formulations and spraying equipment for home use were also introduced.[82]

Paris green maintained its lead in the pesticide market until the 1890s, when it was dethroned by lead arsenate, a compound made from lead and arsenic, as the name implies. Lead arsenate was a new-and-improved insecticide invented to fight infestations of the gypsy moth, a leaf-eating insect that was imported to the United States from France by an amateur insect breeder in 1869.[83] Following its success in curbing the devastating spread of the gypsy moth, farmers in the northeastern United States began applying lead arsenate to their apple trees in their ongoing battle against the codling moth.[m] The compound was simple to prepare – many farmers mixed it themselves – and very effective, partly because it adhered to the plant's surface longer than its competitors did.[84] In the early 20th century, lead arsenate replaced Paris green as the most popular and widely used agricultural pesticide in the United States. It maintained this position until after World War II, when it was replaced by DDT. In addition, it was also used in England, New Zealand, Canada, Australia, France, and many other countries (especially those where the codling moth was common).[85]

One year after the introduction of lead arsenate, two doctors from Massachusetts General Hospital reported an unexplained rise in paralytic polio cases in the Boston area. In an article published in the *Boston Medical and Surgical Journal* in November 1893, Drs. Putnam[n] and Taylor ask: "Is acute poliomyelitis unusually prevalent this season?" According to data they collected at hospitals in the Boston area, polio incidence in the summer months and early fall of 1893 was four times higher than the previous year (26 cases vs. 6).[86] The two doctors grapple with the issue of polio's high prevalence in the summer and autumn months, but, like so many later doctors and researchers, they miss the fact that this time of year largely coincides with apple-picking season in Massachusetts.[87] Is it merely a coincidence that shortly after the introduction of lead arsenate, an insecticide applied in apple orchards, there was a large increase in polio

---

[m] The worm of the codling moth is the proverbial worm in the apple.

[n] This is the same James Putnam, the Harvard neurologist, who was mentioned earlier.

cases at apple-picking season?[o] Putnam and Taylor provide another clue supporting this hypothesis: most of the polio patients came from the rural areas surrounding Boston, and not from the city itself.[88]

A year later (1894), the first major polio outbreak recorded on US soil, occurred in Rutland County, Vermont (Massachusetts' northern neighbor). Dr. Charles Caverly, president of Vermont's State Board of Health, reported that most of the cases occurred between July and September.[89] Similar to Massachusetts, apple orchards were also very common in Vermont,[90] and the harvest season coincided with the timeframe of the polio outbreak reported by Caverly.[91]

Could there be a connection between the increasing use of arsenic-based pesticides and the paralysis that was reported with increasing frequency during the same period?

Lead arsenate, as its name suggests, contains lead and arsenic, and the latter is also a primary ingredient of Paris green. According to the CDC, exposure to minute amounts of these toxic substances, in combination or separately, can cause a variety of symptoms that includes paralysis and death.[92] Reports of paralysis following exposure to arsenic and lead appeared in the medical literature of the period. Dr. Putnam, in the same 1891 article that presents a description of twelve cases of arsenic poisoning, notes that seven of the patients were paralyzed with what he calls "arsenic paralysis".[93] In a report regarding the Massachusetts polio outbreak of 1907, Dr. Lovett, the orthopedist and polio expert, mentions two cases of "polio" paralysis as a result of lead poisoning and a third case following arsenic poi-

---

[o] Per Axelsson, in an article on the history of polio in Sweden, writes that Swedish parents in the first half of the 20th century would warn their children every autumn, "Do not eat apples that have been on the ground!" lest they contract polio.

Per Axelsson, "Do Not Eat Those Apples: They've Been on the Ground!" 2009

soning.[94] Dr. Onof describes a painter who used lead-based paints and eventually experienced flaccid paralysis in both legs and his right arm. After several days of hospitalization, the painter died, and an autopsy revealed the typical lesions of polio in the gray matter of his spinal cord.[95] Dr. Ralph Scobey also mentions a number of cases of polio-like paralysis caused by arsenic poisoning that he found in the 19th-century medical literature.[96]

The resemblance between paralysis due to synthetic toxins and polio paralysis has confused doctors for decades. Dr. Archibald Hoyne, the Chicago School of Medicine pediatrician, notes in a 1951 paper that lead poisoning is one of the diseases that doctors tend to misdiagnose as polio.[97] Dr. Andrew Braff, a US Navy physician, reports a case of lead poisoning in a soldier who worked as a welder and was exposed to lead, arsenic, and zinc fumes. The soldier suffered muscle weakness, paralysis of his legs and arms, and difficulty breathing.[98] He was diagnosed with polio and died two days after being hospitalized. An autopsy found polio-typical lesions in his spinal cord. In addition to the high level of lead found in his blood, a microscopic examination of brain and spinal cord tissue also pointed to lead poisoning as the cause of death. Although the year was 1952 and much knowledge had supposedly been accumulated about polio, doctors still found it difficult to distinguish between paralytic polio and nerve damage caused by lead poisoning. "Lead poisoning is easily confused with poliomyelitis of the bulbo-spinal type,"[99] Dr. Braff concludes.

The change in polio morbidity from a few cases a year to outbreaks of hundreds or more that began in the 1890s is consistent with the transition from the use of Paris green (which contained only arsenic) to lead arsenate (which was more popular and contained arsenic and lead) to control insects. In addition, lead arsenate had another feature that might have increased the risk of poisoning: It remained on the fruit longer (contributing to both its efficacy and its popularity among farmers). A study conducted in 1931 found that in particularly dry summers, apple orchards that were sprayed several weeks before the harvest season had particularly large amounts of lead arsenate remaining on the fruit.[p] Rinsing or brushing the fruit removed only about a third of the arsenic deposits.[100]

The search for a safer alternative to lead arsenate began as early as 1919, when it was discovered that the rinsing methods used at the time were incapable of removing the arsenic deposits from the fruit. Unfortunately, its potential substitutes either did not confer sufficient insect protection or were found to be even more toxic to plants and animals. Hence, the compound remained in widespread use until it was replaced by DDT following World War II.[101]

The use of lead arsenate for insect control was eventually banned by law in the United States in 1988. However, the top layer of soil in regions that were sprayed for many decades retains large amounts of arsenic to this day. In many regions of northern United States, residential neighborhoods were built on land that was formerly used to grow apples. Soil laced with lead arsenate still poses a serious danger to the health of those living in these neighborhoods.[102] Toxic amounts of arsenic have also been found in well water in many US regions. In Vermont, a hydrological survey conducted in 2010 ranked the various counties by the number of wells polluted with arsenic. Rutland County, the site of the first American "polio" epidemic, topped the list.[103]

---

[p] In the northeastern United States, rains are common in summertime. Rain falling after the last spraying of fruit trees and before the harvest could potentially remove much of the residual material left on the fruit. Incidentally, regarding the 1894 polio outbreak in Vermont, Caverly notes that the summer was particularly dry (p. 1).

Infectious Disease? Contagious Disease?

The supposition that polio is an Infectious and contagious disease – that is, it is caused by a living organism (typically a bacterium or virus) and is transmitted from person to person[q] – has not been in dispute in scientific circles for many decades. The institutional version of polio history has cast a thick layer of concrete around it, and any scientist daring enough to challenge it is likely to be ignored or mocked. The disease, as "everyone knows", is caused by the poliovirus – a highly contagious virus that enters the body through the mouth and is excreted in the feces. But is polio really an infectious and contagious disease? Delving into some of its early history suggests that the answer to this question is not nearly as straightforward or unequivocal as the official polio story would have us believe.

In the early 20th century, before the concrete was laid and the dogma established, doctors were much more reluctant to categorize polio as an infectious and contagious disease. They had, as we shall see, very good reasons for not doing so. Karl-Oskar Medin, the Swedish pediatrician who was the first to report a polio outbreak (Stockholm 1887), concluded that it was an infectious, but not contagious, disease.[104] Other Swedish doctors believed that the disease wasn't even caused by a bacterium or a virus, but rather by "miasma" (toxic fumes rising from decay), and that actions should be taken to improve sanitation and hygiene conditions in order to prevent it.[105] Leegaard, a Norwegian researcher, was not able to prove a single case of patient-to-patient contagion in a polio outbreak of 54 cases in Norway (1899). His conclusion: "Infantile paralysis is of an infectious, but not of a contagious nature."[106]

Putnam and Taylor, in reporting on the Boston-area polio

---

[q] Transmission of the disease's causative agent (pathogen) could be direct (through touch, cough, etc.) or indirect (for example, through a contaminated object).

outbreak of 1893, write that the cause of the disease is "perhaps bacterial in character", but they add that this view's "advocates are still far from having made good their claim."[107] Contrary to what is expected from "epidemic disease" (that is, infectious and contagious), the paralysis cases documented by the two "did not come to any extent, from any one locality, but from different parts of the large area of the suburbs of Boston."[108]

Three years later in Vermont, Caverly notes that no "infectious disease" has been found that could explain the 1894 outbreak and that "it is very certain that it was non-contagious." Caverly, who examined each and every one of the 132 cases of paralysis reported in Vermont, bases his determination on the fact that he found no "single instance in which more than one member of a family had the disease, [though] it usually occurred in families of more than one child, and [...] no efforts were made at isolation."[109] Occasional outbreaks of disease, he writes, suggest the existence of a specific "poison" or "toxin", but so far no progress has been made in isolating a particular microorganism to which the cases of paralysis can be attributed.[110] Emerson reinforces Caverly's views in his report of the 1908 Massachusetts polio epidemic: "With regards to the contagiousness of the disease, the investigation of this group of cases suggests that the disease is but mildly contagious to say the most. A large number of children were in intimate contact with those that were sick, and of these children an insignificant minority developed the disease."[111] Lovett, who studied the polio outbreak in Massachusetts one year earlier, found (out of 234 cases) only nine instances of illness under the same roof, eleven instances of illness in extended family members, and twenty instances of illness in acquaintances. "That is, in 40 cases (17%)," Lovett concludes, "there was reason to look into the question of contagion."[112]

Despite the paucity of evidence for direct person-to-person transmission or a disease-causing organism, Emerson and Lovett tend to believe that polio is indeed an infectious disease due to a distribution pattern similar to those of other infectious diseases.[113] Lovett stresses the disease's spread in accordance with transportation routes and its uneven distribution across the various settlements in Massachusetts; these, he claims, indicate the contagious nature of the disease.[114] (On this point he chooses to ignore the fact that the 234 polio cases in Massachusetts were spread among 90 different localities, averaging fewer than three cases per locality.)

The tendency of Lovett, Emerson, and their contemporaries to view polio as an infectious disease, despite the scarcity of supporting evidence, was presumably influenced by the prevailing conceptions of biology in the early 20th century. The groundbreaking work of Louis Pasteur, Robert Koch,[r] and others in the late 19th century put germ theory at the forefront of biological investigation and encouraged scientists and doctors to find links between disease conditions, especially any which occurred in epidemics, and specific causative organisms. A case in point is an article published in 1908 in the *American Journal of Medical Sciences* by Luther Emmet Holt and Frederic Bartlett, New York physicians. Holt and Bartlett reviewed every polio outbreak reported in the medical literature of the time, 35 in all, and paid special attention to reports of multiple morbidity in a single family. Out of the 1,400 polio cases reviewed,[s] only 40 instances of more than one patient in a family were found.[115] Focusing their analysis on those 40 instances and taking into account "the occurrence of epidemics", Holt and Bartlett conclude that polio is "beyond question" an infectious disease.[116] Regarding contagion, the two write that it is an "open question",

---

[r] Robert Koch identified and isolated the bacteria that cause anthrax, cholera, and tuberculosis. Louis Pasteur, the "father of microbiology", developed vaccines against anthrax and rabies.

[s] Only some of the reports included references to multiple morbidity within families. The number of 1,400 patients refers to these reports only.

although they "cannot resist the conclusion that the disease is communicable, although only to a very slight degree."[117]

Thus, despite the obvious inclination of some doctors and researchers reporting them, the early US polio outbreaks did not provide substantial evidence suggesting that it was a contagious disease. Its characterization as an infectious disease was also not based on solid evidence but rather on a distribution pattern that was somewhat reminiscent of distribution patterns of other diseases that happened to be infectious. If polio, like tetanus, is a non-contagious, infectious disease – that is, caused by a live organism but not transmitted from person to person – how was it able to spread far and wide? How could it make its appearance, for example, in a single year (1907) in 90 different communities in Massachusetts?

One plausible explanation is that the bacterium or virus "hitchhikes" with some physical carrier, such as luggage (which Lovett implies when he alludes to polio spreading along transportation routes). The prime suspect is, of course, food. The medical literature is replete with descriptions of mass morbidity as a result of consumption of poisoned food products.[118] The poison was sometimes a bacterium and other times a toxic chemical added to the food for various reasons, such as improving taste or prolonging shelf life. Outbreaks of paralysis due to poisoned food are also well documented. For instance, in 1900 a mysterious epidemic broke in the city of Manchester, England, which paralyzed thousands of people and killed several dozens. After long months of uncertainty, the cause of the disease was identified: high arsenic concentrations in the sulfuric acid used to process sugar in beer production at several of the area's breweries.[119] Ending the use of the toxic sulfuric acid stopped the outbreak in its tracks. Moreover, a subsequent inquiry revealed that the beer brewing process in central and northern England had been contaminating barley kernels with arsenic for decades (albeit at lower levels than those associated with the contaminated sulfuric acid during the 1900 Manchester epidemic). This long-term contamination apparently led to another paralytic disease known as *alcoholic neuritis*, dozens of cases of which were recorded each year in the northwest regions of England in the last third of the 19th century. For years doctors had mistakenly believed the disease was caused by high alcohol consumption, but once the arsenic was removed from the beer's production process, it vanished into thin air.[120]

A similar episode occurred in the central and southern parts of the United States in 1930, where about 50,000 people became paralyzed after drinking an alcoholic patent medicine called Jamaica Ginger. About ten days passed between beverage consumption and the onset of symptoms. As with polio, the paralysis, was caused by damage to the nerve cells in the anterior horns of the spinal cord. After an intensive investigation by law enforcement agencies, the cause of the epidemic was found: a toxic chemical called TOCP that was added to the beverage by one of the manufacturers in order to reduce production costs.[121]

It is clear, then, that disease distribution patterns of early polio outbreaks, with their meager evidence for direct person-to-person contagion, do not support the current view of polio as a contagious disease and also raise questions about its characterization as an infectious disease. These patterns aren't a problem, however, if we ascribe these early paralysis outbreaks in the US to the consumption of agricultural produce sprayed with lead and arsenic. The use of toxic pesticides in agriculture can explain morbidity in a limited or wide geographic area, as well as distribution along transportation routes. It can also accommodate any pattern of familial morbidity – isolated cases, multiple cases, or simultaneous occurrence – since symptom severity would be influenced by the level of exposure and the individual's specific sensitivity to the toxic substances consumed.

The Healthy Carrier: Wickman's Discovery

As we have seen, epidemiological analysis of early polio outbreaks indicates that paralytic polio was not contagious. In
addition, its categorization as infectious was primarily based on
speculation regarding its geographical distribution patterns
rather than on identification of a specific disease-causing organism. How was it, then, that polio was later declared to be both
infectious and contagious, caused by a virus? The medical
world's perceptual shift was largely based on the seminal work of
two researchers – Sweden's Ivar Wickman and Austria's Karl
Landsteiner – who provided the medical establishment with the
evidentiary hook on which polio's virus theory could be hung.

As previously noted, the physicians who reported the first
polio outbreaks failed to demonstrate human routes of contagion
for the vast majority of patients. This lack of evidence for disease
transmission was a considerable headache for polio epidemiologists: How could its distribution patterns be explained if people
weren't passing a virus or bacterium around – from patient to
patient, house to house, and community to community? The
path out of this quagmire was laid by Dr. Ivar Wickman, a
Swedish pediatrician and former student of Karl-Oskar Medin.
Wickman, an energetic and ambitious researcher,[122] studied the
distribution of polio during the epidemic that hit Sweden in
1905 in an effort to trace the chain of transmission.[123] Like his
predecessors, Wickman realized it was impossible to establish
direct links for most of the sick. In addition, about 80% of them
were from families with several children where only one child
had gotten sick, despite the fact that no special efforts appear to
have been made to isolate the patients (at least, Wickman makes
no mention of such efforts).[124] Unlike the seemingly indecisive
researchers before him who had focused on paralytic cases,
Wickman took a bold step forward: He assumed that non-

paralytic patients,[t] and even perfectly healthy people, carried polio's causative agent and could transmit it to others.[125]

Armed with this novel supposition, Wickman set out to map the potential links between patients in a number of Swedish communities that were involved in the 1905 epidemic. In the small and remote village of Trastena, where the first cases of the epidemic were discovered, he was able to link all 49 patients, most of them children, through the village school. As might be expected, most of the affected children attended the local school, or at least occasionally associated with a child who did. This arguably weak association was considered sufficient evidence by Wickman to infer polio transmission, even though most of the "bridge" individuals did not get sick themselves.[126] (Wickman, obviously, did not prove, nor did he have the scientific means to prove, that any person, healthy or sick, was in fact a carrier of the polio causative agent [which wasn't identified at the time, anyway]. Thus, he was unable to provide direct evidence to support the hypothetical transmission routes he describes in his writings.)[u]

Although Wickman's description of the dissemination of polio in the Swedish epidemic of 1905 was largely based on speculation and his theory failed to provide answers to fundamental questions about the epidemic (as will be shown below), in the "official" history of polio, Wickman is said to have "discovered" (or even "proved") that polio is indeed a contagious disease.[127] For this "discovery" he was posthumously inducted to

---

[t] A minority of patients during a polio outbreak experience a mild flu-like illness, with no symptoms of paralysis or permanent damage. This disease was considered a subcategory of polio and was usually referred to as abortive polio.

[u] Wickman typically links polio cases with statements such as "child X visited child Y after the latter became ill" or "person X, whose son contracted polio, worked in the household of family Y in which one of the children contracted polio". He does not provide any evidence that a contagion did occur, or that the potential encounters were sufficient to enable transmission.

the Polio Hall of Fame.[v]

As noted above, the innovative aspect of Wickman's work was largely his assumption that even healthy people could be infected with the polio organism and transmit it to other people. Past polio researchers, he notes, failed to trace transmission chains because they did not account for this fact.[128] But why had Caverly, Lovett, Emerson, and their colleagues, investigators of the first polio outbreaks, emphasized the conspicuous lack of evidence of direct person-to-person contagion? Why had they stressed the importance of finding a direct link between patients? The answer is that then-current knowledge of infectious and contagious diseases suggested that, for most of them, patients were the primary infective agents.[w] Neither Wickman nor his successors offer a persuasive explanation for polio's unique (supposed) ability to spread mainly through healthy people rather than sick people,[129] nor for the fact only a few out of hundreds or thousands of poliovirus carriers are paralyzed.

Wickman also does not provide any explanation for the fact that the 1905 epidemic attacked rural and isolated communities, where houses are relatively far apart, and spared the large and vastly denser urban centers. This fact conflicts with his allegation (seconded by other European colleagues mentioned in his book) that roads and railroads played a central role in spreading the disease.[130] If transportation routes were indeed the primary means of polio transmission, how could one explain the organism's preference for traveling desolate country roads from one remote village to another rather than the much more populous city routes? Why, during its rapid "movement" across Sweden in

---

[v] Wickman is just one of four Europeans who were inducted into the Polio Hall of Fame in Warm Springs, Georgia. The rest, thirteen in number, are Americans. Wickman's bronze bust is displayed right next to the one of his mentor, Karl-Oskar Medin.

[w] A notable exception are diseases spread by non-human carriers, malaria, for example, which is transmitted by mosquitoes.

the summer of 1905, did polio attack such isolated villages as Trastena (49 patients), and avoid large cities such as Malmo (zero patients), Gothenburg (zero patients), and Stockholm (a meager ten patients)?[131]

The institutional explanation for this phenomenon is that in cities, where the population density is higher, all the inhabitants – rich and poor, children and adults – were infected with the virus at a young age, and thus acquired immunity to the disease.[132] This, however, does not explain why morbidity in Sweden's large cities was practically nil, even though most of the population was supposed to be infected with the virus, while morbidity in rural population was substantially higher. It also crudely lumps all city residents together – luxury neighborhoods with slums – despite marked differences in living conditions. Like other important aspects of the institutional story of polio, this explanation seems little more than a "plausible" speculation, lacking any scientific basis, coarsely stitched together in an effort to close up large holes in the infectious-and-contagious theory. In any case, experience later demonstrated that the immunity supposedly gained from living in crowded urban centers didn't protect the residents of New York City during the great epidemics of 1907 and 1916 (nor those of numerous other cities in the first half of the 20th century), in which thousands of people died or became paralyzed.

Notwithstanding the notoriety Wickman's theory had garnered, many of his contemporaries did not accept his ideas. In a lecture at the 1926 conference of the American Medical Association, Dr. Lloyd Aycock of the Department of Preventive Medicine and Hygiene at Harvard Medical School spoke on the epidemiology of polio and its means of distribution. In his remarks, Aycock points out that the perception, derived from Wickman's theory, that greater dissemination of poliovirus in cities, compared to rural areas, leads to higher immunity to the disease and not to higher morbidity contradicts what is known about common infectious diseases.[133] He adds that "there is no theoretical reason why persons in rural life should be more prone to exhibit the paralytic form of the disease."[134]

Aycock also emphasizes the lack of evidence for direct contagion among polio patients (thus confirming the reports of Caverly and others from the early polio outbreaks). In a study conducted the year before (1925), he found that only 5% of affected families reported more than one polio patient. If one deducts from this number, he adds, the cases which broke simultaneously (indicating a common source rather than patient-to-patient transmission), only a "small figure" of cases remains for which direct contagion can even be considered.[135] These remarks were approved by several physicians present.[136] In addition, Hoyne notes in 1951 that isolating patients or maintaining strict hygiene in handling their secretions was not required to prevent disease transmission. During the 35 years Hoyne worked in infectious disease wards of Chicago hospitals, no doctor, nurse, staff member, or hospitalized non-polio patient was ever infected with polio.[137]

Thus, Wickman's theory of polio's spread does not adequately explain its nationwide distribution in the 1905 Swedish epidemic. But how does it fare in establishing the chain of transmission within communities? Wickman's assumption that healthy people can transmit the disease allowed virtually unlimited possibilities for tracing a theoretical chain of contagion between cases. In every village there are common institutions – a school, a shop, a church – where adults and children meet, and may, ostensibly, spread the poliovirus. But even with the help of this mitigating assumption, Wickman was unable to tie all the cases together in the communities he examined. In one of them, he failed to find a possible contagion link for 6 of the 18 children who fell ill.[138] In another outbreak in an island community, he was able to link all 16 patients but found no plausible explanation for how the disease had reached the island in the first place.[139] Wickman was not alone, it seems. He mentions at least three other European polio epidemics for which researchers, despite their best efforts, had been unable to link cases, even though they had included healthy people as potential carriers of the virus.[140]

The disparity between Wickman's "discovery" of the contagious nature of polio and the reality of the early epidemics continued to bother researchers for years. Caverly, for one, although well aware of Wickman's ideas, continued to characterize polio as a "mildly contagious" disease, well into the second decade of the 20th century.[141] Aycock, who also had extensive research experience and a special interest in the way the disease was spread, writes that there is substantial evidence that polio is also transmitted by non-human routes. As an example, he cites Knapp's 1925 report, mentioned earlier, of a polio outbreak apparently spread through milk.[142]

The fact that Aycock refers to milk as a transmission medium is particularly interesting in light of Wickman's own report of a similar case: In one of the villages he studied in 1905, ten polio cases were recorded in six families who lived about a mile apart. In five of these cases the disease broke out on the same day. Wickman found that all families had consumed milk from the same farmer and notes: "Under these circumstances it seems to me extremely probable that the milk conveyed the infection."[143] Could that farmer's milk have contained some toxic substance, to which the cows were exposed, which caused the paralysis? Was that specific substance used by other farmers in that village, and in other villages where the paralytic disease broke out? Wickman did not follow this potential line of investigation, and these questions are likely to remain unanswered forever.

Landsteiner's Virus

At the same time that Wickman was gathering evidence allegedly indicating that polio was a contagious disease, Karl

Landsteiner[x] was toiling in his laboratory in Vienna attempting to prove that it was an infectious disease. In a late-1908 experiment, he and colleague Erwin Popper took the spinal cord of a nine year-old boy who had died days before from polio and ground, filtered, and injected it into various laboratory animals. After failing to paralyze mice, guinea pigs, or rabbits, they finally found success with monkeys. The two injected the solution into the abdominal cavity of two monkeys; one of them, a rhesus monkey, became paralyzed in both legs. Post-mortem evaluations of the monkeys revealed the typical human polio lesions in their spinal cords.[144]

The news about Landsteiner and Popper's groundbreaking experiments quickly took off. For the first time, researchers were able to "isolate" polio's causative organism in their laboratory.[145] Moreover, since the spinal cord taken from the deceased child was filtered through a special filter that was believed to remove bacteria, the two determined that the organism must be a virus. The experiment was replicated within a few months by other researchers around the world, some of which even managed to pass the "virus" from monkey to monkey (something that Landsteiner and Popper had not managed to do[146]). These researchers injected the ground and filtered spinal cord of a person who had died of polio into the brain of a monkey, which later became paralyzed. The spinal cord of that monkey was ground, filtered, and injected into the brain of another monkey who also became paralyzed, and so on.[147] Henceforth, "polioviruses" were supposedly grown in research laboratories for decades, passed from monkey to monkey dozens and hundreds of times, using the procedure described above. Most lab studies from 1910 to the early 1950s used rhesus monkeys, which were injected with what researchers assumed was poliovirus grown in laboratories (i.e., the ground and filtered spinal cord of laboratory monkeys suffering from polio-like paralysis). Thus, polio research sparked

---

[x] Karl Landsteiner was a renowned biologist who first identified the blood groups. For his work in this field he won the Nobel Prize in Medicine in 1930.

a new industry of supplying monkeys to research labs. It is estimated that more than 100,000 monkeys were sacrificed during this period.[148] For the most part, this endeavor was founded on the supposed "isolation" of the virus by Landsteiner, who, for this contribution, was also inducted to the Polio Hall of Fame.[149]

The institutional story of polio regards the work of Landsteiner and Popper, and the researchers who followed in their footsteps, as conclusive proof that polio is an infectious disease caused by a virus. But what exactly did these scientists isolate, and to what extent did they manage to reproduce human polio in laboratory monkeys?

As noted above, the substance injected into lab animals was not purified virus, but rather a portion of spinal cord taken from a person who had died from a paralytic polio-like illness, which was then ground and filtered using a Berkefeld filter, the standard method of that time. In retrospect, it is impossible to know how pure the injected solutions were or to what extent they contained viruses, bacteria, or residual toxic chemicals that managed to pass through the filter. Furthermore, if the solution did contain some virus that caused paralysis in monkeys, how could we know that it was the poliovirus alone, another virus altogether, or possibly even several viruses at once? Because reliable techniques for identifying viruses were not yet available, scientists in the first half of the 20th century had no answers to these questions.

Successful induction of flaccid paralysis in laboratory animals was not unique to polio research. Robert Lovett, for example, describes a number of studies in which researchers injected bacteria, and even pollen, into dogs and rabbits, resulting in polio-like paralysis and the characteristic injury to the spinal cord.[150] At the same time, most attempts to induce paralysis in animals by "infecting" them with the "poliovirus" were unsuccessful. Those included guinea pigs, rabbits, mice, rats, cats, dogs, goats, pigs, cows, and horses.[151]

Another difficulty for early polio researchers was the way laboratory monkeys were "infected". The poliovirus is assumed to enter the human body by mouth, but virtually all attempts to infect monkeys in the natural way failed. Scientists fed them a variety of bodily fluids obtained from human polio patients – saliva, sneeze droplets, throat swabs – but were almost never able to paralyze them. Attempts to induce paralysis in monkeys by injecting the spinal fluid of polio patients (rather than the ground cord) into their brains also failed[152] (although the virus should have been present in the spinal fluid; its presence there serves as one way to diagnose the disease).[153] The only reliable way to paralyze monkeys in the lab was to inject the spinal cord solution of a polio patient directly into their bodies, usually in the abdominal cavity (as Landsteiner did) or the brain (as did most subsequent researchers). Moreover, even this method worked only in a small number of species, mainly rhesus monkeys.[154] And even after becoming paralyzed, the monkeys were unexpectedly not contagious. Milton Rosenau, professor of preventive medicine and hygiene at Harvard, notes (1918) that "monkeys have so far never been known to contract the disease spontaneously, even though they are kept in intimate association with infected monkeys."[155] John Toomey, a veteran polio researcher, reinforces this observation (1941): "no animal gets the disease from another, no matter how intimately exposed."[156]

Another important distinction between the behavior of the "virus" in the lab and in the real world stemmed from the apparent contradiction between Wickman's theory and Landsteiner's experiments. Wickman argued that the poliovirus was spread mainly by healthy people, and that only a fraction of those infected would proceed to develop the paralytic disease. But in the experimental model constructed by Landsteiner and his successors, it was assumed that injecting the virus directly into the monkey's body would paralyze it (indeed, the rate of rhesus monkeys paralyzed with this procedure was quite high). In those cases where the monkey wasn't paralyzed, it was taken to mean that the injected compound did not contain the poliovirus or that the virus was inactive (e.g., neutralized by the animal's antibodies). This conflicts with both Wickman's theory and the current official story of polio, which assert that the poliovirus, even after infecting the gut or the bloodstream, only induces paralysis in a small minority of individuals.

This accepted technique of injecting substances into monkeys as a means to "isolate the poliovirus" led to a series of experiments that, in retrospect, seem quite bizarre. John Paul and colleagues (1940), for example, used it to prove that the poliovirus could be found in sewage. During a US epidemic they collected samples from sewage pipes located in the vicinity of hospitals that treated polio patients, and injected the smelly stuff directly into the brains of rhesus monkeys. Some of the monkeys came down with "laboratory polio", and an autopsy found the typical lesions in their spinal cord. Although some of the samples collected from sewers in different cities during epidemics did not paralyze the monkeys, the researchers determined that the samples that did indicate that the poliovirus is transmitted through sewage systems.[157] Two years later (1942) Kling and colleagues conducted a similar experiment during a polio outbreak in Stockholm.[158] They collected samples from a sewer pipe that served a district of about 100,000 residents in which only twelve cases of polio were recorded that year. In addition, the researchers took only six liters of samples (1.5 gallons) from a sewage system through which about twenty million liters (5.2 million gallons) flowed every day.[159] The samples collected were kept in the refrigerator for about two months and then injected into the abdomen and brain of rhesus monkeys. The polio-like paralysis the monkeys developed and the autopsy findings convinced the researchers they had succeeded in "isolating the virus of poliomyelitis in [the] sample of sewage collected",[160] and they declare with confidence that the sewer is a "vehicle" for polio transmission.[161]

Similarly, Trask (1940)[162] and Horstmann (1944)[163] "proved" that the feces of polio patients contained poliovirus by injecting fecal samples into monkeys' abdominal cavities, brains, and spines. Sabin (1941) "isolated" the poliovirus from flies by injecting monkeys with a solution that included about 500 ground flies retrieved from a Cleveland neighborhood where a number of polio cases were reported.[164] Sabin states emphatically that "the distinctly positive results which we obtained with collections of insects consisting only of flies, leaves no doubt that they are carriers of the virus,"[165] although the solution paralyzed only cynomolgus monkeys, but not the standard rhesus monkeys.[166] Trask (1943) scattered flytraps near the homes of polio patients and injected the dead flies into lab monkeys. In this experiment, too, only the cynomolgus and not the rhesus monkeys were paralyzed.[167]

The most bizarre experiment of this group, it seems, was conducted by Ward and colleagues.[168] The researchers were attempting to determine whether the poliovirus could also be transmitted via food contaminated by flies. They placed food near the homes of polio patients in North Carolina in the summer of 1944 so that it would be accessible to flies. The food, which the flies left their distinct marks on, was flown to a laboratory where it was eaten in part by two chimpanzees. The chimpanzees themselves were barely affected by eating the contaminated food – one of them had a slightly elevated temperature – but when their feces were injected into rhesus monkeys, about a third of those were paralyzed. "Poliomyelitis virus," Ward and colleagues conclude, "has been detected in food exposed to flies at homes of poliomyelitis patients within an epidemic area."[169]

In all of these experiments, and in many similar ones conducted in the first half of the 20th century, the specific agent (or agents) that actually induced paralysis in laboratory animals was never isolated. These experiments did not prove that the poliovirus was present in the sewage samples, in the carcasses of flies in polio-stricken areas, or in human feces, nor did they prove that the virus caused the monkeys' paralysis. The virus was never actually isolated in any of them.

Furthermore, the relevance of these laboratory experiments in monkeys to natural polio morbidity in humans has never been established. This fact did not go unnoticed by some contemporary polio investigators: "Most of the experiments described during this period," Toomey wrote in 1941, "have been made in animals given the disease by [...] artificial avenue of approach. If the virus enters the human being by way of the gastrointestinal tract, practically all [these experiments] have to be discarded in toto."[170] Lumsden notes that the results of the monkey experiments contradict the epidemiological findings: "The views as to the [virus] portal of entry and communicability rest fundamentally and entirely on findings from experiments on monkeys. To some of us it does not appear to square with the facts obtained by epidemiological studies of the disease among human beings. It seems too elastic, too restful. On epidemiological grounds alone, it appears conceivable that poliomyelitis is not caused by a living microorganism or a virus, but by a toxin."[171] Smith and colleagues add in 1945: "In spite of the comparative ease with which poliomyelitis may be experimentally transferred to monkeys [...], it has not been established that the virus in such form gives rise to the human disease. The possibility undoubtedly exists, but direct proof is still lacking."[172]

Even today, more than sixty years after these words were written, "direct proof" of that "possibility" is still lacking.

Although Landsteiner and his successors were never able to reconstruct polio's purported mode of transmission in their lab and hadn't really isolated the poliovirus, these experiments provide solid proof that polio is an infectious disease according to the institutional story. Thus, despite the lack of direct and sufficient evidence from Wickman on the one hand and Landsteiner on the other, the virus theory of polio was established, and it determined the path for the next hundred years of research on the disease.

Polio in Domestic Animals

As mentioned above, most of the attempts to infect lab animals of different species with polio were unsuccessful. Even for those animal species that did exhibit a polio-like disease, the "infection" could hardly be called natural. The "virus" had to be artificially injected into the abdominal cavity or brain in order for the animals to come down with paralysis. The outcomes of these experiments, which were consistent from researcher to researcher, led scientists to believe that polio was unique to humans, that is, it doesn't naturally exist in animals.[173] This perception may have been the reason that science ignored a remarkable phenomenon frequently mentioned in reports of the early outbreaks: Domestic animals were frequently paralyzed at the same time humans were struck by "polio".

Paralysis in farm animals was reported as early as the first major outbreak on US soil. In his report of the outbreak in Vermont in the summer of 1894, Dr. Charles Caverly notes that "During this epidemic and in the same geographical area, an acute nervous disease, paralytic in its nature, affected domestic animals. Horses, dogs and fowls died with these symptoms."[174] A pathological examination of a horse that died subsequent to paralysis of its hind legs found spinal cord lesions typical of polio. A pathological examination of a fowl with paralyzed legs and wings revealed findings of "acute poliomyelitis of the lumbar portion of the cord."[175] "That domestic animals suffered with human beings in our epidemic," Caverly adds, "is a noteworthy fact and one, so far as I can learn, hitherto unobserved. That such was the case cannot be doubted."[176] Caverly, who served on Vermont's board of health for another 24 years following the 1894 outbreak, also reports paralysis in farm animals during polio outbreaks in the state in 1910 (calves and pigs)[177] and 1914 (cows, chickens, dogs, and pigs).[178] He concludes: "Instances of paralysis among domestic animals have always been noted as accompanying our outbreaks of human infantile paralysis."[179]

Dr. Robert Lovett, who authored reports on polio outbreaks in Massachusetts, also mentions instances of paralysis in farm animals. In his report of the 1908 outbreak, he mentions a mother and daughter who contracted polio "shortly after an epidemic of 'leg weakness' in the chickens of the household."[180]

Two years later in a report on the 1910 outbreak, Lovett notes that out of 110 families affected by polio who kept farm animals "34 [families] had illness, paralysis or death in 82 animals near the time of the human paralysis."[181]

In their voluminous 1914 book on polio, Frauenthal and Manning devote several pages to morbidity of pets and farm animals that occurred in parallel with the disease in humans. In addition to Caverly and Lovett's reports reviewed above, they mention 15 other polio outbreaks – in the US, Sweden, England, and Brazil – that also involved paralysis of domestic animals. Among the animals affected were horses, cows, chickens, cats, dogs, pigs, and sheep.[182] For example, during a 1909 polio outbreak in Minnesota, Dr. Hill, the state's chief epidemiologist, described a paralytic illness in three colts that was "strongly analogous in clinical history and symptoms to the disease in the human."[183] Dr. Shore, the veterinarian who treated these colts, writes, "In my veterinary practice of the past five or six years I have found a disease appearing among one- or two- year-old colts that shows a line of symptoms corresponding closely to anterior poliomyelitis in children. I have had from 5 to 10 cases a year during this time, always occurring during the summer months, and the majority of them during the month of August. The affected colts are usually found in the pasture unable to stand."[184]

In California, Frauenthal and Manning write, there were 100 cases of polio in humans in 1910, most of them in San Joaquin County. At the same time, according to a California State Board of Health bulletin, there were numerous reports from veterinarians describing "a considerable number of puzzling paralyses of colts in San Joaquin County."[185] A report of a polio outbreak in Iowa in 1910–1911 describes a large number of cases of paralysis in chickens concurrent with paralytic disease in humans. In a pathological examination of the spinal cord of a fowl with paralysis in two legs and one wing, "The histological picture was that of acute poliomyelitis in man."[186]

Even Wickman himself reports that in the polio outbreak in

Sweden (1903) there were many cases of dogs being paralyzed along with children.[187] In his 1913 book he notes that he and others reported simultaneous morbidity in animals and humans but that "the futile inoculation of [animals] shows their affliction has nothing in common with that in man."[188] With a flick of his pen, Wickman dismisses abundant evidence of both simultaneous paralysis in animals and humans and the striking resemblance between them, even though he could not provide any alternative explanation for this phenomenon.

Wickman's commitment, and that of his fellow researchers, to the suppositions that the poliovirus is the sole cause of polio and that the disease is unique to humans induced them to dismiss the relevance of the simultaneous onset of paralytic disease in humans and domestic animals and regard it as mere coincidence.[y] This was not the first time in the history of science, nor the last, that rigid adherence to scientific dogma led researchers to completely ignore a significant body of evidence that was inconsistent with their current beliefs.

Thus, because the institutional story of polio holds that the disease is caused by a virus and attempts to "infect" animals with the virus failed, the disease in its natural form must exist only in humans. Therefore, paralytic disease in domestic animals, even if it appears simultaneously with human polio and exhibits identical symptoms, must be purely coincidental and of no scientific significance.

Could there be a better explanation for the co-occurrence of animal and human outbreaks of paralysis than the dismissive (and illogical) "coincidence"? Was there, perhaps, a common

---

[y] Contributing to this was a study by a researcher named Carl Ten-Broeck (1914) who tried to infect laboratory monkeys by injecting into their brains the spinal cord (or other parts of the body) of a number of domestic animals – some healthy, some sick with various diseases, and some paralyzed. Tan-Brock failed to induce paralysis in monkeys, but his experiments did not really examine the relationships between paralytic morbidity in humans and animals: None of the animals he used had polio-like paralysis and only one or two were paralyzed in close temporal proximity to a polio outbreak.

causative agent to which both animals and humans were simultaneously exposed?

The alternative theory we presented earlier – the use of toxic pesticides, which became common in the late-19th century – is one such explanation. The use of insecticides such as Paris green and lead arsenate exposed humans to toxic residues through the processing and consumption of sprayed fruits and vegetables. Similarly, pets and farm animals were also exposed to these compounds in the field, orchard, and yard. If pesticides caused polio-like paralysis in humans, it's reasonable to assume they could cause similar illness in animals.

Unfortunately, this important line of inquiry has hardly been investigated. Were the outbreaks of polio-like paralytic disease reported in domestic animals in the early 20th century a new and unique phenomenon, or were such events previously documented in the medical literature? Have similar cases of unexplained paralysis in animals been reported in the absence of nearby polio outbreaks? Was there a common environmental denominator between paralyzed domestic animals and humans in polio outbreaks? Had researchers tried to answer these questions, polio's mysteries might have been solved a century ago.

Polio and Pesticides

In retrospect, clues connecting the emergence of polio in the US in the late-19th century to the increasing use of toxic pesticides in agriculture have been there since the beginning. Epidemics peaked during the harvest season, rural areas were most affected in the early days, simultaneous outbreaks of polio-like paralysis occurred in domestic animals and humans, lead and arsenic were known to cause paralysis – all these facts point to the same suspects: lead arsenate and Paris green. How, then, can one explain the complete disregard of this line of investigation by the doctors and researchers of the era?

An answer to this question is indirectly provided by the historian James Whorton, who researched the history of pesticide use in agriculture in the United States before World War II.[189] In his book, Whorton, who scoured FDA archives, describes how the authorities initially ignored, and then actively hid, the health dangers of consuming food sprayed with the toxic chemicals routinely used by US farmers.

In an 1861 speech to medical students at Harvard University, Dr. Oliver Wendell Holmes, the renowned physician and author, illustrated the irrationality of prescribing drugs with toxic ingredients by noting that "The farmer would be laughed at who undertook to manure his fields or his trees with a salt of lead or arsenic."[190] Less than six years passed before an unnamed Colorado farmer dusted his potato plants with Paris green powder and initiated a new era in agriculture. Because they killed insects so effectively, American farmers embraced the new synthetic pesticides quickly and enthusiastically. As far as safety was concerned, farmers took the manufacturers' assurance that the compounds were completely safe to use at face value. Although acute pesticide poisoning has indeed been rare, and was most often due to careless handling, the health impact of sustained consumption of arsenic and lead residues was never investigated by anyone. This was, in part, because in the 19th century United States no government body was responsible yet for monitoring food quality and safety.[191]

It was not until 1906, with the enactment of the Food and Drugs Act, that the Bureau of Chemistry was authorized by the US Department of Agriculture to oversee agricultural sprays. The primary mission of the Department of Agriculture was to support the farming sector and help it increase its productivity. Thus, it is no wonder that the studies conducted by Bureau of Chemistry researchers, as well as those conducted by entomologists (insect researchers) at agricultural experimental stations, focused on farmers' needs, and not on consumer health. The calculations made by these researchers regarding the safety of the consumption of sprayed fruits and vegetables relied on optimistic and unrealistic assumptions regarding the spraying practices actually implemented by farmers.[z] Worse, the researchers didn't even consider the potential health risks to consumers from constant exposure to tiny amounts of arsenic and lead.[192] The chief entomologist of the US Department of Agriculture exemplified this disregard in 1892 by emphatically noting "how utterly groundless are any fears of injury from sprayed produce."[193]

Overseas, the scientific establishment and the authorities took a more cautious approach. Following the previously mentioned paralysis outbreak in Manchester in 1900 caused by high arsenic concentrations in beer, British authorities appointed a royal commission to investigate the dangers of arsenic in food.[194] The committee, which consisted of prominent scientists and doctors, recommended a maximum threshold that severely limited the amount of arsenic allowed in food and beverages.[195] The committee's recommendation became a de facto standard in Britain and was adopted by other countries as well (but not the United States).[196] In Germany, the Imperial Health Commission opposed the use of lead arsenate, and the compound was prohibited from use in agriculture for a while. Other arsenic-based pesticides were allowed, but only under close supervision, as was customary in other European countries.[197] In France, laws were enacted in 1846 and 1916 prohibiting the use of arsenic as an agricultural insecticide, and the dangers of arsenic were often debated in academia.[198] Although these laws did not effectively prevent French farmers from using arsenic-based insecticides, the situation was considered superior to that of the United States, where no effort was made to restrict agricultural application of arsenic.[199] Unlike their French counterparts, English farmers were in no hurry to use arsenic-based compounds, despite repeated attempts to persuade them to do so.[200] Incidentally, polio morbidity in the UK remained very low (compared to the United States) during the first half of the 20th

---

[z] The farmer in the field often deviated from the official recommendations that specified the number of annual sprayings allowed, the interval between last spraying and harvesting, and so forth.

century and soared only after World War II, when DDT replaced arsenic and lead-based pesticides in industrialized
countries.[201]

Although the amount of spray residue left on fruit marketed
to American consumers steadily increased from the end of the
19th century onward,[202] federal authorities made no effort in the
early 20th century to control or limit the amount of arsenic or
lead in agricultural produce.[203] It was only in the 1920s that the
Bureau of Chemistry at the US Department of Agriculture began
testing arsenic levels in fruit and vegetable shipments. The high
levels found in some of the shipments led the Bureau to set, for
the first time, maximum thresholds allowed for arsenic in agricultural produce. At the same time, the Bureau collaborated with
farmers' organizations in advocacy and persuasion efforts to get
growers to restrict the use of pesticides. Unfortunately, the
inherent conflict of interest between the Bureau of Chemistry's
role (overseeing the use of pesticides in agriculture) and its
Department's stated mission (promoting agriculture) limited the
Bureau's actions and hampered its ability to enforce its own
recommendations.[204] Attempts to impose maximum thresholds
for lead and arsenic content in fruit met, as expected, with fierce
opposition from farmer organizations and elected officials who
acted on their behalf.[205] This state of affairs lasted until 1940,
when the Bureau of Chemistry, now known as the FDA, escaped
the authority of the Department of Agriculture and became an
independent agency.[206]

Knowledge of the intensive use of arsenic and lead-based pesticides in agriculture was confined to the agricultural sector and
its scientists for many years. The growers and their representatives had no wish to disclose to the public that the produce it
consumed was sprayed with toxic pesticides, compounds whose
deadly effects on humans were already widely known. As noted
earlier, the handful of studies examining the amount of arsenic
and lead deposits in fruit were conducted by researchers from
the agricultural sector, and their results, if they were ever published, appeared exclusively in agricultural journals. Even in the

1920s, when the Bureau of Chemistry began its attempts to enforce maximum thresholds for these toxins in fruit,[aa] all involved parties colluded in concealing from the public the fact that agricultural produce was sprayed with toxic compounds in concentrations greater than the thresholds set by the regulator.[207] American growers' associations also went out of their way to suppress occasional international scandals caused by apple exports to Europe. In Britain, for example, sanctions were imposed in 1925 against American apples sprayed with arsenic.[208] In Czechoslovakia and Austria in 1931, newspapers warned the public against eating American apples, and in Poland the import of US apples was completely banned.[209] Years later, an FDA executive admitted that the agency's goal was "to persuade all departmental agencies to cooperate in working out the [spray residue] problem and to refrain meanwhile from creating public alarm."[210] This concealment policy lasted until the mid-1930s and ceased, to the dismay of the agricultural sector, only when muckraking journalists unveiled the truth to the public.[211]

In view of the systemic cover-up operation by federal authorities and the agricultural sector, it isn't surprising that doctors failed to link the outbreaks of paralysis to the growing use of pesticides. Arsenic and lead poisoning had numerous and varied symptoms. A doctor was unlikely to diagnose either condition, and all the more unlikely to trace it back to consumption of specific food[212] (doctors testifying on behalf of the FDA attested to this in court in the late 1920s).[213] Over the years, agricultural application of lead arsenate intensified, adding to the dyes, drugs, household pesticides, and coal vapors that exposed the population to the toxic effects of arsenic and lead. As a result, Whorton notes, the environment in the first third of the 20th century became so saturated with arsenic and lead that "all members of industrialized populations carried at least traces of the metals in

---

[aa] The threshold the Bureau of Chemistry tried to promote in the mid-1920s was 3–4 times higher than the British one (Whorton 1974, p. 79 [p. 140 in the book]).

their tissues." This, in turn, led to "some serious scientific consideration being given the notion that these were normal physiological constituents."[214] Thus, even if arsenic or lead were found in a paralytic patient's tests, this was not considered abnormal and unlikely to catch the attention of a contemporary physician or polio researcher.

Over time, as the virus theory of polio gained prominence, it became even less likely that any scientist would associate a case of flaccid paralysis with lead or arsenic poisoning. As we've seen, Wickman and Landsteiner's semi-speculative publications laid the scientific foundation for polio's virus theory. In the United States, Dr. Simon Flexner, a renowned researcher at the Rockefeller Institute of Medical Research in New York, expanded and elaborated on Landsteiner's initial findings in a series of experiments on monkeys in 1909–1910. Flexner, a vocal and staunch supporter of the unorthodox notion that the poliovirus induces paralysis by entering the body through the nasal passages, made a crucial contribution to the establishment of polio's virus theory in American science circles. By the time the veil concealing the dangers of toxic pesticides was lifted in the 1930s and papers demonstrating pesticides' harms began appearing in medical journals, the virus theory of polio was already well established. Thus, the odds that a scientist or a doctor would look for or recognize a link between lead arsenate and paralytic polio was quite slim. A polio researcher who went against the established dogma was liable to be sharply criticized by his peers and ignored by the National Foundation for Infantile Paralysis, which in those days sponsored virtually all polio research. Moreover, this hypothetical maverick researcher would likely have been the object of brutal attacks by the agricultural lobby and the big pesticide-producing chemical companies.[bb]

Although the code of silence on the harms of pesticides was

[bb] A similar attack was mounted against Dr. James Putnam and his colleagues, the Boston doctors who in the late-19th century put forth the health harms of the domestic use of Paris green. (Whorton 1974, pp. 58–59).

broken in the 1930s and the FDA became an independent agency several years later, the government did not conduct a thorough and comprehensive study of the use of toxic substances in the food production process until 1950.[215] The use of lead arsenate declined only after World War II, when it was replaced by a new generation of pesticides.[216]

Polio Outbreak Patterns: Four More Mysteries

The official story of "the victory of science over the dreaded polio" creates the impression that the disease is well understood by science. Polio's cause, diagnosis, course, and means of prevention – all have been thoroughly researched and explicated by the men and women in the white coats. In fact, even today, more than a hundred years after Wickman and Landsteiner, polio science contains many more question marks than exclamation marks.

The peculiar outbreak patterns of polio posed a unique challenge to researchers. Polio epidemiologists had difficulty explaining, for example, why the disease broke out mainly in the summer and early autumn months,[cc] even though this pattern of morbidity was identified as early as the beginning of the 20th century.[217] Sabin writes (1951) that this is "one of the important unsolved problems in poliomyelitis."[218] John Paul (1952) labels it "mysterious".[219] Nathanson (1979) acknowledges that morbidity in peak months (August–September) is 35 times higher than in the low month (April), but he also has no explanation for the phenomenon. He writes, "The regularity of this pattern over many years suggested that it was governed by a mechanism which should be ascertainable. Nevertheless, the underlying explanation has remained elusive."[220] Thirty-one years later (2010), in a review of the current state of the epidemiology of polio, Nathanson still cannot offer a viable evidence-based

---

[cc] Most cases of polio were recorded in the months of July–September in the northern hemisphere, and January–March in the southern hemisphere.

explanation for the seasonality the disease, but only a "speculative hypothesis".[221]

The increased morbidity in the summer and fall months also raises concerns about the characterization of polio as an infectious and contagious disease. "It is remarkable," Sabin writes in 1947, "that, unlike certain other infections of childhood, the epidemics of paralysis occur during the very months when the children are away from school."[222] Sabin refers to the fact that infectious diseases usually proliferated under conditions of overcrowding, for example, when children are kept together all day in classrooms. But polio's peak morbidity was usually recorded during the summer holiday, when children were out of school.[223] Polio research has never explained this striking deviation from the usual outbreak patterns of infectious diseases in children.

In addition, the majority of cases in the early outbreaks occurred in the less densely populated rural areas, rather than the more crowded urban centers. The Swedish polio epidemic of 1905, reported by Wickman, being a notable example.

Another mystery concerned the irregular timing of polio epidemics. "No good explanation was ever documented for the occurrence of epidemics, although this was one of the most feared features of poliomyelitis and of particular concern to health officers," Nathanson writes in 1979.[224] Sabin, who also struggled with this issue, notes that the morbidity rate in "epidemic years" in the cities of London, Berlin and New York was 10, 20, and 46 times higher (respectively) than the average morbidity in "normal" years.[225] A similar cyclical pattern of morbidity, with a spike occurring every few years, characterizes other childhood infectious diseases. This cycle is due to the yearly increase in the number of young children who haven't been ill in the past and have not yet developed immunity to the disease. These young children get sick in large numbers in the "peak year" and proceed to develop immunity. Thus, between one peak year and another, morbidity drops and is distributed more evenly across ages, rather than concentrated in the very young. But this well-known mechanism is not applicable to polio, Sabin asserts, because in this disease "the age incidence was not found to vary materially from year to year, even during epidemics [...]"[226] Frustrated by the lack of a satisfactory explanation for the irregularity of polio morbidity,[dd] yet another mystery presented to him by the disease, Sabin writes: "The conclusion seems inescapable that poliomyelitis epidemics are the result of the invasion of a community by strains of unusual virulence."[227] Regarding this hypothesis, for which Sabin does not provide any evidence, Nathanson writes 28 years later that no research effort has been made to test it systematically, and therefore it is not possible to determine whether there was a link between virus intensity and the increased polio incidence in epidemic years.[228] Thus, this scientific riddle has also remained unanswered.

Another theoretical challenge for researchers was the emergence of polio at a time when other infectious diseases were on the decline. The improvement in nutrition, hygiene, and sanitation in the late-19th and early-20th centuries took the edge off most infectious diseases, but not polio, which rather intensified and became widespread during this period.[229] What was so special about polio that its incidence increased significantly at the same time incidence of most other infectious diseases was dropping dramatically? The Improved Hygiene theory, which was proposed to explain the sudden rise of polio in late-19th century, is not only factually incorrect (as demonstrated earlier) it also doesn't adequately explain the wide disparity between polio and most infectious diseases. Why does an upgrade of living standards lead to reductions in morbidity and mortality from diseases such as whooping cough, diphtheria, and measles but do the opposite for polio?

If one examines the unsolved mysteries of polio in light of

[dd] Toward the end of this 1951 paper Sabin expresses his frustration by quoting Freud (also quoted earlier in the chapter): "Even lectures I have given up, in order not to be forced to tell something that I only hope to learn some day."

pesticide poisoning, the pieces of the puzzle start to fall in their place. According to this hypothesis, polio first appeared in epidemic form in the late-19th century in parallel with the beginning of the intensive use of agricultural sprays in Western countries. The use of these toxic compounds increased in the 20th century, and so did polio incidence and distribution. The peak morbidity in the summer and autumn months occurred when fruits and vegetables were heavily consumed (and sprayed intensively to protect them from pests) in the temperate regions of the northern hemisphere. If polio were caused by toxic exposure rather than a bacterium or virus, the population density – whether at school or in the neighborhood – would have no effect on its incidence. This would also explain the fact that the age distribution didn't change in peak years, as noted by Sabin, which is atypical of childhood infectious diseases.

Unexplained Surge: Polio Post-WWII

After the turn of the 20th century, polio grew more common, with periodic epidemics a routine part of summer.[230] Until the mid-1940s, the annual morbidity was relatively low, with an epidemic striking every few years. This pattern changed abruptly in the late-1940s, with increased incidence and epidemics appearing every year.[231]

The marked rise in polio morbidity toward the end of the 1940s was not limited to the United States. In England the number of cases leaped in 1947 and maintained its high level for about 10 years.[232] In Germany, South Africa, Japan, Czechoslovakia, and the Netherlands the first polio epidemics weren't recorded until the 1940s. In France, Belgium, and large parts of the Soviet Union, the first epidemics weren't recorded until the 1950s.[233] A similar pattern was observed in Israel as well, with a sharp rise in morbidity in 1949: "...the disease suddenly [occurred] in high numbers," writes Professor Tiberio Swartz, "and [continued] in an uninterrupted series of epidemic events called at that time 'the everlasting epidemic'. This new pattern of the

disease was similar to that observed in Western countries
[...]."[234]

What caused this sudden rise in morbidity – observed in the
United States, England, Israel, and many other countries – in the
late 1940s? The institutional version of the polio story has no
explanation for this phenomenon.[ee] Its theory of Improved
Hygiene cannot explain the change in epidemic frequency in the
US from once every few years as in the pre-WWII era, to year
after year following WWII. It also fails to explain why polio
epidemics suddenly appeared in England in 1947, in Israel in
1949, and in France and Belgium in the 1950s.

Thus, the sudden emergence of an unprecedented wave of
polio epidemics in industrialized nations in the mid-20th century is another riddle in the annals of the disease. A riddle
requiring an answer.

DDT

Dichlorodiphenyltrichloroethane, or *DDT*, is a synthetic insecticide that was widely used in industrialized countries beginning
in the 1940s. DDT was invented in 1874 by a chemistry student
named Zeidler, but was not used at the time. It was not until
1939 that a Swiss chemist named Paul Hermann Müller discovered the compound's insecticidal properties, and Geigy, the
company he worked for, began selling it the following year.[ff] [235]
DDT was a wonder pesticide: very effective, inexpensive to
produce, easy to use, and safe.[236] (At the time, the title "safe" was

---

[ee] Nathanson (2010) argues that morbidity in the US in the late 1940s doubled due to the inclusion of non-paralytic cases in the statistics after WWII.
However, even after deducting these cases, the level of morbidity increased
significantly in the post-war years. In any case, this argument does not explain
the emergence of polio epidemics in other Western countries in the late 1940s
and early 1950s, as mentioned above.

[ff] The Swiss chemical corporations Geigy, CIBA, and Sundoz did business
with Nazi Germany during World War II. The companies operated factories in
Germany and even employed forced laborers. Eventually, these three companies
merged to create the vaccine and drug giant Novartis.

given to any compound that did not cause a severe reaction in a person who came in contact with it).[237] The compound attacked the insects' nervous system and tiny amounts were sufficient to kill them.[238] In addition, it was highly durable: A surface sprayed with DDT killed insects for many months.[239]

DDT was first used in the United States during World War II. In 1943, the military began using it after it was discovered to be highly effective in killing malaria-transmitting Anopheles mosquitoes and body lice that carried the typhus bacteria. The compound was generously sprayed in army camps – in barracks, kitchens and dining rooms, showers and toilets, and the like. Soldiers and civilians were dusted with DDT powder under their clothes. Millions of American soldiers were equipped with their own personal cans of DDT powder to protect against mosquitoes, lice, and other disease-carrying insects.[240]

Following DDT's resounding success in insect control for the US military in World War II, the compound was quickly adopted by the civilian sector as well. Thus, in the second half of the 1940s, DDT became the pesticide of choice for the American people. Its civic uses were myriad: in fields and orchards, in animal husbandry, at home, on city streets, in trains and buses, in public buildings, and more.[241] Soon, many other industrialized countries began using it as well. The "Flit" hand sprayer became an indispensable accessory in every office and household (the "Flit" spray material contained about 5% DDT in the 1940s and 1950s).[242] Exposure to DDT through the consumption of sprayed food was almost inevitable during this period. Its residues remained in fruits and vegetables, in cow's milk,[243] and in meat.[gg] The compound was used in all phases of food production and distribution: farming, storage, processing, packaging, and transportation. An American researcher who analyzed the composition of dairy and meat products in a Texas market for a

---

[gg] Cows were sprayed with DDT to kill insects and some even ate sprayed food. In addition, dairies were frequently sprayed with DDT for hygiene purposes.

period of six months found DDT residues in each and every one of the samples.[244]

From the very beginning, some safety studies indicated DDT was toxic to humans. As early as 1944, John Drayze and colleagues at the FDA's Department of Drug Research, examined its effect on laboratory animals by applying it directly to their skin. Their paper concludes, "The [...] data indicate that the unlimited use of DDT solutions on the skin is not free of danger; however, some solutions of DDT have been found safe for restricted use."[245] Another team in that department tested DDT's toxicity for oral consumption (that is, in food). The researchers write, "DDT is capable of causing subacute toxicity when given in small amounts in the diet for periods of from 3 days to 20 weeks."[246] They also note that "characteristic of DDT poisoning is the wide variation in individual susceptibility, making the estimate of a safely tolerated dose extremely difficult."[247] Smith and Stohlman of the National Institute of Health (NIH) conducted a comprehensive study of the aggregate toxicity of DDT. They write, "The toxicity of DDT combined with its cumulative action and absorbability from the skin places a definite health hazard on its use."[248]

It didn't take long for the first report of DDT poisoning in humans to appear. In a 1945 paper published in the *British Medical Journal*, Dr. Wigglesworth of the London School of Hygiene and Tropical Medicine reports on a lab worker harmed by DDT. The worker applied DDT powder to his hands for several minutes in order to test the compound's toxicity. Within a few days, he developed pain in all four limbs, weakness in his legs, and spasms and tremors throughout his body. He was confined to bed for several weeks and could not go to work for several months. "Even at the end of a year," Wigglesworth notes, "recovery was not quite complete."[249] Four more cases of DDT poisoning in soldiers were reported a year later by Dr. Mackerras of the Australian Medical Corps. Mackerras estimates the injured soldiers were exposed to tiny amounts of DDT and notes that the first signs of poisoning were muscle weakness, headache, and vomiting.[250] In 1949 Dr. Campbell, a physician at the Royal Hospital in Bristol, England, describes a case of chronic fatigue and muscle aches in an employee of the Department of Agriculture who demonstrated the use of DDT for a number of years.[251]

Dr. Case, a researcher at the British Navy's Physiological Laboratory, reports an experiment, conducted in England in 1945 to test the health effects of adding DDT to paint. In the experiment two soldiers stayed in a room painted with a regular paint for 48 hours and then for the same period of time in a different room painted with paint that was mixed with DDT to create insect-repellent walls.[252] Staying in the first room, the soldiers did not report any health issues. When they moved to the second room, however, they began experiencing fatigue, pain in joints and limbs, weakness in their legs, and other symptoms. These problems persisted even after the end of the experiment and gradually diminished over about a month.[253] "It is likely," writes Dr. Case, "that a substance known to be toxic to mammals, shown to be toxic to man under certain conditions, and in wide use, may produce subclinical manifestations, not at present recognized [...]. The rapidly growing use of DDT will extend into circumstances where human intoxication is likely to occur."[254] Regarding the results of the experiment, he writes, "It should be stressed that these experiments [...] do not form the basis for any condemnation of the widespread use of DDT, if proper precautions are taken [...]. They do, however, emphasize that DDT intoxication in human beings is a hazard to be considered and guarded against."[255]

Dr. Fred Bishopp from the Bureau of Entomology at the US Department of Agriculture describes the benefits of DDT in eradicating insects at home and in agriculture in a paper published in 1946.[256] However, Bishopp is also aware of the toxicity of the compound to the nervous system[257] and states emphatically that "DDT must not be allowed to get into foods."[258] Because the substance remains active for many months after spraying, Bishopp writes, great care should be taken in spraying crops or produce intended for human or animal consumption.[259] A few years later (1951) the American Medical Association's (AMA) Council on Pharmacy and Chemistry reiterates Bishopp's warnings,[260] stating that the substance is toxic to the nervous system of animals and humans and can cause various serious symptoms, including flaccid paralysis.[261] The council further notes that poisoning may be caused by ingestion or exposure to small amounts of DDT, and since individuals' reaction to the compound may vary, it is difficult to set a universal safety threshold.[262]

Despite the clear warning signs and question marks that emerged in these early reports and other studies conducted at the time, DDT was not banned in the post-war period, nor was its use restricted. Most researchers were of the opinion that the compound did not harm humans if its usage guidelines were followed.[263] Amazingly, FDA regulations did not even require manufacturers to add the word "poison" or the skull and crossbones symbol on the packaging[264] when it was approved for commercial use on August 1, 1945, just a few months after the end of the war.[265]

Dr. Biskind Goes into Battle

It was not long before Dr. Case's prediction ("the rapidly growing use of DDT will extend into circumstances where human intoxication is likely to occur") began to materialize. The man who broke the news to the science world was an American physician named Morton Biskind. Dr. Biskind, a physician at Beth Israel Hospital in New York City, published a series of papers on DDT harms between 1949 and 1953. These papers were based on his experience treating poisoned patients and extensive research on the health effects of DDT and several other pesticides.

Biskind became intrigued with this subject in 1946 after seeing numerous patients displaying similar symptoms, which could not be attributed to any known illness. This condition, which had become prevalent throughout the United States, was dubbed "virus X syndrome" as doctors surmised it was caused by an unknown virus.[266] Armed with information he had gathered treating upwards of 200 patients with the mysterious syndrome, Biskind began looking for the possible cause of the illness.[267] It wasn't long before he concluded that virus X syndrome, which had appeared shortly after the end of World War II, was caused by DDT poisoning.[268] Symptoms – including headaches, vomiting, nausea, muscle weakness, and paralysis – were consistent with those recorded in the medical literature following exposure to DDT.[269] In some cases they subsided or disappeared completely after the patient's exposure to the compound was reduced.[270]

When he searched the scientific literature for DDT's pre-approval safety tests, Biskind discovered that, although the compound was found to be toxic to animals, investigation of toxicity to humans was minimal at best. The scientific consensus maintained that "normal" exposure to DDT could not cause any harm. This assumption was based on a handful of observations of workers routinely exposed to the material during their work, the experience gained in World War II, and three clinical trials involving only five volunteers (three of whom – as reported in the Wigglesworth and Case papers mentioned above – experienced severe effects).[hh] Almost all of the subjects of these trials and observations were young, healthy men. The compound, Biskind realized, had not been tested on any other segments of the population, even though it was widely accepted that toxic susceptibility varies considerably between individuals. Moreover, the level of exposure from actual DDT usage was often much higher than researchers had assumed in their calculations.[271] "To anyone with even a rudimentary knowledge of toxicology," he concludes, "it exceeds all limits of credibility that a compound lethal for insects, fish, birds, chickens, rats, guinea pigs, rabbits,

---

[hh] Biskind interrogated soldiers returning from overseas service and found out that some who were exposed to DDT actually suffered from the symptoms described. However, those were attributed to other causes by army medical personnel.

dogs, cats, goats, sheep, horses, cattle and monkeys, would be nontoxic for human beings."[272]

Virus X syndrome was not the only novel illness to appear shortly after DDT was approved for general use, and humans were not the only ones affected. Almost 60 years after Charles Caverly reported paralysis in farm animals during the polio outbreak in Vermont, Biskind describes a similar phenomenon: "Since the last war there have been a number of curious changes in the incidence of certain ailments and the development of new syndromes never before observed. A most significant feature of this situation is that both man and all his domestic animals have simultaneously been affected."[273] In humans, he notes, among other things, a sharp increase in polio morbidity and conditions of extreme fatigue and muscle weakness. As for domestic animals, he lists a number of diseases that became common after the war that were not mentioned in the *Keeping Livestock Healthy* handbook published by the US Department of Agriculture in 1942. "This coincidence alone," he writes, "should have been sufficient to rouse a suspicion that something new that is common both to man and his domestic animals, has been operating in their environment during the period these changes have occurred."[274]

Alluding to polio, Biskind mentions the studies of Lillie and colleagues at the National Institutes of Health who found that DDT can damage the anterior horns of the spinal cord (leading to the lesions typical of polio). This injury, he writes, has occurred irregularly in animals exposed to DDT, similar to its uncommon appearance in humans.[275] As an example he cites a documented case of a cat that began convulsing a few hours after being dusted with DDT and died several days later with its hind legs paralyzed.[276] "When the population is exposed to a chemical agent known to produce in animals lesions in the spinal cord resembling those in human polio, and thereafter the latter disease increases sharply in incidence and maintains its epidemic character year after year, is it unreasonable to suspect an etiologic relationship?" he asks.[277]

Biskind proceeds to present epidemiological evidence for a link between polio and DDT: In the United States, the incidence of polio rose sharply following 1946, when DDT was introduced for civilian use. Morbidity remained high in the following years as well, in stark contrast to pre-DDT outbreak patterns, when epidemics occurred only once every few years. In Mexico, polio morbidity was rare until 1945, but increased significantly after that. In 1950, almost a thousand cases were recorded in Mexico City alone. In Israel, where DDT was introduced a few years later, polio epidemics appeared only after 1950, and incidence is lower in the Arab population which maintains a more traditional way of life. In the Philippines and other Far East regions, the incidence of polio among American soldiers – who frequently use large amounts of DDT – is very high, while it is extremely low in the local population.[278]

Ironically, one of the justifications for using DDT was to fight polio by exterminating insects. Although there was no conclusive evidence that flies or mosquitoes played a significant role in the spread of the disease,[279] municipal authorities in many cities initiated extensive spray operations to eradicate "disease-carrying" insects. Systematic spraying of cities and towns with DDT (and other insecticides), including from airplanes,[280] did not prevent polio epidemics, nor did it stop or slow them down.[281] But it did have an apparent effect on the health of the residents in sprayed areas. Dr. Robert Mobbs, a North Carolina physician, told Biskind of his comprehensive tour of the southern US in the 1950s: "Wherever DDT had been used extensively against polio, not only was there an epidemic of the syndrome I have described but the incidence of polio continued to rise and in fact appeared where it had not been before."[282] To this, Biskind adds, "This is not surprising since it is known that not only can DDT poisoning produce a condition that may easily be mistaken for polio in an epidemic but also being a nerve poison itself, may damage cells in the spinal cord and thus increase the susceptibility to the [polio]virus."[283]

DDT was the most popular insecticide of the post-war years,

but it was certainly not the only one. Shortly after it was introduced, insects began acquiring resistance to it. This, Biskind writes, led to the development of newer, and more potent, compounds,[284] some of which were more toxic than DDT.[285] In 1951, more than 252 million pounds of various pesticides were used in the US agricultural sector alone. In 1952 the quantity was even higher.[286] Safety studies, he warns, have never examined the aggregate effect of these compounds on the human body, although people are exposed to many of them on a daily basis. "How many simultaneous insults can the human body take?" he wonders.[287]

Biskind's call for a thorough investigation of the health effects of pesticides remained unanswered. His campaign was hopeless from the get-go. The inconceivable systemic failure he had exposed – that the safety of DDT and other insecticides had only been superficially examined and the use of these compounds was likely responsible for a great deal of severe illness – was greater than federal health agencies could ever publicly admit. An article published in the *New York Post* in March 1949 that echoes Biskind's claims does not mince words: "DDT the great bug-killer may turn out to be one of the most devastating biological weapons ever loosed by a people upon themselves [...] DDT is slowly poisoning large numbers of Americans, especially children."[288] The government response to these harsh accusations was not long in coming. A joint committee for the Department of Health, the Department of Agriculture and the US military issued a formal response, flatly denying Biskind's claims. In an editorial in the *American Journal of Public Health* of July 1949, the (unnamed) author cites the committee's findings that "the toxicity of DDT for man 'has been given full consideration in making recommendations for its use'" and "there is no evidence that the use of DDT in accordance with the recommendations of the various federal agencies has ever caused human sickness due to DDT itself." In addition, the committee's report states that claims that DDT is responsible for the onset of virus X syndrome in humans, and "X disease" in cattle, are fundamentally flawed, as these diseases were identified even before the use of DDT.[289] Shortly after disingenuously issuing this unequivocal and decisive denial of the potential harms of DDT, the US Department of Agriculture recommended ending the use of the compound in the dairy industry. DDT accumulates in adipose tissue and is excreted in cow's milk, the department said; therefore, it is recommended "that safer materials be used for insect control [...] in places where the milk might be contaminated, such as dairy barns, milk rooms, rooms containing dairy feed, or in similar situations on the farm." However, the public can be reassured that "all in all, the situation seems to be well in hand and the public adequately protected."[290]

In subsequent papers published in 1950 and 1953 Biskind answered the accusations made against him by the authorities, noting that they did not provide any evidence supporting their claims. "The relationship [between DDT and 'virus X' diseases]," he writes, "was promptly denied by government officials, who provided no evidence to contest the author's observations but relied solely on the prestige of government authority and sheer numbers of experts to bolster their position."[291]

Although federal authorities outright denied the allegations against DDT, their response actually confirmed Biskind's assertion that the compound was but superficially tested. As Biskind had pointed out, government agencies had presented no data on the overall level of exposure of the US population to DDT (and other toxic chemicals), and specifically for susceptible groups such as infants, children, and pregnant women. In addition, no studies had been conducted to examine the effects of exposure to the new insecticides on these susceptible subpopulations. The few studies and observations that were performed were confined to young, healthy men. Those, according to the government, were sufficient.

Despite authorities' attempts to dismiss Biskind's claims, there were those who took them seriously. In 1950, the US Congress appointed a special committee headed by Congressman James Delaney to "investigate the use of chemicals in food and cosmetics." The committee's letter of appointment authorized it to investigate "the extent and the effect of the use of chemicals, synthetics, pesticides, and insecticides in the production and preparation of food products and to determine the effects of such use on the public and upon agricultural stability."[292] The committee convened for a period of two years, during which it summoned no less than 217 witnesses, including Dr. Morton Biskind himself.[293] The committee's work met with strong opposition from the chemical manufacturers who joined the government agencies in an attempt to conceal the damage caused by the compounds they marketed. "Virtually the entire apparatus of communication, lay and scientific alike," Biskind writes in 1953, "has been devoted to denying, concealing, suppressing, distorting and attempts to convert into its opposite, the over-whelming evidence."[294] The rich and powerful pesticide companies employed an army of lobbyists and public relations officers whose mission was to torpedo the committee's work, and they did not pull any punches. Defamation, derogatory nick-names, and even threats were aimed at the chairman of the committee, Congressman Delaney, and at the witnesses who testified to the lack of evidence for the safety of the new pesticides.[295]

Despite the immense pressure and fierce opposition that Dr. Biskind and the committee endured, their efforts were not in vain, as we shall see later in the chapter.

Interim Summary: Polio in the Early 1950s

More than forty years after Ivar Wickman and Karl Landsteiner laid its epidemiological and virological foundations, and after decades of intensive research involving thousands of physicians and researchers, polio science of the early 1950s seemed to be going nowhere fast. In terms of understanding the disease and providing practical means to combat it, science hadn't made much progress. Most of the mysteries and open questions that baffled early polio investigators were still unanswered (and, in fact, remain so to this day). The sudden emergence of consecutive epidemic years following WWII, even as living conditions continued to improve and infectious disease incidence continued its sharp drop, only underscored the helplessness of science to curb the disease that had been the recipient of more research investment than any other in history.

Medical professionals, whose daily work involved dealing with the immense human suffering that polio inflicted, were particularly frustrated. Dr. Archibald Hoyne, a veteran and experienced pediatrician from the University of Chicago who had been treating paralytic patients for decades, summarized the state of the medical knowledge of polio in 1951. In a paper titled "Poliomyelitis Problems", he lists the main theoretical and practical gaps in the understanding and treating of the disease:[296]

1. Still unknown etiologic [causative] agent.

2. Warm weather prevalence, unusual for a communicable [infectious] disease.

3. Undetermined manner of transmission.

4. Susceptibility in the exceptionally well nourished.

5. Variability of symptoms.

6. Lack of a practicable laboratory diagnostic test.

7. Diagnostic difficulties added by the "new virus" [other viruses causing polio-like illness, see later in the chapter].

8. Reliable measures for prevention.

9. Dependable methods for treatment.

10. Question whether isolation of poliomyelitis patients is an effective means of controlling the disease.

Hoyne's list, although not exhaustive, reflects the dismal state of polio research in the early 1950s: The causative agent of the disease was unknown; the pattern of epidemics and mode of transmission were unclear; diagnosis was inaccurate; there were no reliable means of prevention or treatment; and more.

The scientific confusion that prevailed regarding some of the fundamental aspects of polio is typified by the dispute concerning its method of transmission. In addition to its theoretical significance, the mode of transmission was also of great practical importance, as public health officials would derive their preventive measures from it. Every year as summer neared, municipal health officers had to decide on which active measures to take, and the rules of conduct to be enforced, in order to try and blunt the sting of polio. Should children be allowed to go to the movies? Should they be allowed to attend public swimming pools? Would it be advisable to send children out of town if outbreaks occurred? Should houses where inhabitants had come down with polio be quarantined? If so, for how long? Should patients be isolated from their family and friends?

Disagreements among official bodies over how polio is spread are evident in a paper published by Dr. Sabin in 1951.[297] In the paper, Sabin tries to find middle ground between the position of the New York City Department of Health, which states that "the exact methods of transmission of the disease are not known," and that "in the present state of our knowledge this cannot be answered," and the opinion of experts attending the National Conference on Recommended Practices for the Control of Poliomyelitis conducted that year, which concluded that the disease was transmitted from person to person in the vast majority of cases and that "there has been no reliable evidence of spread by insects, water, food or sewage."[298] Sabin, who authored some of the studies that "isolated" the poliovirus in flies and sewage, eventually rejects both of these positions. In his view, current research suggests that the poliovirus is transmitted primarily through the fecal–oral route, and may therefore be transmitted directly from person to person (through hand contact, for example) or indirectly through intermediaries, such as flies or food.

Despite his own conviction, evident in his writings, and de-

spite his reputation as one of the most prominent polio researchers, Sabin was unable to convince many of his colleagues on this
crucial issue. John Paul, for one, notes a year later (1952) that
"there is agreement among students of poliomyelitis that not
enough is known about the factors responsible for the spread of
poliomyelitis to enable elimination of the virus from a community."[299] Dorothy Horstmann, a decade later (1963), writes that "as
with so many contact infections, the exact manner in which
polioviruses are transmitted from one person to another is
imperfectly understood."[300] She even points to the apparent
contradiction (of which Sabin himself is aware)[301] between the
researchers' findings – that the virus is secreted in the feces for
many weeks (and sometimes even several months) – and the
epidemiological evidence that polio patients infect mainly in the
days leading up to the disease.[302] In other words, if the main
route of transmission is through fecal contact, as Sabin claims,
and a sick person secretes the virus in the feces for a long period
of time, patients should be expected to infect close contacts even
weeks after getting sick, but the evidence says otherwise. The
scientific dispute on this issue has never been settled. Thus, even
with regard to the fundamental question of disease transmission
– problem #3 on Hoyne's list – polio science of the early 1950s
could not offer an adequate answer.

The helplessness of polio science, then and now, to provide
convincing answers to the disease's mysteries is hardly surprising
if one examines the groundwork on which it was founded. Since
its early days, polio epidemiological research was based on
Wickman's assumptions, while its biological research has followed the path set forth by Landsteiner. Wickman's assumption,
that polio's causative agent was primarily transmitted by healthy
carriers, provided a flexible theoretical framework that could
explain almost any case of illness as a result of direct or indirect
contact with another person. Thus, polio researchers were able
to "squeeze" polio's atypical distribution patterns into the familiar transmission model of common infectious diseases. But in
doing so, they confined themselves to a model that was incon-

sistent with much of the reality of the spread of the disease. Indeed, countless studies were conducted in the first half of the 20th century based on Wickman's assumptions about polio transmission, yet they had not translated into practical measures that could curb the spread of the disease.

If Wickman had stamped polio as "contagious", Landsteiner was the one who classified it as "infectious". The purported "isolation" of the virus by Landsteiner wedded polio research to the idea that a virus was its causative agent. Landsteiner's laboratory model, which was based on injecting material taken from patients' spinal cords directly into monkeys' brains or abdomens, did not match the way humans were supposedly infected. Hence, it too was unsuccessful in providing practical tools for dealing with the disease in the real world. "One must still admit," writes Dr. John Paul in 1952, "that there are no more immediate measures available for the prevention and cure of the acute disease than existed in the times of Medin and Wickman."[303] And Hoyne writes, "Notwithstanding the intensive studies of investigators, very little information of practical value has been added to our knowledge of poliomyelitis during the past forty years." He adds, "One might almost be tempted to make the contradictory statement that the more we learn about poliomyelitis, the less we know."[304]

Thus, in the early 1950s, while science was decisively winning the battle with most of the deadly infectious diseases of the 19th century, it stood helpless in the face of relentless and merciless polio epidemics striking yearly in the industrialized world.

But this dire predicament was soon to change.

The Salk Polio Vaccine

In 1949, the research trio of Enders, Weller, and Robbins from the Boston Children's Hospital were the first to grow the poliovirus in a culture of human embryonic skin and muscle tissue.[ii] This technological breakthrough triggered a flurry of inventions and improvements in lab techniques that paved the way for the development of Salk's polio vaccine, just five years later. Virological studies of polio were previously conducted, for the most part, with live monkeys, and as a result progress was slow, expensive, and cumbersome. Growing the virus in a Petri dish or test tube was relatively simple, quick, and inexpensive and enabled faster and better lab procedures, such as virus detection in fecal samples or measurement of blood antibody levels.[305]

Jonas Salk swiftly adopted the new techniques and even refined some of them in his laboratory, and in 1954, in cooperation with US health authorities, he conducted a large-scale trial of a polio vaccine. About a year later (1955), the authorities announced that the trial was successful and promptly launched a large-scale vaccination campaign with the new vaccine.

Within a few short years, the vaccine's apparent success in curbing the disease swept away all the uncertainties, question marks, knowledge gaps, and unresolved mysteries that had plagued polio research since its inception. The Messiah in the white coat had arrived, and inconvenient questions that might have spoiled the euphoria of "science's victory over the accursed disease" were pushed aside. The institutional story of polio began to crystallize, omitting those parts that were inconsistent with the heroic message that health authorities and other stakeholders sought to establish in the public consciousness. Polio science, limping and full of holes as it was, was clad in an impenetrable suit of armor after the vaccine's alleged success; the unsolved mysteries that had unsettled researchers for decades ceased to be worthy of discussion or research (henceforth, if they were ever mentioned, it was typically in the retrospective publications of veteran polio researchers such as Horstmann or Nathanson).

[ii] Until then, researchers had been able to grow the poliovirus only in a culture of neural cells (for example, brain cells) that could not be used, for safety reasons, as a substrate for a vaccine virus.

The alleged success of the vaccine in banishing polio to the history books serves the medical establishment in two ways – as conclusive proof that polio is caused by the poliovirus and as the foundation for the public perception that science had learned everything there was to learn about polio. If it weren't for the vaccine's alleged heroics, the story of polio would have remained as it was in 1951, when Archibald Hoyne listed his "ten problems" of polio research (most of which remain unanswered to this day).

As this chapter demonstrates, even if one accepts the vaccine's apparent success in eliminating the disease without question, the institutional story of polio remains incoherent and unconvincing, while its mysteries remain unresolved. Moreover, a thorough examination of the official story of the vaccine uncovers even more question marks and enigmas. As we will see, the supposed success of the vaccine doesn't just fail to solve the old puzzles of polio – it adds even more on top.

The Polio Vaccine: A Prior Morbidity Decline

The Salk vaccine, we're told, was the main reason polio disappeared from the Western world in the mid-20th century. The great epidemics of the 1950s, the official story tells us, all but vanished in the second half of the century thanks to universal vaccination campaigns. But this description oversells any role the vaccine may have had in curbing the disease. In fact, the data show that a major decline in polio morbidity in the 1950s occurred before the vaccine was put to use.

The United States was the first country to introduce the Salk vaccine. Figure 10-1 (next page) shows that the peak year for polio morbidity was 1952 (with almost 60,000 cases), followed by a consistent decline over the next few years. By 1955, when vaccination was launched, morbidity had already dropped to about half of its peak level (29,000 cases). Mortality data followed a similar pattern: a steady decline from the 1952 peak (over 3,000 deaths) to about a quarter of that number in 1955.

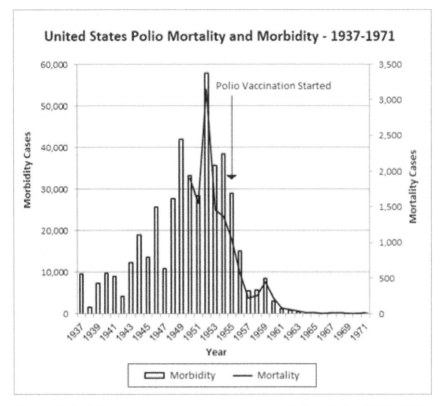

Figure 10-1: Polio mortality and morbidity in the United States (1937–1971)

The post-1955 drop in morbidity, which was attributed to the vaccine, was also affected by two other factors: a change in diagnostic procedures and the introduction of new laboratory tests. Until 1955, a diagnosis of "polio" was made when complete or partial paralysis was observed following patients' hospitalization. From 1955 onward, patients were examined again sixty days later, and only those who were still paralyzed at that time were diagnosed with paralytic polio. This procedural change led to an artificial decrease of unknown magnitude in the number of "paralyzed" patients after the introduction of the vaccine.[306] In some localities, public health officials made another important diagnostic change after 1955: Blood and fecal samples taken from suspected polio patients and tested for the presence of the poliovirus. No poliovirus was found in many of the samples that were analyzed (and sometimes no other known virus either). In such cases, patients who would formerly have received a diagnosis of polio were diagnosed with other diseases instead and not included in polio statistics (more on this later).[307]

The consistent pre-vaccine decline in polio morbidity observed in the United States was also reported in other Western countries. Israel, for example, recorded its highest morbidity in 1950. A year later morbidity dropped by more than half, and in four of the next five years it continued to decline. In 1956, a year before vaccination started in Israel, only about a quarter of the number of cases were recorded compared to the peak year of 1950. In 1957, the year in which the vaccine was introduced, there was a large decrease in morbidity. According to the experts, however, the vaccine's contribution to the drop is unclear, since the following year (1958) incidence rose back to the 1956 level despite the fact that mass vaccination continued in full force.[308]

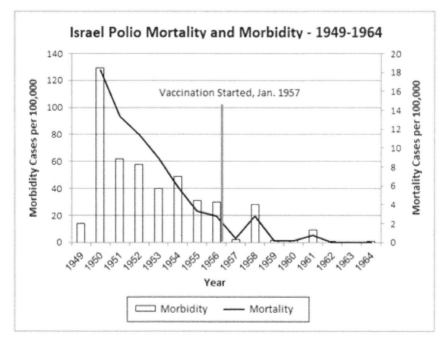

Figure 10-2: Polio mortality and morbidity in Israel (1949–1964)

Similar to the US, following the vaccine's introduction only paralytic cases were included in Israel's polio statistics, which probably contributed to the decrease in numbers.[309] In the United Kingdom, too, polio morbidity dropped by more than half between the peak year (1947) and the year the vaccine was introduced (1956).[310]

The Polio Vaccine: Doubtful Efficacy

Health authorities in the US and elsewhere usually present the graph of declining polio morbidity in the 1950s as "proof" that the vaccine eliminated the disease. By itself, though, the temporal proximity between the use of the Salk vaccine and the drop in polio incidence in the late-1950s is not conclusive proof of the vaccine's efficacy. Demonstrating a correlation between two events, as we all know, is not enough to prove a causal link between them. As noted earlier, the incidence of polio had been steadily declining in some countries even before the vaccine was introduced. This declining trend continued, indeed, after the introduction of the vaccine, and in the early 1960s the disease all but disappeared in the industrialized world. But was it the Salk vaccine that eliminated polio? As we shall see below, the answer to this question is much more equivocal than you might think.

The US recorded its greatest annual decline in polio incidence in 1955, the year mass vaccination with the Salk vaccine began. Those leading the national charge regarded this large decline in morbidity as evidence of the vaccine's efficacy. But was their optimism based on evidence? Although polio had acquired an early reputation as a disease of infants and young children (thus, the name *infantile paralysis*), US morbidity in the 1950s was actually distributed over a wider age range – infants, children, adolescents, and even many adults contracted the disease. The vaccination campaign that began in April 1955, was limited to only two cohorts that year – first and second graders.[311] Hence, it is unlikely that the dramatic reduction in polio seen that year was due to vaccination alone. Even if the vaccine completely eliminated polio in the two vaccinated cohorts, that could not explain the sharp morbidity decline recorded in 1955.[jj] Polio incidence had already dropped by about 50% between the peak year of 1952 and 1955. While health authorities didn't attribute this decline to any specific factor, they attributed the continued decline, from 1955 on, to the vaccine.

Similar events were reported in Sweden, where vaccine use began in 1957. Dr. Sven Gard, a world-renowned Swedish virologist and polio expert, notes that the decline in morbidity in Sweden following the introduction of the Salk vaccine also occurred in those who were not vaccinated.[312] Gard fails to provide an adequate explanation for this phenomenon.

While a number of reports by US health officials recounted the vaccine's success in reducing polio morbidity in specific cities,[313] other studies in the late 1950s indicated that it wasn't very effective. Poos and Nathanson, for example, report a polio outbreak in the winter of 1955 at the US naval base in Hawaii, wherein the Salk vaccine was used extensively. The two conducted a comprehensive and meticulous epidemiological investigation and found that although morbidity was slightly lower among the vaccinated than the unvaccinated the difference was not statistically significant.[314]

Dr. Herman Kleinman, an epidemiologist at the Department of Health in Minnesota, participated in a panel discussion with other polio experts in 1960 where he described his frustration in determining the overall effect of the vaccine. Studies he had conducted in Minnesota using data from 1955 and 1956 had indicated that receiving two doses of Salk vaccine was 83% effective in preventing paralytic polio. However, when he examined the 1957 data using the same method, he found that two doses were only 24% effective in preventing paralytic polio.[315] In retrospect, Dr. Kleinman argues in 1960, the results of

---

[jj] As will be shown later in the chapter, the Salk vaccine does not provide herd immunity. Therefore, vaccination of one age group cannot significantly affect the morbidity level in another.

these studies cannot be relied upon because accurate computation of vaccine efficacy is impossible due to the complexity of the calculations and the lack of accurate data. "I believe [the Salk vaccine] has some degree of effectiveness," he says, "but I do not know the extent because I cannot get proper denominators."[316] And it's not just the difficulty in calculating the vaccine's efficacy that bothers Dr. Kleinman. Antibody tests for children vaccinated in Minnesota showed that more than half did not produce antibodies to common poliovirus strains (1 and 3). "If polio antibodies mean anything, in respect to protection, then I am forced to conclude that much of the Salk vaccine we have been using is useless," proclaims Dr. Kleinman.[317]

Dr. Sumner Berkovich and colleagues reported similar issues in a paper summarizing the Massachusetts polio outbreak of 1959. In Massachusetts, too, the vaccine appeared to be largely ineffective: Nearly half of those stricken had received three or more doses of the vaccine. The majority of cases were in children between the ages of 5 and 19, and in this age range, three-fourths of the patients had been vaccinated three or more times.[318] Like Kleinman in Minnesota, the Massachusetts researchers found that the vaccine's efficacy could not be accurately calculated due to unreliable vaccination data for the various age groups. "However," they note, "that [the Salk vaccine] did not provide the expected protection is apparent."[319] In addition, Like Dr. Kleinman, Berkovich and his colleagues found that the vaccine did not produce an adequate level of antibodies in many of the vaccinated.[320]

The low level of polio antibodies found in many of the vaccinees in Minnesota and Massachusetts is consistent with the findings of several studies that examined the potency of the Salk vaccine in the second half of the 1950s.[321] The vaccine was supplied by a number of commercial companies that were supposed to manufacture it uniformly according to a method specified by Dr. Salk. In practice, though, researchers found tremendous variation – as much as factor of 600 – in vaccine potency across manufacturers and batches.[322] In addition, when safety issues were discovered shortly after the vaccine was introduced in 1955 (this was dubbed the *Cutter Incident* and will be described later), changes were made to the manufacturing process that significantly reduced the potency of vaccines produced in 1956 onward.[323]

The 1960 panel of experts, which included two other biostatisticians, a renowned virologist, and an Illinois Director of Public Health in addition to Dr. Kleinman, highlights additional failures in the production process of the Salk vaccine, as well as the marked difference between its actual efficacy and how it was presented to the public by the health authorities. Dr. Herbert Ratner, panel facilitator and professor of Preventive Medicine and Public Health at the University of Chicago, concludes: "A scientific examination of the data, and the manner in which the data were manipulated, will reveal that the true effectiveness of the present Salk vaccine is unknown and greatly overrated."[324]

A year later, the Salk vaccine was replaced by the Sabin vaccine in the United States.

In Israel, the experience with the Salk vaccine was largely similar to that of the United States. The Salk vaccine was introduced in Israel in early 1957, and that same year a sharp decrease in polio morbidity was recorded (37 cases in 1957 compared to 550 cases in 1956).[325] This was, seemingly, convincing evidence of the success of the national vaccination campaign. But here, too, the data tell a different story. Dr. Michael Davies and colleagues from the Health Ministry's Polio Advisory Committee found that the decline in morbidity in 1957 was observed in all age groups, not just those who were vaccinated.[326] And despite the fact that ongoing mass vaccination significantly increased the proportion of vaccinated children in the population, polio incidence soared to 573 cases a year later (1958). That was slightly more than the number of cases reported in 1956, the year before the vaccine was introduced.[kk]

In his essay on the history of polio in Israel, Professor Tiberio Swartz of the Israeli Ministry of Health notes that the 1957 vaccination campaign "was probably not associated with the low morbidity recorded during the year."[327] In Israel, as in the United States, production problems impaired the quality of the vaccine. "The polio vaccine produced in Israel in 1957 and used until mid-1958," writes Swartz, "performed poorly in potency tests and induced low seroconversion rates."[328] Although its quality supposedly improved after mid-1958, Swartz seems reluctant to attribute the full morbidity reduction in 1959 and 1960 (only 36 and 38 cases, respectively) to the vaccine: "The role of vaccination in the prevention of poliovirus activity at that time cannot be excluded," he writes.[329]

In 1961, polio morbidity in Israel rose again, albeit to a lesser extent than in 1958. In a study conducted by Jacob Yofe and colleagues, the data again indicated that the Salk vaccine was largely ineffective. An examination of the age distribution of paralytic cases found that among the children included in the vaccination campaign (ages 1–8 years) 51 were paralyzed. Of those 51 children, 40 had received three or more doses of the vaccine, another 5 had received two doses, and only 6 had one or zero doses.[330]

Like their American counterparts, Dr. Davies and his colleagues note the difficulty in calculating the 1957–59 efficacy of the Salk vaccine accurately. Polio morbidity during this period, they claim, was influenced by many factors, such as the distribution of polio strains from year to year, changes in vaccine composition and potency, and variance in seasonal morbidity and morbidity rates across age groups. In the absence of complete and accurate data, the researchers could not determine what specific effect the vaccine had on disease incidence.[331]

[kk] Remember that from 1957 onward the diagnostic criteria were tightened and only paralyzed polio cases were included in the official statistics in Israel. Hence, it is likely that the 1958 incidence was similar to that of 1953.

Thus, even as they were publicly demonstrating unreserved support for the vaccine, government health authorities had to take the multiple studies indicating that it was not very effective into account. Eventually, American and Israeli health authorities alike acknowledged the failure of the Salk vaccine, albeit implicitly: In 1961, just six years after it was globally heralded as the "miracle cure" for polio, the Salk vaccine was replaced by Sabin's vaccine in both countries. And if this decision alone does not seem sufficient evidence of public health authorities' true assessment the Salk vaccine's role in curbing the disease, this should be considered as well: In late 1961 and early 1962, after the Sabin vaccine replaced Salk's, health authorities in both the US and Israel strongly recommended that all children be vaccinated with the full course (three doses) of the new vaccine, even those who had already received three or more doses of the former vaccine.[332]

The obvious lack of trust US and Israeli health authorities had in the Salk vaccine contradicts their official statements lauding its success in stopping polio. In 1961, the year the Salk vaccine gave way to the Sabine vaccine, incidence of polio in the United States was about 5% of its level in 1955.[333] In Israel, morbidity among the Jewish population in 1960 was about one percent of the peak rate of 1950 (1.5 cases per 100,000 vs. 147 cases per 100,000).[334] There was no question that polio morbidity had dropped dramatically since the beginning of the decade, but – judging by health authorities' actions – the Salk vaccine was not the primary reason for that drop.

Echovirus, Coxsackievirus, and No-Virus

In the summer of 1958, three years after polio vaccination was launched in the US, a sizeable polio outbreak, considerably larger than any that had hit the state since 1952, occurred in Michigan. Some 1,200 cases were reported, mostly in and around the city of Detroit and most of them paralytic. The outbreak lasted from the beginning of July until the end of October, with peak morbidity recorded in mid-September. In an attempt to curb the disease, health authorities initiated a vaccination campaign that began in mid-August.[335] During the epidemic, 1,060 fecal and blood samples of hospitalized patients were sent for virological testing to the University of Michigan's state-of-the-art virus laboratory.[336] In addition, clinical histories were taken for each of the patients.

Analysis of the outbreak's epidemiological data indicated that the Salk vaccine was effective in reducing paralysis (most of the paralyzed were unvaccinated);[ll] however, its effectiveness in preventing non-paralytic polio was very low – or even negative![337] But analysis of the lab tests revealed the most intriguing finding: Poliovirus was only found in about 70% of the blood and fecal samples from the paralytic patients and 13% of those from non-paralytic patients.[mm] A small proportion of the samples that did not contain poliovirus contained other viruses, of the ECHO or coxsackie families, but in the rest of the samples no known virus was detected. (It is worth noting that the University of Michigan's Virus Laboratory used the most advanced technology of the time, developed by Enders and his colleagues and perfected by Salk. In addition, the laboratory tested the samples from paralytic patients a second time when poliovirus was not detected in the first test.[338])

Laboratory tests of fecal or blood samples from polio patients were also performed for other US outbreaks in the late 1950s, with similar results. In a large polio outbreak in Chicago in 1956 (1,100 cases, of which 75% were paralyzed), Bundesen and colleagues found poliovirus in about 63% of the samples ob-

---

[ll] The researchers do not present data on the vaccination rate in the population (stratified according to age group, ethnicity, place of residence, etc.), and therefore the effectiveness of the vaccine could not be calculated.

[mm] According to the data, an inverse correlation was found between the level of vaccination and the poliovirus in the samples. The poliovirus was found in higher rate in samples of unvaccinated patients and in lower rate in samples of those vaccinated with three or more doses. Similar findings were also obtained in studies from California (see below, Magoffin 1962, table 2, p. 4).

tained from paralytic and non-paralytic patients.[339] Melnick and colleagues took samples from 126 paralytic patients in a 1958 Houston outbreak. The poliovirus was not found in 20% of the samples (in one sample an ECHO virus was detected and in another a coxsackie virus). Poliovirus was also not found in over 80% of the samples taken from non-paralytic patients in Houston.[340] Dr. Robert Magoffin and Dr. Edwin Lennette of the California Department of Public Health's Viral Diseases Laboratory published a paper summarizing the issue in 1962. In their paper the two note that studies conducted in California found poliovirus in 80% of paralytic polio patients under the age of 5 and about 60–65% of patients over that age.[341] An official report from the US Public Health Service's Polio Surveillance Unit cites similar numbers regarding national polio morbidity in 1958–1961: The poliovirus was found in about 75–80% of the paralytic cases, and in about 30–50% of the non-paralytic cases.[342] Similar reports came from Israel (poliovirus was not found in nearly 20% of paralytic patients in 1958)[343] and Kazakhstan.[344]

Thus, consistent findings from polio outbreaks in various US cities and other countries in the late 1950s, indicate that no poliovirus was found in the blood or stools for more than 20% of paralytic patients (and a much higher rate for non-paralytic patients). What, then, had caused polio-like disease in these patients?

Investigators of the period, for the most part, looked for another virus to blame. The primary suspects were ECHO and coxsackie viruses, which were occasionally found in samples from "polio" patients. Viruses from those two families could cause polio-like paralysis in lab monkeys (including the typical spinal cord injury).[345] However, these viruses were found in only a small proportion of the poliovirus-free samples and could, therefore, be blamed for only a fraction of the cases.

Dr. William Hammon of the Department of Epidemiology and Microbiology at the University of Pittsburgh, a prominent American polio expert of the 1950s, also weighed in on this subject. In a paper published in 1958, Hammon describes a number of cases of paralytic and non-paralytic disease that were diagnosed as polio by "experienced poliomyelitis clinicians" but tested negative for the poliovirus. These cases were dubbed "paralytic poliomyelitis-like", Hammon writes, "because of the formerly held concept that this type of paralytic disease is only caused by one of the three types of poliovirus."[346] Although tests found strains of ECHO and coxsackie viruses in some of the cases examined, it is not possible to determine unequivocally that those were the cause of the disease, says Hammon.[347] On the other hand, the possibility that these viruses can cause disease that is not clinically distinguishable from paralytic polio cannot be ruled out.[348]

The uncertainty as to the cause of these "polio-like" cases leads Hammon to write cautiously. However, when discussing the significance of these findings in relation to the Salk vaccine, he concludes decisively that "These paralytic and nonparalytic illnesses cannot be expected to be prevented by the present poliomyelitis vaccine and may be considered vaccine failures [...]."[349]

Out of all the polio researchers mentioned above, Hammon is the only one to point out the obvious: It is unlikely that the Salk vaccine had an impact on disease that wasn't caused by the poliovirus. If so, how could poliovirus vaccines (Salk and Sabin) have completely eliminated polio in the United States when poliovirus couldn't be the cause of about 20% of paralytic cases? As with many of the other polio riddles addressed in this chapter, no convincing answer has been offered to this day. The institutional story of polio disregards it altogether.

Salk Vaccine: Cannot Prevent Spread of Virus

Another problem the official story of polio has a hard time with is the fact that the Salk vaccine does not prevent a vaccinated person from contracting the poliovirus and passing it to another person. The Salk vaccine produces antibodies in the vaccinated person's blood, which allegedly protect against the invasion of the poliovirus from the gut into the bloodstream. These antibodies are supposed to eliminate the invading virus from the blood, thus preventing it from reaching the central nervous system and causing paralysis. However, the injected Salk vaccine does not stimulate antibody production in the gut; therefore, it cannot prevent poliovirus infection in the digestive tract of a vaccinated person. Once settled in the gut, the poliovirus can then infect other people through the feces.[350] The Sabin vaccine, on the other hand, is given by mouth and purportedly builds resistance to poliovirus in the digestive tract ("gut immunity"), and therefore constitutes an effective barrier to the spread of the virus in the population.[351] Infection with the natural poliovirus ("wild virus") is believed to produce similar resistance.[352]

As previously discussed, after the introduction of the Salk vaccine, polio morbidity declined even further than expected in some countries (US, Sweden, Israel). The large morbidity reduction in those who hadn't been vaccinated led researchers to suggest that the vaccine induced herd immunity. Theoretically, herd immunity would occur if the vaccinated could not transmit the virus. This would severely reduce the disease's ability to travel through the population, thereby reducing infection in the unvaccinated as well. But most studies examining the issue found that the Salk vaccine did not prevent the spread of the poliovirus. One such study was conducted by Dr. John Fox and colleagues from the Department of Epidemiology at the Tulane University School of Medicine in New Orleans. The researchers found that the Salk vaccine had no significant effect in preventing contagion.[353] Vaccinated and unvaccinated children infected their family members equally.[354] In addition, no significant differences were found between vaccinated and unvaccinated children with respect to the length of time the virus was excreted in the stools or the amount of virus excreted.[355] "It is concluded," the researchers write, "that widespread use of Salk vaccine should not by any reasonable mechanism influence poliovirus dissemination."[356]

A study by Drs. Lepow, Woods, and Robbins of the Department of Pediatrics and Contagious Diseases at Cleveland Metropolitan General Hospital gave similar results. The researchers found that the Salk vaccine does not create gut immunity, and therefore cannot significantly reduce the number of people infected with the poliovirus.[357] In addition, no correlation was found between the level of poliovirus antibodies in the blood and resistance to poliovirus infection in the gut.[358] "It is concluded," they write, "that immunization with killed poliomyelitis vaccines cannot be expected to decrease the numbers of persons in the community with alimentary poliovirus infection. Thus, vaccination, while of value to the persons immunized, is unlikely to provide protection to those not vaccinated."[359]

These studies by Fox, Lepow, and other researchers contributed to acceptance of the scientific maxim that the Salk (or IPV) vaccine does not prevent the spread of the poliovirus. An official World Health Organization document (1997) expresses the scientific consensus on this issue: "Inactivated polio vaccine (IPV) works by producing protective antibodies in the blood – thus preventing the spread of poliovirus to the central nervous system. However, it induces only very low-level immunity to poliovirus inside the gut. As a result, it provides individual protection against polio paralysis but only marginally reduces the spread of wild poliovirus. In a person immunized with IPV, wild virus can still multiply inside the intestines and be shed in stools. Because of this, IPV could not be used to eradicate polio."[360]

The idea that his vaccine did not prevent the spread of the poliovirus and therefore did not provide protection for the unvaccinated, bothered Salk considerably. If the vaccine did not confer herd immunity, then it could not account for the full decline in morbidity observed in the United States and other countries in the late-1950s. In an attempt to protect his invention's reputation, Salk suggested that his vaccine decreased poliovirus concentration in nasal and oral secretions and that contributed to its ability to prevent disease. But as you may recall, the scientific consensus was that poliovirus is largely transmitted through contact with feces (the fecal–oral route) and negligibly through contact with oral or nasal secretions (hence-forth, the *nasopharyngeal route*). While the vaccine does not affect poliovirus excreted in feces, some studies had indeed found that the vaccine significantly reduces viral secretion in the nose and mouth, and it was on this finding that Salk based his defense. In countries with a high level of sanitation, he argued, the virus could be expected to spread mainly through the naso-pharyngeal route; therefore, the protection conferred by the vaccine against contagion in this pathway could certainly limit the spread of the virus and thus generate herd immunity.[361]

In the absence of supporting evidence, Salk's hypothesis re-mains a speculative claim and nothing more, as Gard points out.[362] In the American studies that examined the issue (some of which were mentioned above), no evidence was found to sup-port the idea that the nasopharyngeal route had become the dominant pathway of contagion. And, in fact, the studies con-firmed the established perception that the fecal–oral route is the main pathway of contagion.[363]

The Salk vaccine's inability to significantly limit the spread of the poliovirus has important consequences, as will be described shortly. Thus, it is not surprising that even today there are those who try to ascribe herd immunity capabilities to it, at least in industrialized countries. Dr. Stanley Plotkin, a veteran polio researcher and editor of the textbook *Vaccines*,[364] repeats Salk's above claim in the chapter devoted to the inactivated polio vaccine (IPV, or Salk's vaccine).[365] Like Salk before him, Plotkin does not provide convincing evidence to support his claim and defers to vague wording.[366] In fact, some of the papers he cites in the chapter – studies in the US, Finland, and Cuba that found that nearly all Salk-vaccinated children excreted the poliovirus in their stools after being exposed to it – actually reinforce the understanding that even in industrialized countries the oral-fecal route is the dominant pathway of contagion.[367]

The inability of the Salk vaccine to stop transmission of the poliovirus raised unanswered questions regarding the decline in polio morbidity in the US in the 1950s. The decrease in morbidity among the unvaccinated, one that could not be attributed to the vaccine, implies that another factor was contributing to the gradual disappearance of polio.

A similar issue exists for countries in which Salk's was the only vaccine ever used. In the US and Israel, where the Sabin vaccine replaced Salk's, the ultimate elimination of the disease and the supposed disappearance of the virus could ostensibly be attributed to the Sabin vaccine (which allegedly confers herd immunity). But in countries such as Sweden, Finland, and the Netherlands, where the population was vaccinated exclusively with the Salk vaccine,[368] the official story cannot explain the complete elimination of the disease. The Salk vaccine does not prevent the virus from spreading, and thus cannot even theoretically prevent all paralytic morbidity (as evidenced by the numerous times paralytic polio was reported in people who were vaccinated with three or more doses).[369] Thus, the best outcome that could be expected from exclusive use of the Salk vaccine would be a large reduction in morbidity (as had ostensibly happened in the United States and Israel before the introduction of the Sabin vaccine), not its complete disappearance.[370]

By the same token, it is hard to reconcile current polio vaccination policy in the vast majority of Western countries. In the early 2000s, most European and North American countries reverted to exclusive use of the inactivated Salk vaccine.[nn] The reason for this change was the realization that the Sabin vaccine sometimes causes paralysis in the vaccinated, and since polio has been eliminated in the Western world, it is safer to use the Salk vaccine.[371] But the fact that the Salk vaccine does not prevent transmission of poliovirus should mean that using it exclusively is a "ticking time bomb" in the global village of the 21st century: Every day numerous flights from African and Asian countries where polio is still prevalent land at European and American airports. Because screening passengers for the poliovirus is not

---

[nn] The US switched to exclusive use of the Salk (IPV) vaccine in 2000, the UK in 2004, Israel in 2005 (until early 2014).

practical – most carriers do not show any symptoms, as Wick-man "discovered" – it should be assumed that the virus routinely infects Western countries.[372] Thus, exclusive use of the Salk vaccine would presumably increase the likelihood that a single traveler excreting the virus would lead to poliovirus infection of an entire country and the re-emergence of paralytic polio. (Similar considerations purportedly guided the Israeli Ministry of Health in 2014 when it decided to re-introduce the Sabin vaccine after nine years of using the Salk vaccine exclusively.[373])

Are Western health authorities relying on good fortune alone to prevent the entry and spread of what they deem to be a highly contagious and dangerous virus that could potentially arrive as a covert passenger on any incoming international flight? If so, luck has apparently been on their side, at least as of this writing: No polio cases have been reported in Western countries in the past fifteen years.

The Cutter Incident: A Turning Point

On April 12, 1955, a press conference was held in Ann Arbor, Michigan, to announce the successful outcome of the large-scale clinical trial of the Salk vaccine. On the same day, the vaccine received expedited approval from Oveta Culp Hobby, the US Secretary of Health, Education, and Welfare. The next day, five manufacturers began sending vaccine shipments (manufactured in advance and stored in anticipation of the vaccine's approval) all over the United States.[oo] Only two of the five companies had provided vaccines for the clinical trial. These vaccines were also tested by the Biological Laboratory of the National Institutes of Health (NIH) and Salk's Laboratory at the University of Pitts-burgh. Following approval, however, safety testing of the vaccines was left to the five manufacturers. In addition, the

---

[oo] Even before the results of the trial were announced, the NFIP purchased $9 million worth of vaccines from the five preselected manufacturers to ensure immediate delivery upon licensing.

manufacturers were instructed by Salk to make some modifica-
tions in the production process of the vaccine intended for mass
distribution, compared to the vaccine used in the trial.[374]

On April 25, barely two weeks into the vaccination campaign, reports of paralysis in vaccinated children and/or their
families began appearing in Illinois, and later in California and
Idaho. These cases were attributed to the vaccine because the
paralysis happened within 11 days of vaccination and occurred
in the injected limb. In addition, it seemed that all the paralyzed
children received vaccines manufactured by Cutter Laboratories
of California, one of the licensed manufacturers of the Salk
vaccine. Reactions to this sequence of events – later dubbed the
Cutter Incident – were "predictable and unedifying":[375] None of
the people or organizations involved – not the National Foundation for Infantile Paralysis, the US Department of Health,
Education, and Welfare (henceforth, the DoH), the local health
authorities, the vaccine manufacturers, or Salk himself – assumed responsibility for the disaster. Though it's debatable
exactly who was responsible, it was soon agreed by all that the
only entity that could handle a crisis of this magnitude was the
DoH. Under the guidance of Leonard Scheele, the US Surgeon
General, Cutter promptly recalled its vaccine from the market.
Vaccine shipments from other manufacturers were suspended
for a week and then slowly renewed. The DoH gathered a committee of experts to implement new production regulations and
more stringent safety inspections. The manufacturers, with the
exception of Cutter, eventually resumed production at full
capacity. Scores of lawsuits filed against Cutter Laboratories on
behalf of the "incident's" victims moved through the courts for
decades.

The Cutter Incident is an important landmark in United
States vaccination history. It marks the specific point in time
when federal health authorities assumed a leadership role in
vaccination.[376] Until April 1955, for the most part, vaccination
efforts were in the hands of private organizations (like the NFIP
or the AMA) or the responsibility of state and municipal health

departments.[377] The long scientific research and development process that led to the polio vaccine was financially supported and directed by the NFIP, a nonprofit organization funded by donations from private citizens. The vaccine's clinical trial was also funded by the Foundation, and even after its successful results were announced, the vaccine was approved, and the manufacturers began to meet the huge demand, the DoH still stood on the sidelines.

Secretary Hobby initially refused to issue formal federal policies for the urgent questions of the day: who should get the vaccine first, how much it should cost, and whether or not federal funds should be set aside to purchase vaccines for those who could not afford them.[378] But the Cutter Incident quickly reversed this policy of non-intervention, and the DoH began playing a key role in managing vaccines and vaccination.[379] Thus, the government's Laboratory of Biologics Control, which was responsible for the quality control of vaccines, was reorganized and expanded.[380] The Communicable Disease Center (the precursor of today's CDC) established a national system for monitoring polio morbidity, as well as vaccination data.[381] Congress allocated funds to the CDC to purchase vaccines and supply them to states and municipalities that required financial assistance.[382] In the early 1960s, government funding was also extended to smallpox and DTP vaccines.[383]

The government's central role, first assumed in 1955, has completely changed the balance of power in the field of vaccines. The federal government went from being a largely neutral external auditor to being a major stakeholder. Until 1955, health authorities had only indirect supervisory responsibility for any defects in vaccines manufactured and marketed by private pharmaceutical companies. But after assuming responsibility for the nationwide vaccination campaign, federal health authorities knew they would be the first to be blamed for any problems detected in the vaccines provided by the business sector. As would be expected, then, vaccine manufacturers – no longer simply the objects of government auditing and supervision –

became allies to be supported, nurtured, and even protected if the need should arise.

Too much overlap between governmental and commercial interests in any field of activity typically leads to a state of imbalance with potentially devastating consequences to the public. One such example is federal agencies' (including the Department of Agriculture, the FDA, and the US military) steadfast support for DDT and the aggressiveness with which they attacked Dr. Morton Biskind and anyone else who dared to speak of the dangers of using the compound in the late 1940s. DDT, which was produced by for-profit commercial companies, enjoyed unwavering government support following its massive military use in World War II. Similar government protection had been provided to lead arsenate and the pre-DDT pesticides: For decades the US Department of Agriculture and farmers' organizations systematically concealed the fact that most fruits and vegetables were sprayed with large amounts of arsenic and lead.

It wasn't long before the new alliance of the federal government, polio vaccine manufacturers, and the National Foundation – whose members all shared a common interest in publicly presenting polio vaccination as a great success – began affecting what the public was allowed to hear.

In a 1957 paper Paul Meier, professor of epidemiology at the Johns Hopkins University School of Public Health, describes the faulty safety testing of the Salk vaccine and how this information was prevented from reaching the general public (and even the medical profession). Most of the professional publications that appeared before and after the Cutter Incident, Meier writes, blurred any facts that might have exposed the vaccination campaign to criticism. "Perhaps the most disturbing element of the entire program," he notes, "has been the disparity between the risks that were known to be involved and the repeated assurances of safety."[384] The National Foundation, in a memo sent to doctors, also stated emphatically that the vaccine was completely safe and that the risk of ensuing paralysis was "zero".[385] When participating in the expert panel convened by Dr. Ratner three years later, Professor Meier's opinion on the subject was no different. "How is it that today you hear from the members of this panel that the Salk vaccine situation is confused; yet, what everybody knows from reading the newspapers, and has been known since the vaccine was introduced, is that the situation as far as the Salk vaccine is concerned was and is marvelous?" he asks. He then answers, "The best way to push forward a new program is to decide on what you think the best decision is and not question it thereafter, and further, not to raise questions before the public or expose the public to open discussion of the issue."[386]

The health establishment took pains to prevent open debate on the merits of vaccination by blocking any information with the potential to erode the public's confidence in federal vaccine policy. In his book *The Cutter Incident*, Dr. Paul Offit, an infectious disease expert at the Children's Hospital of Philadelphia and a vaccine inventor, exposes a 1955 CDC secret report, authored by Dr. Alexander Langmuir, the CDC's chief epidemiologist, and Dr. Neil Nathanson, who at the time headed the CDC's polio surveillance unit. The two conducted a follow-up investigation into the Cutter Incident and discovered that Wyeth's vaccine had also caused several cases of paralysis.[387] Following their report, the company silently recalled the allegedly "hot lot" from the market.[388] No one other than senior US health officials ever saw that report. "It was never released to the media," Offit writes, "never shown to polio researchers, never shown to the National Foundation, never shown to polio vaccine advisers, never distributed to health care professionals, never published in medical journals, and never made available to defense attorneys in subsequent lawsuits against Cutter Laboratories. As a result, only a handful of people knew about the problem with Wyeth's vaccine."[389] Years later, Nathanson said he thought the report had been buried due to officials' wish to maintain public confidence in the Salk vaccine: "As long as the problem was with one manufacturer [i.e., Cutter] and a couple of lots of vaccine, it would be viewed as an aberration due to sloppy manufacturing or testing procedures and not an intrinsic problem. Once it was extended to a second manufacturer, it would be seen as intrinsic to the product." In this scenario, Offit further clarifies, "people would be afraid to use any polio vaccine."[390]

The Cutter Incident illustrates the ease with which health authorities in the second half of the 20th century – before the age of the internet and social networks – were able to conceal critical medical information from the public that had the potential to damage vaccination's reputation, and thus their own as well.

Five years after the Cutter Incident, and after the Salk vaccine had been given to tens of millions of people in the US and around the world, another serious problem emerged. In 1960, Bernice Eddy, a researcher at the NIH Biological Laboratory, discovered that injecting hamsters with a small amount of the substrate used in the Salk vaccine's production process led to the development of cancerous tumors in many of them.[391] Though she was explicitly ordered not to publish her discovery – her managers were concerned that the publication could severely harm the vaccination program – Eddy presented her findings at a scientific cancer conference in New York anyway. Her manager's response was swift. Her lab was taken away from her, and she was demoted and moved to another position. Soon thereafter, her findings were corroborated by other researchers, and the carcinogen in the substrate was identified by two Merck researchers: A previously unidentified virus found in rhesus monkey kidneys, which had been used to grow poliovirus for the vaccine. The new virus was named SV-40;[pp] further tests confirmed its presence in a significant portion of both Salk and Sabin vaccines produced in the United States.

In an attempt to prevent public panic (or criticism), health authorities kept the vaccines' contamination with this potential-

---

[pp] SV stands for *simian virus*, a virus of monkey origin. SV-40 was the fortieth monkey virus that had been identified.

ly cancer-causing virus under wraps, and polio vaccination proceeded as usual. It was not until 1963, three years following Eddy's original discovery, that US health authorities ordered vaccine manufacturers to modify their production processes in order to purge the SV-40 virus from the vaccine. Rhesus monkeys were replaced by African green monkeys, which were free of SV-40 in their natural habitat. In that three-year time span, however, as health authorities secretly weighed their options, tens of millions more people were vaccinated with the contaminated polio vaccines, bringing the total number of Americans potentially infected with SV-40 to 98 million (a similar number presumably existed outside the United States). Later on, after publishing a number of questionable epidemiological studies, US health authorities declared in the mid-1970s that, "fortunately," the SV-40 virus does not actually cause cancer in humans. The issue was buried, and research ceased for the next twenty years.[qq]

Regardless of whether SV-40 causes cancer in humans or not, there is no doubt that health authorities concealed its presence in polio vaccines in order to maintain public confidence in the vaccine. By concealing details of the Cutter Incident, the dubious effectiveness of the Salk vaccine, and the SV-40 contamination, US health authorities of the '50s and '60s proved that when it came to the polio vaccine, presenting the public with the truth, the whole truth, and nothing but the truth was never an option. Judging by their actions, their top priority was always protecting the vaccine program, not the public.

Polio and Pesticides: A Re-evaluation

In a 1951 paper, Dr. Albert Sabin, future inventor of the second polio vaccine, discussed what was then known about polio

---

[qq] Interest in the SV-40 virus resurfaced in the 1990s, when researchers discovered the virus in human cancerous tumors. This time, too, the authorities did everything in their power to bury the story. That affair is described in Debbie Bookchin and Jim Schumacher's excellent book *The Virus and the Vaccine*.

distribution patterns. Among other things, the unresolved issue of simultaneous morbidity in a single household held Sabin's attention. Researchers had grappled for many years with the fact that when several members of the same family came down with polio it was usually at the same time, rather than one after another, as is typical of infectious diseases. "One of the most striking facts in the epidemiology of poliomyelitis is the regularity with which most members of a family either succumb within a few days of one another when there are multiple [paralytic] cases, or are found to be simultaneous carriers of the virus," Sabin writes. "While there are a number of possible explanations for this, all of which may apply at different times," he adds, "the consumption of a common article of food or drink, contaminated [with the poliovirus] before or after it reaches the home, is as plausible and possible as any other."[392]

Polio researchers have never considered contaminated food and water to be significant factors in the spread of the disease,[393] and that is the case even today. Nevertheless, Sabin's explanation for simultaneous polio morbidity may have hit the mark, though not in the way he intended. If one replaces the contaminant Sabin was assuming (the poliovirus) with a toxic pesticide (lead arsenate or DDT), a fairly coherent and reasonable hypothesis emerges: Joint consumption of contaminated food can certainly cause concurrent illness in several members of a household.

The Pesticide Theory provides plausible explanations for additional mysteries which the official story of polio cannot adequately resolve: Polio outbreaks appeared in the Western world in the late-19th century due to the surge in pesticide use in agriculture. Most of the cases occurred during the summer and autumn months because that was fruit-picking season. Early epidemics naturally hit rural areas, where the pesticides were used, occasionally paralyzing domestic animals as well as humans. In countries such as the UK or France, where pesticides were more strictly regulated, polio incidence was relatively low and outbreaks began much later. In developing nations, where pesticides were not commonly used by the population, no polio outbreaks occurred among the locals. The European inhabitants of these countries, on the other hand, who likely used their trusted pesticides against local insects, contracted polio at much higher rates. This would also have been true for WWII military personnel stationed overseas, who used DDT heavily and were paralyzed at rates much higher than their peers back home. Officers, who were likely to be more actively protected from insect-borne illness by army procedures, were sickened significantly more often than enlisted men.

Following WWII, DDT replaced the older generation of pesticides in industrialized countries. DDT was very cheap and very effective. In addition, unlike pesticides based on arsenic and lead, it was initially believed to be completely safe for humans. As a result, it quickly gained unprecedented popularity and was used more intensively and expansively than its predecessors.[394] Thus, annual polio epidemics began appearing in many countries where low incidence had been the rule, such as the UK and Israel. In the United States, too, the disease changed pattern: Rather than every few years, epidemics now occurred year after year after year.

The sudden onset of polio epidemics in industrialized countries after World War II clearly coincides with the sudden explosion in DDT use, but how would polio's disappearance from these countries be explained?

The official story holds that the fight against the disease was won by the vaccine – and the temporal proximity between introduction of the vaccine and the elimination of the disease some 5–10 years later (reiterated in many countries) appears to supports this. However, as we have seen, a closer examination of the facts raises serious doubts about the efficacy of the Salk vaccine, the one credited with most of the apparent drop in polio morbidity. As you may recall, some countries began using the Salk vaccine at a time when polio incidence had already been declining for several years. Additionally, American and Israeli studies indicate that the vaccine's efficacy was dubious and about a fifth of the paralysis cases (that the poliovirus vaccine supposedly eliminated) could not have been caused by the poliovirus. Furthermore, reduced polio morbidity in the unvaccinated population was attributed to herd immunity from use of the Salk vaccine, an effect that studies repeatedly showed the vaccine could not have had.

Thus, the institutional story, which attributes the disappearance of polio to the vaccine, doesn't explain many of the historical facts. But does the Pesticides Theory fare any better? Does the drop in polio morbidity correlate to a reduction in pesticide use in relevant countries? Unfortunately, this question cannot be definitively answered due to the lack of reliable data on pesticide use in the 1950s. Unsurprisingly, any link between pesticide use and polio incidence was never investigated at the time, though in retrospect there appear to have been many sound reasons to conduct in-depth and comprehensive inquiries into the matter. The use of pesticides was backed by the powerful farmers lobby as well as the Department of Agriculture, health authorities, chemical companies, and – specifically for DDT – the US military. The government, which was in charge of licensing the compounds and ensuring their safety, was not keen to conduct studies that could highlight the dangers of pesticides and bring them to public attention, and certainly not any looking for a link between pesticides and polio. Government agencies' cover-ups of the Cutter Incident and SV-40 contamination, as well their active collusion in concealing the health hazards of lead arsenate and other toxic pesticides, attest to this.

After four years of meticulous research, Rachel Carson published *Silent Spring* in 1962, publicly exposing the harmful environmental effects of DDT for the first time. Carson's book raised awareness of DDT's impact on wildlife instantaneously, initiating public debate and a legacy of environmental activism that lasts to this day. While the destructive effects of DDT were new to the public, government authorities, however, had no need for such an introduction. They had been aware of the compound's dangers for years and, as we shall soon see, had already taken steps to monitor, and even reduce, its use.

As early as 1946 Dr. Fred Bishopp, from the Bureau of Entomology of the US Department of Agriculture, was writing about the toxicity of DDT to the nervous system.[395] In a paper published in the *American Journal of Public Health*, Bishopp warns that "DDT must not be allowed to get into foods"[396] and care must be taken when spraying it on crops intended for human or animal consumption.[397] In 1949, the same journal published the authorities' response to Dr. Morton Biskind's claims regarding DDT toxicity. Paradoxically, after vigorously denying Biskind's allegations, they admit that DDT accumulates in adipose tissue and has been found in the milk of cows sprayed with the compound. In fact, an official recommendation not to use DDT in dairies or any other facility where milk was processed or stored had been issued in April of that year (1949).[398]

In 1951, the US Public Health Service stated that "DDT is a delayed-action poison. Due to the fact that it accumulates in the body tissues, especially in females, the repeated inhalation or ingestion of DDT constitutes a distinct health hazard. [...] The deleterious effects are manifested principally in the liver, spleen, kidneys and spinal cord [...] DDT is excreted in the milk of cows and of nursing mothers after exposure to DDT sprays and after consuming food contaminated with this poison. Children and infants especially are much more susceptible to poisoning than adults."[399] The American Medical Association's Council on Pharmacy and Chemistry convened that year and declared, "It is not reasonable to expect that human beings can avoid injury if they are exposed year after year to a toxic agent in atmospheric concentrations that kill insects in a few hours. [...] The resultant injury may be cumulative or delayed, or simulate a chronic disease of other origin, thereby making identification and statistical comparison difficult or impossible."[400] Identifying the source of the injury could have been made even more challenging by the fact that in the post-war era almost everyone was exposed to DDT in one way or another (similar to the widespread exposure to arsenic- and lead-based substances in the pre-war period).

Growing concerns about the toxicity of chemical pesticides also reached the US Congress. As you may recall, in 1950 Congress set up a special committee to "investigate the use of chemicals in food and cosmetics." The committee, chaired by Congressman James Delaney, summoned over 200 witnesses and devoted much time to examining the toxicity of pesticides.[401] Its final report, published in 1952, contained a recommendation to Congress to "pass legislation to control the flow of chemical substances into the nation's food supply."[402] Congress complied with the committee's recommendation, and relevant laws were indeed enacted in 1954 and 1958. The 1954 law, among other things, authorized the Department of Health, Education, and Welfare, and even obliged it, to set a maximum threshold for the amount of pesticides allowed in food.[403] The Department of Agriculture, as well as state and local health authorities, acted as early as 1952 to limit exposure to DDT, for example, by discouraging the use of household devices dispersing DDT.[404] In addition, it became apparent around that time that certain types of insects, both in the field and home, had developed resistance to DDT, and more effective insecticides began replacing it.[405]

Thus, the evidence shows that US authorities were well aware of the dangers of DDT in the early 1950s and took active measures to limit its use, especially in food production. Due to the lack of relevant data it is impossible to say whether, and to what extent, these actions contributed to the reduction of polio morbidity in the US and overseas; however, the United States at least, experienced a consistent and unexplained decline in polio morbidity after the peak year of 1952 until 1955, when the Salk vaccine was introduced.[rr]

Later in the 20th century, after disappearing from industrialized countries, polio reappeared in developing countries. Could pesticides also have played a major role in the sudden emergence

---

[rr] Incidentally, the last natural polio case in the United States (as opposed to vaccine-induced paralysis) was recorded in 1972 (Nathanson 2010, p. 8), the same year DDT use was banned.

of polio in these countries in the last third of the 20th century?

Polio in the Developing World

In the mid-1960s, with polio on the brink of extinction in industrialized countries, public preoccupation with the disease died down. After decades of intensive research, two vaccines, and successful elimination of the disease in Western countries, it was time to divert the resources that had been allocated to polio to more pressing needs. Government research budgets were redirected to fighting other infectious diseases, and even the National Foundation for Infantile Paralysis changed its focus to reducing the occurrence of birth defects. The age of polio in industrialized countries was over.

For the next twenty years, polio garnered little public or scientific interest.[406] This dormancy ended abruptly in the mid-1980s with the publication of the results of "lameness" surveys that had been conducted in developing countries since the mid-'70s.[407] More than a hundred surveys, conducted between 1974 and 1983, found high incidence of polio-like paralysis in numerous developing nations. Many reported rates between 500 and 1,000 paralytic cases per 100,000 children (that is, one case of paralysis per 100 to 200 children),[408] similar to rates recorded in the US and Israel during the peak epidemic years of the early 1950s.[409] It seemed that polio, which had all but disappeared from industrialized nations, had surprisingly resurfaced in developing countries. Thus, the age of polio in the developing world had officially begun.

The surprising data from the lameness surveys changed the scientific perception regarding polio morbidity in developing countries. Recall that polio had been considered a disease caused by "too much hygiene" ever since the post-WWII period, that is, prevalent only in nations which enjoyed high standards of living. That was how epidemiologists explained the sudden emergence of the disease in epidemic form in the West in the late-19th century and its absence from developing countries thereafter.

Once paralysis surveys of the 1970s indicated high levels of polio-like paralysis in developing countries, researchers had to explain how the disease had unexpectedly reared its head in parts of the world that had hitherto been considered immune due to poor sanitation and hygiene.

Once again, the Improved Hygiene theory could not provide a coherent explanation that was consistent with the evidence. Living conditions in the countries where polio was newly prevalent were rarely comparable to those of the West in the 1940s and 1950s. Polio in these countries was largely associated with poverty and poor sanitation[410] in contrast to its familiar "middle-class" characterization in industrialized countries. But if living conditions in the developing world hadn't changed much during the 20th century, why hadn't polio been there before the mid-1970s?

To solve this dilemma, polio epidemiologists had to turn the historical record of the disease on its head. Outbreaks, they now asserted, had always been prevalent in these developing nations, but, alas, past polio researchers hadn't identified them.[411] Obviously, this contention contradicts the Improved Hygiene theory – its central tenet being that the disease first appeared in the West due to improved living conditions and was absent from places where standards of living remained poor. Now, the official story insisted that polio has always been prevalent in the Third World – because of its poor sanitation. But one cannot hold this epidemiological stick from both ends, as the Israeli adage goes: Either paralytic polio thrives in conditions of good hygiene (as in the industrialized world in the late 19th century) or it is linked to conditions of poor sanitation and hygiene (as in the developing world in late 20th century). One can't have it both ways.

Thus, the supposition that polio has always been prevalent in developing countries, if true, would blatantly contradict the accepted epidemiological theory of the disease. But is there even any convincing evidence for this claim? Let's see.

There is nothing in the surveys of the 1970s that implies or even suggests that polio was always common in the developing world, or even that it was common in the middle or early 20th century. Contemporary researchers do not provide new evidence that would retroactively negate the findings of previous researchers who had consistently failed to find significant polio morbidity in these countries. The surveys of the 1970s found particularly high paralysis rates in some countries: 1 in 83 children in Côte d'Ivoire, 1 in 77 in Niger, and 1 in 53 in Burma (Myanmar).[412] Could past polio researchers, both Western and local doctors who had lived in these countries for decades, really have missed such high incidence of a very conspicuous health condition? Extraordinary claims require extraordinary evidence, as Carl Sagan was wont to say, and such evidence in this case is certainly lacking, if not completely absent.

Thus, with no factual basis for the supposition that polio has always been common in developing countries, its sudden emergence there in the last third of the 20th century is yet another baffling mystery that the official story cannot explain. But how does our alternative Pesticide Theory fare? Can it explain what the institutional story cannot?

DDT began to be widely used in developing countries less than a decade after the end of World War II. The recently established World Health Organization (WHO) launched a global malaria eradication initiative in the early 1950s that used massive amounts of DDT to kill disease-carrying mosquitoes.[413] This initiative was preceded by successful malaria eradication operations in Brazil in the late 1930s and Egypt in the mid-1940s[ss] in which Paris green was used extensively to kill malaria-carrying mosquito larvae[414] (a high incidence of polio was correspondingly reported in Egypt by John Paul and colleagues as early as 1944).[415] Several years after massive DDT spraying operations commenced in developing countries, polio outbreaks made their first appearance. As Horstmann reports in 1963, "the disease is only now beginning to appear for the first time in

---

[ss] In Egypt, DDT was also used to a limited extent during this period to disinfect train cars, aircraft, and boats (Killeen 2002, p. 6).

epidemic form" in many tropical and subtropical areas.[416] [tt]

Although the dangers of DDT were widely known as early as the 1960s, and scientists specifically warned against using it to control malaria,[417] the WHO ignored the warnings and continues to use it still in the 21st century.[418] A World Bank report (2002) reveals that high concentrations of DDT were found in food samples from developing countries where it is still in use, and even in some countries where it was banned many years ago. Significant amounts were also found in human samples – in adipose tissue, blood, and breast milk.[419]

At the same time public health campaigns began using DDT in the fight against malaria, farmers in developing countries began using imported pesticides in their battles with crop-destroying pests. Insecticide use in developing countries, negligible until the end of WWII, grew rapidly in the 1980s to about a quarter of the total world consumption and continues to expand rapidly.[420] Science recognizes some of the pesticides used in developing nations, in particular those based on arsenic and lead, as causes of polio-like disease.[421]

This growing use of toxic pesticides in the developing world was not accompanied, as it was in industrialized countries, by effective government measures to minimize their inherent health risks. Thus, the population, approximately 60% of whom depend directly on agriculture for their livelihood, is exposed to these toxic chemicals to a greater extent than in industrialized countries:[422] Farmers in poorer regions typically use older and cheaper chemicals (including DDT,[423] as well arsenic and lead-based compounds[424]) that are more hazardous than their newer substitutes.[425] In addition, they don't tend to be well schooled in safe handling of these compounds, and governmental oversight and enforcement of regulations is ineffective.[426] Exposure to pesticides occurs in several ways: Through living next to sprayed

---

[tt] Note that Horstmann describes a transition period, which also contradicts the notion that older generation polio researchers "missed" polio in the developing world.

fields, working in sprayed fields, and consuming agricultural produce shortly after it was sprayed. Poor living conditions and nutritional deficiencies intensify the detrimental effects of toxins on people's health.[427] It should hardly be surprising, then, that developing nations are ranked first in global incidence of pesticide poisoning.[428]

Thus, while the institutional story of polio cannot adequately explain its sudden emergence in the developing world in the late-20th century, an apparent correlation exists between the rapid increase of pesticide use and the emergence of the disease in these regions. Polio-like paralysis was quite rare in developing countries in the first half of the 20th century and became very common in the second half, coincident with the use of DDT to fight malaria and pesticides (including DDT) in agriculture.

One Up, One Down: Polio and AFP in the 3rd World

Following the results of the Third World paralysis surveys in the late 1970s and early 1980s, the WHO embarked on a global polio eradication campaign. The operation, which began in 1988 and was dubbed the *Global Polio Eradication Initiative* (GPEI), set a goal of eradicating polio from the face of the earth by the year 2000.[429] Since the 1990s, vaccination campaigns have been carried out annually in developing countries, where millions of children receive the oral polio (Sabin) vaccine. When the initiative began, the WHO set up a global monitoring system to track incidence of polio-like paralytic disease.[430]

Although the stated goal of the initiative has not been achieved – at the time of writing, polio has not yet been globally eradicated – the WHO claims its efforts have been very successful: Worldwide incidence of polio dropped from 350,000 cases in 1988 to only 403 in 2013 (a 99.9% reduction).[431]

At first glance this seems an impressive achievement indeed, but a closer examination of the facts reveals that this dramatic reduction is due in part to an artificial inflation of the data. The stated incidence of 350,000 polio cases in 1988 – which repeatedly appears in the publications of the WHO, CDC, UNICEF, and other agencies[432] – is merely an estimate, rather than a concrete figure. In fact, the number of polio cases actually reported in 1988 was less than a tenth of the official number (32,419 cases).[433] Thus, the claim that global polio morbidity has declined by 99% since 1988 compares a speculative estimation on the one hand to a precise number of reported cases on the other (more on that below).[uu]

Recall that from the late-19th to mid-20th century flaccid paralysis was diagnosed by default as polio.[434] Following improvement in virus identification in the late 1940s, reports of polio patients with no detectable poliovirus in their blood or stool began surfacing. Over time, more and more cases of non-polio flaccid paralysis were identified and placed under the newly formed umbrella of *acute flaccid paralysis* (AFP) *syndrome*. AFP syndrome, like polio, is characterized by muscle weakness that develops rapidly and reaches maximum severity within a few days to a few weeks.[435] This umbrella category includes an assortment of diseases known to cause muscle weakness and paralysis and unexplained conditions that present the same symptoms: Guillain-Barré syndrome, various viral and bacterial diseases, conditions induced by toxic chemicals, drugs, and vaccines, and, of course, paralytic polio.[436] Because the course and symptoms of many of the myriad AFP diseases and conditions are quite similar,[437] it can be very difficult to distinguish between them (and even more so in developing countries, where advanced diagnostic tools are typically in scarce supply). They are also easily confused with paralysis caused by exposure to pesticides.[438] Thus, an official WHO diagnosis of polio depends on lab tests positively identifying the poliovirus in the patient's stool or blood.[439] The rule of thumb for polio diagnosis is as follows: If the symptoms of the paralytic patient meet the defini-

---

[uu] Moreover, the paralytic "polio" cases reported in 1988 did not appear to be laboratory confirmed, as were the 2013 cases. Laboratory tests would likely have found that many of the 1988 cases were not caused by the poliovirus.

tion of AFP and the poliovirus is isolated from the patient's stools (or blood), it is considered a polio case. If the poliovirus is not found in the samples, the case is diagnosed as non-polio AFP. This procedure also applies in Western countries.[440]

You can view the WHO's data on paralytic morbidity on the organization's website. Examination of this data reveals an astonishing finding: Not only have the WHO's polio eradication efforts failed to reduce the worldwide incidence of polio-like paralysis, they appear to have increased it – and to a considerable extent. While reported polio morbidity dropped to almost zero between 1988 and 2010, the global incidence of AFP has risen to about 100,000 cases in 2010, three times the global level of paralytic illness recorded in 1988.[441]

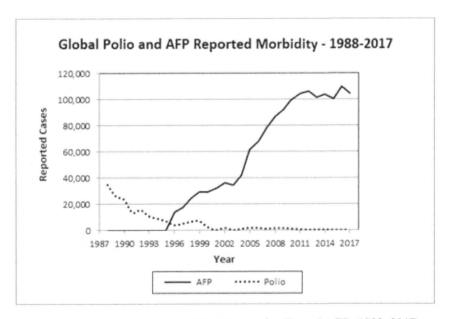

Figure 10-3: Worldwide reported incidence of polio and AFP (1988–2017)

As depicted in Figure 10-3 above, the number of cases of non-polio acute flaccid paralysis has been steadily rising, in parallel with the decrease in polio incidence. The data for individual countries such as India (Figure 10-4, next page), where polio was highly prevalent, follow a similar trend.

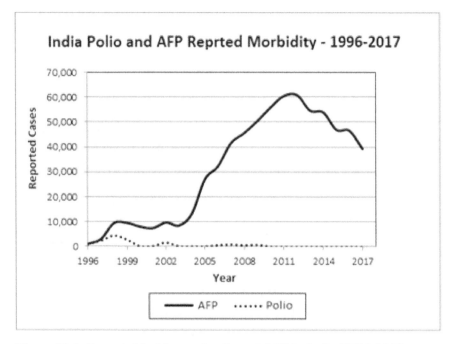

Figure 10-4: Reported incidence of polio and AFP in India (1996–2017)

Although the marked increase in the rate of paralytic morbidity since the mid-1990s has been documented by the WHO itself, nothing seems to have been done to study or mitigate it. "It is sad," write Drs. Vashisht and Pulliel in the *Indian Journal of Medical Ethics* (2012), "that even after meticulous surveillance, this large excess in the incidence of paralysis was not investigated as a possible signal, nor was any effort made to try and study the mechanism for this spurt in non-polio."[442] According to media reports in India, "the cases of children with non-polio AFP were not being monitored by either the polio eradication programme or the larger state health care system. As a result, there was no clear picture of what was causing the AFP, the kind of diseases these children displayed, or how many of them were seriously affected."[443]

One suggested cause for India's surge in paralytic morbidity is the oral polio vaccine itself. Frequent vaccination campaigns in India have resulted in many children receiving as many as ten or fifteen doses of the vaccine within a short period of time – well beyond the three or four doses that were recommended for children in industrialized countries.[444] This hypothesis is supported by the findings of the Indian doctors Vashisht and Pulliel, who found a correlation between the number of polio vaccines dispensed in a region of the country and the region's incidence of non-polio AFP.[445]

In a lecture he gave at the School of Public Health at the University of Michigan in 1951, Dr. Albert Sabin described the primary objective for the study of polio in his day: "The goal of poliomyelitis research," writes Dr. Sabin, "is not the elimination of poliomyelitis infection but of the paralysis which is the important consequence of that infection."[446] Seventy years later, the World Health Organization and its polio eradication initiative seem to have set themselves the opposite target: to eradicate poliovirus at all costs, even if the cost is substantially increasing paralytic disease. Whether the oral polio vaccine itself is to blame for the leap in the incidence of paralysis in the developing world or whether another factor is at play, it is quite clear that the WHO is not much bothered by this state of affairs and is taking no action to reverse its course. This bizarre disregard for the suffering caused by rising rates of paralysis raises serious questions about the credibility of both the WHO and its Global Polio Eradication Initiative.

Nineteen Polio Mysteries

Poliomyelitis has undoubtedly received as much attention from epidemiologists as any other viral disease of man. Yet in spite of intensive study over a century, many of the salient epidemiologic features of this infection must still be considered enigmas. Even some of the accepted dogmas about poliomyelitis can be debated as perhaps erroneous.[447]
Neal Nathanson, 1979

The list below summarizes the polio "mysteries" discussed in this chapter. For each, we present explanations (if any) according to both the officially sanctioned history of polio and the Pesticides Theory.

1   Why did polio epidemics emerge in the United States specifically in the late-19th century?

Institutional
Due to better hygiene, first exposure to the poliovirus occurred later in life, often when people no longer had protective maternal antibodies. This is the *Improved Hygiene* theory, which, as the chapter shows, is inconsistent with the biological evidence and flatly contradicts most of the epidemiological evidence as well.

Pesticides
Pesticides (particularly, lead arsenate) began to be widely used in the US in the late-19th century.

2   Why did polio epidemics strike industrialized countries in the first half of the 20th century, when almost none occurred in the developing world?

Institutional
According to the (senseless) Improved Hygiene theory, in the Third World sanitation and hygiene remained poor, so polio incidence also remained very low.

Pesticides
Before WWII, pesticides were rarely used by indigenous people in developing countries.

3 Why did polio hit hardest in the summer and early autumn?

Institutional
No explanation.

Pesticides
In the northern hemisphere, the majority of (sprayed) fruits and vegetables were picked and consumed in the summer and autumn months.

4 Why did polio's incidence peak in the summer, when most children are not attending school, even though the disease's purported mode of transmission (person to person) favors crowded conditions?

Institutional
No explanation.

Pesticides
Person-to-person transmission is largely irrelevant for pesticide-induced morbidity.

5 Why did most of the early polio outbreaks occur in sparsely populated rural areas rather than in the large and crowded metropolitan areas?

Institutional
No explanation.

Pesticides
Farming communities were the first to be poisoned by the use of toxic pesticides.

6   Why were many of the early polio outbreaks in rural areas accompanied by concurrent outbreaks of paralysis in domestic animals?

Institutional
No explanation.

Pesticides
Farm animals and pets, like humans, were also exposed to pesticides in their food and environment.

7   Why did polio emerge and intensify during a historic period when mortality and morbidity of most infectious diseases were dramatically declining?

Institutional
Polio emerged due to better sanitation and hygiene (while other diseases declined for the same reason).

Pesticides
Paralysis epidemics weren't caused by an infectious agent but rather by pesticide intoxication. Pesticide use increased during this period.

8   Why were high polio rates observed in European residents of developing countries, while local residents rarely experienced acute flaccid paralysis?

Institutional
According to the Improved Hygiene theory, Europeans were not exposed to the poliovirus as infants and got sick when first exposed to the virus (which was ubiquitous in developing countries) at an older age.

Pesticides
European residents in developing countries were protecting themselves from local insects with pesticides that the locals didn't use.

9 Why was polio incidence much higher in Western soldiers stationed in different parts of the world during and after World War II than in their comrades back home?

Institutional
According to the (senseless) Improved Hygiene theory, these soldiers were more exposed to poliovirus in foreign countries than their peers at home.

Pesticides
The overseas military environment was heavily sprayed with pesticides to fight disease-carrying insects.

10 Why was polio incidence among WWII British officers in India, North Africa, and Italy five to ten times higher than that of British enlisted men?

Institutional
No explanation.

Pesticides
Officers' barracks, clubs, etc., were presumably sprayed more extensively, to protect the officers even more than enlisted men.

11 Why were polio's disease patterns (for example, the age distribution of patients being similar in epidemic and low-prevalence years) so different from those typical of other childhood infectious diseases?

Institutional
No explanation.

Pesticides
Epidemics were dependent on various factors related to pesticide use.

12 Why did polio incidence suddenly skyrocket in many industrialized nations after World War II?

Institutional
No explanation.

Pesticides
Many countries which had not used pesticides much prior to WWII began using DDT extensively in the post-war years due to its safety reputation, low price, and high efficacy.

13 Why did polio epidemics in post-WWII United States begin occurring in consecutive years, rather than once every few years as in the pre-war period?

Institutional
No explanation.

Pesticides
DDT use in the post-war years far exceeded that of the pesticides in the pre-war era.

14 Why, contrary to other infectious diseases, are polio patients virtually non-contagious, while the disease is presumably spread so easily by healthy people?

Institutional
No explanation.

Pesticides
Morbidity wasn't due to an infectious agent, so these questions are irrelevant.

15 Why do several members of the same household tend to contract polio at the same time, rather than one after the other, as usually happens with infectious diseases?

Institutional
No explanation.

Pesticides
Morbidity wasn't due to an infectious agent. Several members of a household could easily be simultaneously exposed to toxic compounds from food or other sources, such as spraying devices in the home.

16 How did the Salk vaccine manage to nearly eradicate polio in the US (and other countries), even though at least 20% of the paralysis was not caused by the poliovirus?

Institutional
No explanation.

Pesticides
Polio-like morbidity was mainly caused by exposure to pesticides. The drop in morbidity started before the Salk vaccine and continued in all segments of the population, regardless of the vaccine.

17 How did the Salk vaccine manage to completely eliminate the spread of the poliovirus in countries where it was given exclusively, even though the vaccine essentially does not confer herd immunity?

Institutional
No explanation.

Pesticides
Same as above.

18 Why didn't polio epidemics appear in the developing world until the second half of the 20th century?

Institutional

Polio thrives in conditions of poor sanitation and hygiene that are prevalent in the developing world (never mind the fact that this contradicts both the Improved Hygiene theory and epidemiological evidence from the earliest polio outbreaks).

Pesticides

After WWII, the use of pesticides in developing countries expanded rapidly, especially DDT and lead- and arsenic-based compounds.

19 Why is polio in the developing world associated with a poor standard of living, while in the West it was linked to the opposite?

Institutional

No explanation.

Pesticides

Polio-like paralysis is mainly caused by pesticide use and has little to do with standards of living (in the broad sense).

* The list above, for the most part, presents unresolved questions concerning the epidemiological aspects of polio that the chapter focused on. In addition to those, numerous mysteries also surround the physiological aspects of the disease, for example: How does the virus pass from the gut to the central nervous system? What prevents this transition in the vast majority of those infected with the virus? Why does paralysis develop in some people and not in others?

Summary

The way health authorities present the story of polio creates the impression that science has figured it all out, and researchers and doctors have a very good grasp of its various characteristics – clinical, epidemiological, and virological. Scientific knowledge of polio, the institutional story holds, was accumulated over decades of painstaking and rigorous research carried out by thousands of researchers and physicians who dedicated their lives to fighting the disease. Building on this foundation, Salk and Sabin were able to develop the vaccines that led to the disappearance of the disease from the industrialized world (and, sometime in the near future, from the rest of the world).

Most physicians and researchers today are only familiar with this version of polio's history and are completely unaware of the vast body of evidence that casts serious doubt on its validity. The institutional story of polio presents the public with a veneer of distinguished scientific theory, but when one looks "under the hood" one discovers that its central tenets are largely based on hypotheses, speculation, and poor evidence. Contrary to polio's portrayal as a "closed case" in the history of science, the door has never fully shut on polio, as the official scientific explanation is full of holes, contradictions, and mysteries which have not been resolved to this day.

Epidemiologically, polio theory rests on Ivar Wickman, whose theory of disease distribution relied on hypothetical transmission routes between (healthy) carriers of the poliovirus. Recall that Wickman did not provide solid evidence to prove his theory and ignored its marked inconsistency with the national morbidity patterns in the epidemics he studied. The categorization of polio as a contagious disease relies, to this day, on Wickman's shaky arguments, despite a conspicuous lack of solid evidence accumulated in the past hundred years to back it up.

The characterization of polio as an infectious disease is based on the work of Karl Landsteiner and the researchers who followed in his footsteps. But, as we have seen, the experimental model developed by Landsteiner, which provided the blueprint for polio research for decades, never really isolated the poliovirus and was not even able to satisfactorily reconstruct the natural disease mechanism in laboratory animals. As a result, this model's relevance to polio in humans was, and remains, rather dubious.

Polio's clinical definition is also ambiguous and imprecise. Flaccid paralysis has always been caused by numerous and varied agents, and was given dozens (or even hundreds) of different monikers in the medical literature. Physicians in the first half of the 20th century did not have tools at their disposal for accurate differential diagnosis. Even today, physicians are unable to diagnose polio with certainty based on the patient's clinical symptoms or the course of the disease, and must rely on virus-detection lab tests to arbitrarily differentiate between polio and "polio-like" disease (AFP).

The foundations of polio science are so inadequate and sketchy, despite more than a hundred years of intensive research effort, that it's small wonder it does not provide convincing solutions to most of the mysteries and question marks surrounding the disease since it became a public health threat in the late-19th century.

The alleged success of polio vaccines in eradicating the disease has all but eliminated scientific interest in polio theory's numerous shortcomings and limitations. The vaccines "worked", the disease was "eradicated", and that's all that mattered. But as we have seen, there are substantial reasons to doubt the role polio vaccines played in the disappearance of the disease. The Salk vaccine managed to miraculously reduce paralytic morbidity from non-polio diseases and seemingly provide herd immunity, despite its known limitations in this respect. Disregarding the vaunted success of the Salk vaccine in industrialized nations, most of these nations rushed to replace it with the Sabin vaccine as soon as it was approved by US health authorities, and those already vaccinated with the Salk vaccine were urged to be revaccinated at once with the new vaccine. The alleged success of the Sabin vaccine in eliminating the remnants of paralytic morbidity in industrialized countries contrasts with its notable failure to do so in developing countries in the early 21st century. Recall that while polio has almost disappeared in the developing world, the incidence of polio-like paralysis has increased by a factor of three or more during the same period.

The story of polio also includes an important milestone in the history of vaccines: In 1955, after the first cases of paralysis were reported in the newly vaccinated (the Cutter Incident), federal US health authorities assumed responsibility for vaccination and vaccines. From that day onward, anything that could jeopardize vaccination efforts by damaging the public's impression of vaccines became their business. It is hardly surprising, therefore, that these authorities have consistently and continuously withheld information about the dangers and ineffectiveness of the vaccine from the public, and sometimes even from medical professionals and scientists. This withholding follows a precedent that government agencies began when they concealed information about arsenic- and lead-based pesticides in food and DDT's insufficient safety tests and potential health harms.

Today, several decades past the point of no return, the institutional story of polio occupies such a central role in the larger myth of vaccines that the medical establishment has no interest whatsoever in reopening the closed file – or more aptly perhaps, the Pandora's Box of polio.

11

THE VACCINE HOAX

"Welcome to the real world."

Morpheus, The Matrix

You may recall, dear reader, that a few days or weeks ago, we promised you a definitive answer to the greatest vaccine question of all: "Who is right in the vaccine debate?" If you made it this far – seven chapters dedicated to the science of vaccine safety and three to vaccination myths – we are quite certain you won't be too surprised when we wrap everything up and present you with our bottom line. However, before doing that, let's revisit the main points presented in each of the book's chapters.

Book Summary

Chapter 1 – Turtles All the Way Down: Vaccine Clinical Trials

❖ Each and every one of the vaccines on the US CDC-recommended childhood schedule has been tested in clinical trials against another vaccine (or vaccine-like compound) that has a similar scope of side effects. Not a single one was tested against a true placebo, a neutral compound with no significant side effects.

❖ The clinical trials' designers use this technique to cover up the high rate of adverse events expected with each new vaccine. Thus, the new vaccine can be declared "safe" and its side effects proclaimed "normal", as the recorded side effects do not substantially exceed those of the other vaccine.

❖ When every new childhood vaccine is tested for safety against another vaccine, which was itself tested against yet another vaccine, which was tested against another vaccine – well, you get the picture – it's turtles all the way down.

❖ The use of this intentionally flawed trial methodology means that every vaccine on the US childhood schedule received FDA approval without a true measurement of the actual magnitude of its adverse events.

❖ In their quest to hide the true rate of vaccine adverse events, some vaccine manufacturers resorted to a trial methodology that blatantly violates the medical research code of ethics (*the Helsinki Declaration*). In those specific trials, control-group infants were given a new compound (the vaccine-sans-antigen) that had *no* potential health benefits for them and an unknown safety profile, which could (and probably did) cause serious and persistent injuries. Such an unethical and immoral action has no rational explanation other than the interested parties' desire to hide the true extent of the side effects of the tested vaccines.

❖ All of the above has been carried out by medical professionals employed by vaccine manufacturers and was fully approved by the regulating health agencies in the US and Europe (including the FDA, CDC, and EMA).

Chapter 2 – The Science of Adverse Events: A Missing Link and an Empty Toolbox

❖ Even after more than sixty years of modern medical research, medical science has yet to lay a methodological foundation for vaccine-safety science.

❖ The lack of basic research on vaccine side effects is hardly accidental. Health authorities rarely allocate funds to physiological research on vaccine safety, nor do they require manufacturers to perform such studies. Instead, institutional vaccine safety research largely settles for epidemiological studies which can only produce statistical correlations with little theoretical or practical value. These studies, which are unable, by design, to prove a causal link, do not push the boundaries of vaccine-safety science and contribute almost nothing to the development of new medical tools for prevention, diagnosis, and treatment of vaccine injury.

❖ Due to the lack of sound vaccine-safety science, the physician's toolbox for handling vaccine injuries is virtually empty. Doctors have no diagnostic tools for prescreening vaccine-injury-susceptible individuals. They do not have sufficient safety information to customize vaccine schedules for susceptible children. They cannot verify or rule out potential links between vaccine(s) and subsequent adverse health events, which means they cannot make informed recommendations regarding future vaccination. And they cannot offer effective medical treatments to negate severe and chronic health issues potentially caused by vaccines.

❖ In addition, the virtually nonexistent scientific foundation of vaccine safety has a negative impact on health authorities' and manufacturers' motivation to improve vaccine safety, as well as their capacity to do so.

Chapter 3 – Deficient by Design: Vaccine Adverse Event Reporting Systems

❖ Current vaccine adverse event reporting systems, which do not actively solicit case reports or mandate reporting by medical staff, suffer from severe underreporting.

❖ In stark contrast, many Western countries, including the US, have been operating active and mandatory systems for infectious disease reporting for many decades.

❖ Due to their severe underreporting, these systems cannot fulfill their formal mission of post-marketing monitoring of vaccine safety.

❖ In addition, these systems cannot actually measure, nor can they provide meaningful insight on, the true extent of side effects for any vaccine.

❖ US health agencies, though fully aware of the severe limitations of current reporting systems, still fund and publish meaningless statistical safety studies based on their deficient data to bolster the public perception of vaccine safety.

❖ Despite these reporting systems' severe limitations, health authorities discourage initiatives aimed at improving reporting accuracy and completeness.

Chapter 4 – Epidemiology 101

❖ Epidemiological research cannot prove, or disprove, a causal link between two events. At most, it can confirm or refute the existence of a statistical correlation between them.

❖ In order to prove a causal link, a physiological mechanism must be demonstrated experimentally.

❖ Epidemiological research cannot invalidate the results of physiological research.

Chapter 5 – Purposely Biased Science: Epidemiology and Vaccine Safety

❖ Since it is relatively easy to skew their results, epidemiological studies are the primary tool health authorities and drug companies use to maintain the illusion of vaccine safety.

❖ There are many techniques scientists can use to adjust the outcome of an epidemiological study to align with a predetermined conclusion.

❖ The prevailing research bias in the field of vaccination safety is the inevitable result of the way medical science is funded. This budget-allocation system ensures that researchers are completely dependent on funding sources, whether government entities or pharmaceutical companies, which are staunch proponents of vaccination.

❖ Purposely biased epidemiological vaccine-safety studies are published regularly in leading medical journals and enjoy favorable coverage in mainstream media.

❖ Although these studies often exhibit glaring biases and conflicts of interest, the medical journals' flawed peer-review process doesn't (or won't) expose them. Following their publication, flawed as they are, critical scientific discussion of their fraudulent content rarely, if ever, takes place.

❖ These biased studies are frequently cited in the medical literature and health agencies' official publications as proof of vaccine safety. Their flaws, biases, and researchers' conflicts of interest are never mentioned.

❖ The broad institutional legitimacy granted to these purposely biased studies and their authors exemplifies the fundamentally flawed modus operandi of vaccine-safety research.

❖ The medical establishment is able to get away with this deception because the public, still under the spell of The Pure Science Myth, is unaware of the inherent defects in the way medical science is conducted and is mostly unable to detect the flaws of vaccine-safety science published in medical journals.

Chapter 6 – The Studies That Will Never Be Done

- ❖ Health agencies often proclaim that the current childhood vaccine schedule has been thoroughly tested by the appropriate professional bodies and found to be the best available. Contrary to this claim, the vaccine program as a whole has never been tested for efficacy or safety. This was unequivocally confirmed by the Institute of Medicine (IOM) in a 2013 special report.

- ❖ The impact that key aspects of the vaccine program have on children's health has also never been examined. Although numerous vaccines have been added to the childhood schedule over the past thirty years, no studies have ever examined the ramifications of the growing number of vaccines infants receive, the ages at which they are received, the frequency and order in which they are received, as well as other key aspects of the schedule. Nor has anyone studied the effects on susceptible sub-populations.

- ❖ This lack of scientific evidence makes it impossible to quantify the overall benefit (positive or negative) of the childhood vaccination program. Hence, the sweeping institutional claim (and widely-held belief) that the vaccine program has a positive effect on the health of the vaccinated is scientifically unfounded.

- ❖ The establishment steadfastly refuses to conduct vaccinated vs. unvaccinated studies, though these studies could potentially reveal important clues regarding the dramatic rise of chronic disease in recent decades. Performing these studies is economically feasible, as well as ethically and methodologically sound.

- ❖ The establishment's continued refusal to commission vaccinated vs. unvaccinated studies that assess the overall impact of the vaccine program on children's health has no rational explanation other than reluctance to publicly disclose the inconvenient truth: Unvaccinated children are far healthier than their fully vaccinated counterparts.

Chapter 7 – Unsubstantiated Vaccination Guidelines

❖ There is also a glaring lack of adequate science supporting the safety of certain vaccination guidelines implemented by US and international health authorities.

❖ The authorities' claim that simultaneous administration of multiple vaccines poses no additional risk is based on inadequate research, at best. Some of the vaccine combinations given routinely in the US (for example, 9 injections against 13 diseases at 15 months) have never been tested for safety.

❖ There is no empirical scientific basis for asserting that a child can tolerate up to 10,000 vaccines at one time, or that there is no upper limit to the number of vaccines a child can receive in a single day.

❖ The institutional recommendation of vaccinating infants with mild illness is not based on scientific evidence.

Chapter 8 – The Disappearance of Disease

❖ Improvements in living standards (including better nutrition, sanitation, and hygiene) have led to a dramatic reduction in mortality from infectious diseases from the mid-19th to the mid-20th century. In addition many of these diseases saw a sharp decline in morbidity, and some were all but eliminated.

❖ Nearly all the drop in infectious disease mortality in industrialized countries was recorded before the 1930s, when effective medications, and later vaccines, began to be widely used.

❖ Vaccines contributed only marginally to the drastic reduction in mortality (by reducing deaths from a small number of diseases) and had a more significant, though not major, role in reducing overall morbidity of infectious disease.

❖ In the 20th century, at the same time that the intimidating infectious diseases of the past were gradually disappearing from industrialized nations, chronic disease began to rise steadily.

❖ Today, one in twelve American children is disabled due to a chronic illness and one in four takes routine medication for a chronic condition. A similar situation prevails in other industrialized countries.

❖ The "silent epidemic" of chronic disease has become the main threat to children's health, imposing a huge economic burden on society. Presently, its societal costs far exceed those of infectious disease.

❖ Although they are well aware that the bulk of the reduction in infectious-disease burden cannot be attributed to vaccines, health agencies in the US and worldwide continue to publicly promote the myth that "vaccines saved humanity from the horrible diseases of the past."

❖ At the same time, they advance another misleading myth – "our health has never been better" – conveniently ignoring the huge increase in chronic illness in children that has been documented in recent decades.

Chapter 9 – Herd Immunity

❖ The social benefit attributed to vaccines is largely based on the concept of herd immunity, that is, the assumption that vaccinated people, in addition to protecting themselves, also protect the unvaccinated.

❖ Vaccines may provide herd protection, but to do so they

must prevent not only the illness itself, but also infection with the disease pathogen and transmission to another person.

❖ Of the fourteen vaccines on the CDC-recommended childhood vaccine schedule, only five clear the herd immunity bar by targeting diseases for which herd immunity is relevant for children and being capable of actually delivering it. The remaining nine vaccines are either unable to generate herd immunity, or the protection is either partial or inconsequential for infants and children.

❖ In addition, the assertion that vaccines' benefits outweigh their harms is not backed up by solid scientific evidence. Reliable data on vaccines' true rates of short- and long-term side effects do not exist. In the absence of solid scientific proof of net benefit from vaccination, there is no moral justification for mandating vaccines or otherwise compelling their use.

Chapter 10 – The Polio Mysteries

❖ The institutional story of polio presents a semblance of a worthy scientific theory to the public (and even to scientists themselves).

❖ In fact, the scientific theory on which it is based is full of holes, speculations, contradictions, and mysteries which have not been solved to this day.

❖ Despite intensive research efforts over more than a hundred years, the evidence supporting polio science is so incomplete and inadequate that it cannot provide convincing answers to most of the mysteries and question marks that have surrounded the disease since it first became a public-health threat in the late 19th century.

❖ The so-called success of polio vaccines in eradicating the disease, along with the institutional need to protect the vaccine program, has put an end to scientific interest in the fallacies and limitations of polio theory.

❖ Substantial question marks remain regarding the contribution of polio vaccines to the disappearance of the disease from the Western world.

❖ While the World Health Organization's intensive vaccination campaigns in the Third World have supposedly eliminated polio morbidity, the rate of polio-like paralysis has soared to more than three times the paralysis rate reported at the start of the campaign.

And now, off to the summaries...

If Vaccines Were Safe

Let us consider a what-if scenario in total opposition to the picture that emerges from the ten chapters outlined in the previous section. What if the health establishment were actually right about vaccine safety? What if common vaccine side effects were indeed mild and transient and severe vaccine injury as rare as "one in a million"? If so, how would that fit with other aspects of vaccine safety policy? In other words, is the way the health establishment conducts vaccine-safety activities consistent with its categorical assertion that vaccines are very safe?

If vaccines did not cause serious adverse events, as we are repeatedly told, then there would be no rational reason to give control groups in pre-licensure clinical trials another vaccine, as is the current norm. Administering a placebo to the control group in a clinical trial is superior in every relevant aspect: Not only is it cheaper and simpler than using another vaccine, it also provides reliable background rates for both efficacy and safety. Furthermore, there would also be no rationale for giving a control group the vaccine-sans-antigen in a vaccine trial. Why needlessly risk infants by using a compound that has zero potential benefit and an unknown safety profile, when a safe alternative (placebo) is readily available? Why breach basic tenets of medical science ethics for no reason? If the vaccine on trial was expected to have only mild side effects, then what possible reason could there be for employing such a procedure?

If vaccines were indeed safe, it wouldn't make sense to waste valuable resources on building and maintaining a computerized system for reporting adverse events of vaccines with inherent defects, well-known to all concerned, that cancel out most of its theoretical benefits. In a world where vaccines were safe, authorities would establish an active system with mandatory reporting by medical personnel, similar to infectious disease reporting systems that have existed in Western countries for decades. Such a system would provide reliable estimates of the actual (presumably low) rates of vaccine side effects. This, in turn, would confirm the excellent safety profile obtained in clinical trials, and would further bolster public confidence in the vaccine program.

If vaccines were safe, vaccine-safety research would be conducted unreservedly, including physiological studies exploring potential links between vaccines and subsequent adverse health events. Thus, those rare cases of suspected vaccine injury would receive comprehensive and in-depth medical investigations. The specific circumstances of each case would be documented and appropriate laboratory tests conducted. In addition, subsequent biomedical studies would be performed to examine the possible causal association between the vaccine and the ensuing health condition. These studies would lay the scientific foundation required for developing diagnostic tools for prescreening those at risk of vaccine injury, as well as effective treatments for the injured, and for the overall improvement of vaccine safety.

Assuming that vaccines were safe, epidemiological safety studies would not be publicly presented as "conclusive proof", but as they really are – methodologically limited and potentially biased instruments that can neither confirm nor refute a causal link between vaccination and potential side effects. The scientific community would not shy away from discussing the merits

(or lack thereof) of these studies, and bad ones would be criticized appropriately.

If vaccines were indeed safe, health authorities would be
happy to meet parents' growing demand for comprehensive and
frequent epidemiological studies examining the overall benefit of
the vaccine program and its impact on the incidence of various
chronic health conditions. Vaccinated vs. unvaccinated studies
would surely top the establishment's priority list, as the results of
these studies would likely confirm the safety of vaccines and
pacify the concerned parents. In addition, research would be
conducted to scientifically validate vaccination guidelines before
they were actually implemented. Needless to say, all of these
studies would be funded and directed by neutral public agencies
and would be conducted by objective scientists with no conflicts
of interest.

This concludes our little "what if" game. Now, let's get back
to reality.

In the real world, as documented throughout this book, vaccine science is run very differently from the imaginary scenario
described above: The clinical trials are "cooked"; adverse event
reporting systems are rudimentary by design; biomedical research into vaccine injury is virtually nonexistent; health
authorities sponsor biased epidemiological studies, conducted by
researchers with huge conflicts of interest; studies evaluating the
true benefit of the vaccination program are never done and
neither are studies comparing vaccinated and unvaccinated
populations; and key vaccination guidelines are not based on
sound science. Each item on this list, as well as the totality of the
list, testifies to the inconceivable chasm between institutional
claims of safety and the reality of vaccine science. While the
establishment repeatedly declares that the safety of vaccines has
been impeccably tested and proved excellent, its actions convey
a deliberate intention to conceal the true magnitude and severity
of their harms. While they proclaim that the vaccination program is the best and safest possible, the authorities are well
aware that its real net benefit has never been scientifically

studied. While they state that vaccination guidelines are always based on rock-solid science, in reality some were never tested and others are based on shaky scientific foundations. While the establishment's representatives solemnly declare they are doing everything in their power to ensure the safety of vaccines, in practice they are doing anything but. In fact, for decades they have deliberately refrained from doing precisely those studies that could clarify vaccines' association with rising rates of chronic illness.

Institutionalized Fraud

For many years, parents and medical professionals have been harshly criticizing health authorities' deliberate misconduct with respect to vaccination. Most of the points raised above are frequently discussed all over the internet, but due to cyberspace limitations it can be hard to absorb their full meaning and implications. Nuggets of information are scattered across dozens of different websites, and tremendous effort is required of an individual attempting to form a coherent view out of the chaos. Now, however, this body of work is systematically presented and documented in one place, backed up by solid scientific evidence, and it is no longer possible to avoid acknowledging the dire truth.

This book presented a broad and comprehensive analysis of vaccine safety. We scrutinized the field from various angles, and from each of those a similar view emerged: Adequate scientific evidence for the safety of vaccines is severely lacking, and health agencies and pharmaceutical companies are deliberately concealing their true harms from the public. This grim reality cannot be attributed to some local failure, a one-time random deviation from proper procedure, or a "standard" bureaucratic failure of some government entity. The individual parts seem to mesh so perfectly that it is very difficult to view them as coincidental and unrelated mishaps. Thus, one must inevitably conclude that all parties involved are engaged in deliberate and systematic efforts to hide the painful, astonishing, and earth-shattering truth regarding the "safety" of vaccines from the public.

It is imperative to clarify at this point: We are not claiming that vaccines are a complete and utter scam. Diseases are real, and some vaccines protect against contracting disease. The historic record shows that vaccination played a significant role in reducing incidence of some infectious diseases. That said, however, there is no question that the health establishment engages in deceptive propaganda designed to exaggerate and artificially inflate the benefits of vaccines. Thus, it is responsible for maintaining the fiction that vaccines played a primary role in neutralizing the threat of infectious disease, for promoting the falsely heroic story of the polio vaccine, and for manipulatively misusing the concept of herd immunity to justify mandating vaccination.

But wrong as it is to push false narratives that glorify vaccines' benefits, the concerted and institutionalized effort to conceal their harms is a much graver offense. This deliberate policy, employed by the health establishment for decades and supported by other related parties, is the deceptive foundation on which the entire house of cards is built.

At this point, you may be wondering whether doctors are aware of the facts presented in this book. Could they possibly know about the enormous fraud that has harmed so many millions of our children? And if so, what is their reaction to all of this?

The answer is that, apart from a tiny minority, doctors are completely unaware of the vaccine fraud. Most of them have no clue how vaccines are tested in their pre-licensure clinical trials. The vast majority would probably be surprised to hear that the vaccine program they believe to be immaculate has never been tested for safety, or that studies comparing vaccinated and unvaccinated subpopulations have never been done. Doctors do not study vaccines in medical school much beyond memorizing the current schedule and, other than the few who specialize in vaccinology, have no incentive or time to dig deeper into a field that is not their specialty. Even pediatricians and family doctors don't feel a need for further vaccine knowledge, as the vaccine schedule is set by the health authorities and vaccine injuries, they are taught and conveniently believe, are one in a million.

Most of the higher-ups, however, who run the vaccine field – those who license vaccines, monitor their adverse events, set vaccination recommendations, or allocate funding for vaccination research – are fully aware of the consequences of their own actions.

The Third Level of the Discussion

There is no doubt that vaccines and vaccination is one of the most hotly debated issues of our time. It's safe to assume that every day innumerable vaccine-related discussions are taking place in virtually every corner of the internet world. These discussions, whose active participants and readers are usually parents, are typically conducted on one of three levels, and the results can be predicted according to the level on which the discussion is taking place.

On the first (and shallowest) level of vaccine discussion, critics usually have the upper hand. Video clips and photos of children whose parents say were badly injured by vaccines, reports of vaccine manufacturers' corruption and criminal activities, and horrifying stories of malpractice and incompetence within the medical system catch the attention of many parents, often causing them to stop and reconsider their position regarding vaccination.

But that is seldom the end of it. Usually, vaccine proponents, typically science students or professionals in the medical or medical sciences fields, are quick to counter, harnessing the nearest available science to refute the critics. They often provide a plethora of scientific evidence that appears to confirm – unequivocally – the institutional assertion that vaccines are indeed safe and effective. And they do so with self-confidence, scientific proficiency, and apparent expertise in vaccine research. This is the second level of the discussion. Most of the participating parents find it difficult to keep up with the skilled professionals at this point. They typically lack the expertise to critique a scientific paper on vaccines and are only rarely capable of challenging its content or conclusions. Vaccine proponents, who are mostly academically trained, are thus playing on their "home court", and the result, almost always, reflects their built-in advantage over their lay opponents.

Many vaccine discussions end at this point, with the pro-vaccination side coming out on top – but not all. Sometimes, among the vaccine critics there is someone who takes the discussion to the next level – the third one. At this level, the science put forward by the professionals to prove their claims is itself critically scrutinized. Then, the bare and ugly truth is exposed, just as it has been documented in this book: Vaccine science is woefully incomplete and biased, deliberately designed and performed to satisfy the interests of its funders (as opposed to the public), science that willfully refuses to tell the whole truth. This is the final stage of the discussion – when vaccine proponents run out of pertinent arguments. They just don't have answers to the issues raised. Vaccine science is rigged and, although they feel they must deny it, they know it is so.

Game over.

Medical Tyranny: Shutting Down Criticism

When the vaccine debate evolved to the third level, it became an existential threat to the medical establishment. The entire vaccine construction was suddenly in serious jeopardy of being exposed as the giant fraud it is. Something had to be done.

Up until ten to fifteen years ago, the medical establishment didn't exhibit any reluctance to have its representatives participate in public confrontations with vaccine critics. The typical televised debate on the issue, which usually pitted the "dignified and reasonable expert" against the "emotional vaccine-skeptical mother, served the institutional narrative well. The mother described the harm that vaccines had allegedly done to her child, and the expert, while expressing empathy for her child's misfortune, asserted that any link between vaccination and the child's condition had been unequivocally refuted by science. Discussions of this sort perfectly aligned with the institutional desire to define the vaccine debate as "experts versus parents" or "science versus anecdotes". But over time, to the establishment's growing dismay, a new breed of parents began to appear in these debates. These parents, who spent years of their life studying vaccine science, were presenting arguments similar to "turtles all the way down", which the "dignified experts" found very difficult to counter. Doctors and scientists who spoke on behalf of the vaccine establishment came to realize these debates would no longer be the "walk in the park" they'd expected. The parents were winning.

This process, which took place in the US in the first decade of the 21st century, and later in many other Western nations, spelled the end of open vaccine debate in mainstream media. Confronted with the arguments laid down in this book, the medical establishment was quick to realize that in order to keep the great vaccine fraud alive it had but one choice: Squelch the discussion. Winning debates with biased research and appeals to authority, a strategy which had been so successful before, was no longer a viable option.

Everyone in mainstream media seems to have "gotten the memo", as in a few short years vaccine-critical voices completely disappeared from television and the rest of mainstream media. And the era of witch-hunting vaccine critics commenced. No vaccine-choice advocate or parent of a vaccine-injured child was ever allowed to make their case publicly. No vaccine-critical doctor or scientist, attorney or law professor was invited to speak. Anyone who dared criticize any aspect of the vaccine program was re-branded as an "anti-vaxxer", and it was open season from there on: Critics were de-legitimized, marginalized, and derided, no matter their credentials. Leading scientists, accomplished physicians, a Nobel Prize laureate, and even laypeople asking questions – all were branded and brutally attacked by the media, as well as by medical establishment and industry henchmen, the moment they spoke out about vaccine reservations.

In 1976, the CBS network's famed *60 Minutes* show aired its prime-time investigation on the fabricated "swine flu" epidemic. Only one person died of the flu, while millions received a rushed vaccine, which was later withdrawn. More than 450 vaccinated people developed the paralyzing Guillain-Barré syndrome, and at least 25 died. In 1982, NBC aired *DPT: Vaccine Roulette*, an hour-long documentary on children who had been hurt by the DPT vaccine, produced by journalist Lea Thompson. This type of program, which created a public outcry at the time, is unfortunately no longer allowed on US television. The last person to attempt injecting some vaccine truth was talk-show host Katie Couric, who in 2013 interviewed a mother whose daughter died shortly after receiving the HPV vaccine, Gardasil. Following the airing of the show, Couric was immediately attacked by every major news outlet for, in her own words, "[spending] too much time on the serious adverse events that have been reported in very rare cases following the vaccine." She was quick to issue a public apology, thus, presumably, paying the price for her "dire mistake" and saving her career. To date, no one in mainstream media has dared to follow in her footsteps.

Thus, when even the voice of the injured was no longer allowed to be heard, media reporting of vaccine-related issues became completely one-sided: Only vociferous proponents of vaccines are now allowed to speak – as the ordained priests of "Science". Science is the new religion, and the medical establishment is its prophet. Our new god has spoken: *"Vaccines are safe and effective!"* Science, and science alone, should be allowed to speak on the subject of vaccination. Vaccine critics, by virtue of any opinion that is not wholeheartedly supportive of the entirety of the vaccine program, regardless of their scientific credentials or the merits of their arguments, should never be allowed to speak – not even in the name of the once-revered principle of "journalistic balance" – since their "lies" might "endanger" public health.

This is how the public has been brainwashed to believe that, when it comes to vaccines, free and open debate is "dangerous" and unacceptable.

The Vaccine Judgment of King Solomon

Throughout this book we have repeatedly emphasized the wide gap between the medical establishment's portrayal of vaccines and the grim reality. This chasm is perhaps no better exemplified than by the steadfast and hypocritical refusal of prominent vaccine proponents to engage in public debate with vaccine critics.

Top vaccine promoters such as Drs. Paul Offit and Peter Hotez, who frequently appear on media outlets singing the praises of vaccination, consistently decline invitations from leading vaccine-choice advocates to debate the safety of the vaccine schedule or other important related topics. This surprising timidity displayed by premier US vaccinologists, who are otherwise as vocal as can be, seems to be magically shared by establishment vaccine experts all over the world. In fact, it has become a worldwide epidemic: Vaccine champions, purportedly committed to educating the public on the benefits and importance of vaccination, repeatedly refuse golden opportunities to decisively defeat their main opponents!

What would King Solomon have said if two disputants came before him, one willing to debate the merits of his case while the other refused to, claiming that his side was the only one that should be heard because his opponent has been "known to be wrong"? Is there any doubt that the wise and practical king – being free from pharma lobbyists and the medical establishment's political influence – would rule in favor of the party more willing to defend his stance against the one who wished to evade debate?

You may be wondering at this point about the usefulness of

clarifying scientific truths in a public *debate*. You may imagine it like a political debate between two nominees, with its two-minutes-per-topic format, gimmicks, and quips. That is 20th century debate. A 21st century debate, conducted on an internet-based platform such as Facebook, would be the perfect setting to allow a comprehensive, thorough, and productive debate. The two sides could lay down their arguments meticulously, providing references and supporting material as required. The debate could go on for days, or even weeks, elucidating relevant topics as the need arose. The audience could follow at their leisure, weigh the arguments made by both sides, check the references, and make up their own minds. If one side played unfairly – evading questions, refusing to back up their arguments, etc. – this would be noted by the viewers and reflected in their success.

Such a debate would be the perfect mechanism for settling many of the controversies surrounding vaccination. And that is exactly why the medical establishment's spokespersons will NEVER engage in such a debate, wherein substance would speak louder than sound bites. Just imagine a debate where the vaccine "experts" are publicly asked the inconvenient questions this book has presented. They would have no choice but to evade direct replies as they have no adequate answers. Within days, this debate could be viewed by millions all over the globe, spelling a PR mega-disaster for the vaccine establishment.

Vaccine proponents are well aware of this scenario. That's why they flee, like snakes from a bush fire, whenever invited to formal debate. To cope with the ever-increasing flow of invitations, vaccinologists have created a brand new field of thought, which might be termed *vaccine-debate refusology*: the study of potential excuses for refusing a formal debate with a vaccine critic. In recent years, vaccine proponents spent much of their time honing their *refusological* techniques, while providing much-needed emotional support for fellow *refusologists*. State-of-the-art *refusology* has come up with two excuses of quantum-theory-level sophistication: The first is something along the lines of *We are busy scientists/physicians and we don't have time to waste on vaccine debates*, which is ludicrous considering the enormous amount of time these people spend promoting vaccines when there's no capable critic within a country mile. The second rocket-science excuse is *We don't want to give anti-vaxxers the stage to spread their misinformation*, which, if you think about it, is a not-so-subtle admission that they know if they show up they inevitably will lose the debate.

Think about it: The medical establishment's people claim that vaccines are scientifically proven – beyond any doubt! – to be safe and effective. If they are so confident, why don't they welcome public debate where they can prove it – once and for all – to all those "hesitant" parents? Why do they go on spending all those millions of taxpayer dollars on studies that aim to better understand parental attitudes regarding vaccination, when they have numerous opportunities to "get in the ring" with their leaders and beat the hell out of the critics for all the world to see?

If it weren't for the countless lives ruined – and those being destroyed right now even as you read this paragraph – the hypocrisy displayed by vaccination's champions would be comical.

Real Science and Vaccine "Science"

There aren't many things in science that are certain, but there's at least one thing that is: There is no science without open and free discussion. If there is no debate, it is not real science – it is counterfeit science. Call it "government science", "corporate science", "fake science" or just plain "science" (with quotation marks) – whatever you wish. But real science it's not.

Beyond the undemocratic nature of thwarting free debate on vaccines and denying freedom of expression to the very citizens (and their children) whose bodies the medical establishment seeks to control, the no-debate policy blatantly contradicts the scientific ethos itself. Science does not preclude discussion – it encourages it. Science never rejects a point of view just because it opposes the current accepted dogma – true science objectively judges it on its merit. In science, *who* is making an argument is irrelevant – only the argument itself matters.

Science is ever evolving, and free scientific discussion guarantees its progress. True scientists are not afraid of discussion – they are eager for it. A one-sided scientific discussion is a feature of dark historical periods and totalitarian regimes, not free democratic societies.

Science belongs to the people. It belongs to humanity, not to corrupt government agencies and pharmaceutical giants who collude to rewrite the principles of science in order to continue the decades-long cover-up of their crimes against humanity.

The magnitude of these crimes is enormous – these entities are in way too deep to ever be able to admit any wrongdoing. They will do whatever is necessary to protect the great vaccine hoax. For them, it is a matter of life and death – literally.

And so it is for us.